*Roshan Lall Gupta's*

# Recent Advances in
# SURGERY

*Roshan Lall Gupta's*

# Recent Advances in SURGERY

**Volume 19**

*Editor*

**Puneet**

MS DNB (Surg) FACS FRCS
Professor
Department of Surgery
Institute of Medical Sciences
Banaras Hindu University
Varanasi, Uttar Pradesh, India

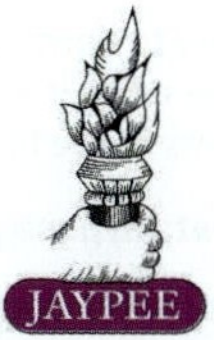


JAYPEE BROTHERS MEDICAL PUBLISHERS
*The Health Sciences Publisher*
**New Delhi | London**

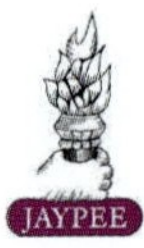

JAYPEE **Jaypee Brothers Medical Publishers (P) Ltd**

**Headquarters**

EMCA House, 23/23-B
Ansari Road, Daryaganj
New Delhi 110 002, India
Landline: +91-11-23272143, +91-11-23272703
+91-11-23282021, +91-11-23245672
e-mail: jaypee@jaypeebrothers.com

**Corporate Office**

4838/24, Ansari Road, Daryaganj
New Delhi 110 002, India
Phone: +91-11-43574357
Fax: +91-11-43574314
e-mail: jaypee@jaypeebrothers.com

**Overseas Office**

JP Medical Ltd.
83, Victoria Street, London
SW1H 0HW (UK)
Phone: +44-20 3170 8910
e-mail: info@jpmedpub.com

**EU GPSR** Authorised Representative

Logos Europe, 9 rue Nicolas Poussin
17000, La Rochelle, France
Phone: +33 (0) 6 67 93 73 78
e-mail: contact@logoseurope.eu

Website: www.jaypeebrothers.com
Website: www.jaypeedigital.com



**Inquiries for bulk sales may be solicited at:** jaypee@jaypeebrothers.com

***Roshan Lall Gupta's Recent Advances in Surgery (Volume 19)***

*First Edition:* **2026**

ISBN: 978-93-7202-154-7

*Printed at: Samrat Offset Pvt. Ltd.*

**Dedicated to**

*My wife, Ritu Ragini*
*Son, Akshat and daughter, Aanya*

# Contributors

**Amir M Parray**
Associate Professor
Gastro-Intestinal Services
Department of Surgical Oncology
Tata Memorial Hospital
Homi Bhabha National Institute
Mumbai, Maharashtra, India

**Anandhi Amaranathan**
Additional Professor of Surgery
Jawaharlal Institute of Post-Graduate
Medical Education and Research
Puducherry (Pondicherry), India

**Apurva Srivastava**
Consultant and Director
Noninvasive Vascular Lab
Institute of Vascular and Endovascular
Sciences
Sir Ganga Ram Hospital
New Delhi, India

**Ashish Verma**
Professor
Department of Radiodiagnosis and
Imaging
Institute of Medical Sciences
Banaras Hindu University
Varanasi, Uttar Pradesh, India

**Asuri Krishna**
Professor
Department of Surgical Disciplines
All India Institute of Medical Sciences
New Delhi, India

**Aviral Srivastava**
Senior Resident
Department of Urology
Institute of Medical Sciences
Banaras Hindu University
Varanasi, Uttar Pradesh, India

**Brijesh Singh**
Assistant Professor
Department of Surgical Disciplines
All India Institute of Medical Sciences
New Delhi, India

**Deeksha Kapoor**
Senior Consultant
GI Surgery, GI Oncology, Minimal
Access Surgery
BLK-Max Super Speciality Hospital
New Delhi, India

**Dhaval Vasa**
Assistant Professor
Department of Surgical Oncology
Tata Memorial Center
Mumbai, Maharashtra, India

**Dinesh Bagaria**
Additional Professor
Division of Trauma Surgery and
Critical Care
JPN Apex Trauma Center
All India Institute of Medical Sciences
New Delhi, India

**Divya Dsilva**
HBNI Fellow
Department of Surgical Oncology
Tata Memorial Center
Mumbai, Maharashtra, India

**Ishan Kumar**
Professor
Department of Radiodiagnosis and
Imaging
Institute of Medical Sciences
Banaras Hindu University
Varanasi, Uttar Pradesh, India

**Kajal Mishra**
Senior Resident
Department of Surgical Disciplines
All India Institute of Medical Sciences
New Delhi, India

**Nikhil Chaudhari**
Consultant
Institute of Vascular and Endovascular Sciences
Sir Ganga Ram Hospital
New Delhi, India

**Poornima Aiswarya Munagala**
Vascular Registrar
Department of Vascular Surgery
James Cook University Hospital
South Tees NHS Foundation Trust
Middlesborough, UK

**Pramod K Singh**
Professor
Department of Radiodiagnosis and Imaging
Institute of Medical Sciences
Banaras Hindu University
Varanasi, Uttar Pradesh, India

**Pranab Dey**
Professor of Oncopathology
Homi Bhabha Cancer Hospital and Research Centre
Tata Memorial Center
New Chandigarh, Punjab, India

**Puneet**
Professor
Department of Surgery
Institute of Medical Sciences
Banaras Hindu University
Varanasi, Uttar Pradesh, India

**Rahul**
Additional Professor
Department of Surgical Gastroenterology
Sanjay Gandhi Post Graduate Institute of Medical Sciences
Lucknow, Uttar Pradesh, India

**Ritu Ojha**
Associate Professor
Department of Radiodiagnosis and Imaging
Institute of Medical Sciences
Banaras Hindu University
Varanasi, Uttar Pradesh, India

**Rohit Kumar Singh**
Assistant Professor
Department of Surgery
Baba Keenaram Medical College
Chandauli, Uttar Pradesh, India

**Ruby Gupta**
Senior Research Scientist
Centre for Chronic Disease Control, New Delhi
Centre for Health Analytics and Trends
Ashoka University
Sonepat, Haryana, India

**Sameer Trivedi**
Professor
Department of Urology
Institute of Medical Sciences
Banaras Hindu University
Varanasi, Uttar Pradesh, India

**Sanjay K**
Senior Resident
Department of Surgical Gastroenterology
Sanjay Gandhi Post Graduate Institute of Medical Sciences
Lucknow, Uttar Pradesh, India

**Satyendra Kumar Tiwary**
Professor
Department of Surgery
Institute of Medical Sciences
Banaras Hindu University
Varanasi, Uttar Pradesh, India

**Shailesh V Shrikhande**
Deputy Director
Tata Memorial Hospital
Professor and Head, Cancer Surgery
Chief, GI and HPB Service
Tata Memorial Center
Mumbai, Maharashtra, India

**Shalaka Joshi**
Professor and Consultant Surgeon
Department of Surgical Oncology, Breast Services
Tata Memorial Center
Mumbai, Maharashtra, India

**Shanto Shila Guha**
Senior Resident
Department of Surgery
All India Institute of Medical Sciences
Raipur, Chhattisgarh, India

**Shristi Rathore**
Senior Resident
Division of Trauma Surgery and Critical Care
JPN Apex Trauma Center
All India Institute of Medical Sciences
New Delhi, India

**Somaiah Aroori**
Consultant HPB and Transplant Surgeon
Honorary Professor, Peninsula Medical School
University of Plymouth, UK

**Subodh Kumar**
Professor of Surgery
Division of Trauma Surgery and Critical Care
JPN Apex Trauma Center
All India Institute of Medical Sciences
New Delhi, India

**Sushant Sorene**
Assistant Professor
Department of Surgical Disciplines
All India Institute of Medical Sciences
New Delhi, India

**Toshita Jain**
HBNI Fellow
Department of Surgical Oncology
Tata Memorial Center
Mumbai, Maharashtra, India

**Tushar S Mishra**
Professor
Department of Surgery
All India Institute of Medical Sciences
Bhubaneswar, Odisha, India

**Vasileios K Mavroeidis**
HPB, Transplant and General Surgeon
Department of Transplant Surgery
North Bristol NHS Trust, Bristol, UK

**Venakt Vineeth Amavasya**
Renal Transplant Fellow
South West Transplant Centre
University Hospital Plymouth NHS Trust
Plymouth, England, UK

**Vikram A Chaudhari**
Professor
Gastro-Intestinal Services
Department of Surgical Oncology
Tata Memorial Hospital
Homi Bhabha National Institute
Mumbai, Maharashtra, India

**Vikram Kate**
Dean (Academic)
Professor of General and Gastrointestinal Surgery
Jawaharlal Institute of Post-Graduate Medical Education and Research
Puducherry (Pondicherry), India

**Vivek Katiyar**
Associate Professor
Department of Surgery
Institute of Medical Sciences
Banaras Hindu University
Varanasi, Uttar Pradesh, India

**Yajnadatta Sarangi**
Assistant Professor
Department of Surgical Gastroenterology
Sanjay Gandhi Post Graduate Institute of Medical Sciences
Lucknow, Uttar Pradesh, India

# Preface

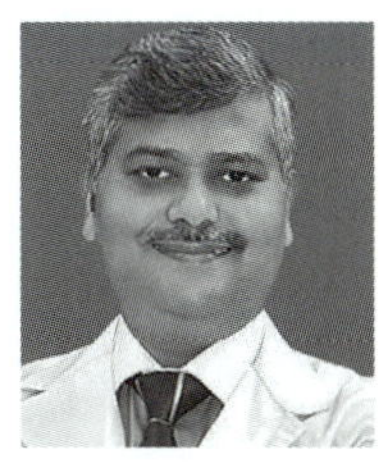

The new edition of *Roshan Lall Gupta's Recent Advances in Surgery (Vol. 19)* provides comprehensive coverage of topics across all surgical specialties. It includes general subjects, recent trends, and advances in the field of surgery, along with insights into future surgical management. Each chapter incorporates the latest guidelines, diagnostic approaches, and management strategies for surgical patients.

This edition also explores several special topics such as radiomics and radiogenomics, biobanking and its relevance in the current era, liquid biopsy, and endovascular treatment. The book thoroughly discusses modern techniques and current developments in the management of general surgical problems.

This book will help the postgraduates and DNB surgery candidates to pass their exit examinations and also enrich them with the recent update in the field of "Surgery." It is also designed to enrich the young practicing surgeons with the latest updates in surgical science. The content is presented in clear, concise, and simple language, complemented by charts, algorithms, and photographs for easy understanding. Each chapter has been authored by renowned and eminent surgeons who have based their contributions on current evidence and clinical practice.

I hope this book not only enhances the knowledge but also improves the clinical practice of surgeons, ultimately contributing to better patient's care.

**Puneet**

# Acknowledgments

I extend my sincere thanks to all the authors for their valuable contributions to this edition. The text has been written in simple and student-friendly language to facilitate easy understanding and is well-suited for young surgeons to apply in their clinical practice. I am confident that this edition will prove to be informative and beneficial to its readers. I also express my gratitude to M/s Jaypee Brothers Medical Publishers (P) Ltd., New Delhi, India, for their continued support and for publishing this book.

# Contents

CHAPTER

# Management of Choledocholithiasis

*Kajal Mishra, Sushant Sorene, Brijesh Singh, Asuri Krishna*

## INTRODUCTION

Prevalence of choledocholithiasis is 10% in patients with symptomatic gallstone disease and 15% in those presenting with acute cholecystitis.[1] Majority of stones in common bile duct (CBD) migrate from the gallbladder (secondary choledocholithiasis). These stones are commonly cholesterol stones or black pigment stones. Less than 10% of CBD stones are formed de novo due to stasis (primary choledocholithiasis) **(Table 1)**. Since the first successful CBD exploration documented by Thornton in 1889, and later catheter-based treatment by Courvoisier and Kehr, open cholecystectomy and CBD exploration has remained the standard of care for nearly a century. However, with advancements in endoscopic techniques and minimal invasive surgery in the last two decades, there has been a paradigm shift in the management of these stones.

## PRESENTATION

Presentation of the patients with stones in CBD depends on their location, size, numbers, and presence or absence of bacterial infection. Common symptoms include pain in the right upper quadrant of abdomen, jaundice, and fever. One-fifth of the stones remain asymptomatic and spontaneously pass into the duodenum. On the other hand, a few patients develop biliary

**TABLE 1:** Types of CBD stones.

| *Characteristic* | *Primary CBD stones* | *Secondary CBD stones* |
|---|---|---|
| Incidence | <10% | 90–95% |
| Origin | Formed de novo in CBD | Migrate from gallbladder |
| Geographical distribution | Common in Europe and America | Common in Asia |
| Association | Associated with gallstones in 90–95% | Associated with intrahepatic stones in >50% |
| Chemical nature | Brown pigmented stones | Cholesterol and black pigmented stones |

(CBD: common bile duct)

**TABLE 2:** TG 18/TG 13 diagnostic criteria for acute cholangitis.

| *Criteria* | *Sub-criteria* | *Parameters* |
|---|---|---|
| Systemic examination | A1: Fever | Temperature >38°C |
| | A2: Laboratory features of inflammatory response | • Leukocyte count <4,000 or >11,000 per μL<br>• C-reactive protein ≥1 mg/dL |
| Cholestasis | B1: Jaundice | Total bilirubin ≥2 mg/dL |
| | B2: Laboratory data—abnormal liver function tests | • ALT >1.5 × STD<br>• AST >1.5 × STD<br>• ALP >1.5 × STD<br>• r-GTP >1.5 × STD |
| Imaging | C1: Biliary dilatation | |
| C2: Evidence of the etiology on imaging (stricture, stone, stent, etc.) | | |
| *Suspected diagnosis*: one item in A + one item in either B or C<br>*Definite diagnosis*: one item in A, one item in B, and one item in C | | |

[ALP: alkaline phosphatase; ALT: alanine aminotransferase; AST: aspartate aminotransferase; CRP: C-reactive protein; r-GTP (GGT): r-glutamyltransferase; STD: upper limit of normal value]

pancreatitis due to ampullary edema. Another dreaded complication is suppurative cholangitis (obstruction with infection)—due to impacted stone in the lower CBD. Classical features include—biliary colic, jaundice, fever (*Charcot's triad*) and in more severe disease, renal dysfunction and mental obtundation (*Reynold's pentad*). Charcot's triad has an excellent specificity (>90%) but poor sensitivity (26%) for choledocholithiasis. Hence, Tokyo guidelines (TG) were laid down in 2007, later revised in 2013 and 2018 with a sensitivity of 92% and specificity of 78% for the diagnosis of ascending cholangitis[2,3] **(Table 2)**.

## EVALUATION

- *Laboratory tests:* Complete blood count to look for anemia and leukocytosis (which may suggest acute cholangitis), liver function tests, and pancreatic enzyme levels to evaluate for concurrent pancreatitis are included in the laboratory workup in a suspected case of choledocholithiasis. Serum alanine aminotransferase (ALT) and aspartate aminotransferase (AST) concentrations are typically elevated early in the course of biliary obstruction. Later, serum bilirubin, alkaline phosphatase (ALP), and gamma-glutamyl transpeptidase (GGT) start rising.
- *Trans-abdominal ultrasonography (TAUS):* It is the initial imaging of choice in a patient with suspected choledocholithiasis. It is universally

**TABLE 3:** Clinical predictors for CBD stones.

| *Probability* | *Predictors* | *Recommended strategy* |
|---|---|---|
| High (>50%) | Any one of the following:<br>• CBD stone on US/cross-sectional imaging<br>• Clinical ascending cholangitis<br>• Total bilirubin >4 mg/dL and dilated CBD on US/cross-sectional imaging | Should be treated with ERCP |
| Intermediate (10–50%) | • Abnormal liver biochemical tests<br>• Age >55 years<br>• Dilated CBD (>6 mm or >8 mm with cholecystectomy) | Should be further evaluated with MRCP or EUS or IOC or intraoperative US |
| Low (<10%) | No risk factors | Can proceed with cholecystectomy with or without intra-operative evaluation of CBD |

(CBD: common bile duct; ERCP: endoscopic retrograde cholangiopancreatography; EUS: endoscopic ultrasound; IOC: intraoperative cholangiography; MRCP: magnetic resonance cholangiopancreatography; US: ultrasound)

available, noninvasive, permits bedside evaluation, and provides a low-cost means of evaluating the CBD for stones. The sensitivity of TAUS alone for choledocholithiasis ranges from 20 to 90%.[4] A dilated CBD (>6 mm in individuals <60 years of age) on transabdominal ultrasound is suggestive of, but not specific for, choledocholithiasis.

*Risk assessment of choledocholithiasis:* American Society of Gastrointestinal Endoscopy 2019 guidelines[5] have stratified the clinical features and laboratory/radiology parameters into three categories to predict the possibility of choledocholithiasis and guide further management **(Table 3)**.

## FURTHER EVALUATION AND MANAGEMENT

### High-risk Patients

In patients with acute cholangitis, and/or definite ongoing evidence of biliary obstruction, preoperative ERCP (endoscopic retrograde cholangiopancreatography) and stone removal is recommended according to ASGE guidelines (2019). If ERCP is not feasible, initially a per-cutaneous biliary drainage can be done in severe cholangitis (presence of organ dysfunction). Stone clearance should be followed by elective (laparoscopic or open) cholecystectomy. Similar results can be achieved by single stage surgery—laparoscopic cholecystectomy with CBD exploration and ductal clearance. A recent Cochrane-based meta-analysis including 16 randomized controlled trials (RCTs) analyzed the outcomes of endoscopic versus surgical clearance of bile duct stones. Single stage laparoscopic surgery (cholecystectomy with CBD exploration) was reported to be more cost-effective and associated with reduced hospital stay in comparison to preoperative ERCP followed by elective cholecystectomy. However, clinical success, morbidity, and mortality were similar in the two groups.[6]

## Intermediate-risk Patients

Intermediate-risk patients have an estimated 10–50% probability of a CBD stone. These patients require additional evaluation [magnetic resonance cholangiopancreatography (MRCP) or endoscopic ultrasound (EUS)] to rule out choledocholithiasis prior to direct ERCP. MRCP is preferred (sensitivity of 87% and specificity of 92%) as it is a noninvasive and a widely available test. If the results are inconclusive, EUS becomes an effective tool with a sensitivity and specificity of 97% and 90% respectively.[7]

*Intraoperative cholangiography* can also be done in patients with intermediate risk of choledocholithiasis, although its feasibility decreases in case of acute inflammation and small caliber cystic duct. *Intraoperative ultrasonography* has over 90% sensitivity and specificity in experienced hands and can be used routinely in laparoscopic cholecystectomies where we suspect CBD stones. However, it has a long learning curve, high equipment costs, and is not readily available. In case of intraoperative detection of CBD stones, either laparoscopic CBD exploration or postoperative (post laparoscopic cholecystectomy) endoscopic CBD clearance can be done.

## Low-risk Patients

These patients have <10% probability of having a CBD stone and can undergo cholecystectomy without any preoperative workup for CBD stones.

*Magnetic resonance cholangiopancreatography*: MRCP is a noninvasive imaging method with an accuracy of >95% in detecting CBD stones. The classical features on MRCP include: dilated CBD (>6 mm), dilated intrahepatic biliary radicals, and filling defect in CBD along with gallstones **(Fig. 1)**. MRCP has been incorporated into the pathway for the investigation of suspected CBD stones as it has a pivotal role in reducing the rate of "negative" ERCP. However, the accuracy of MRCP for stones <5 mm is less.

- *Endoscopic ultrasound:* EUS has the highest sensitivity (95%) and specificity (100%) for CBD stones. Routine use is discouraged as it is an invasive modality. It should be done in intermediate-risk patients **(Table 3)** if MRCP is negative and the clinical judgement continues to suggest the possibility of CBD stone. EUS should preferably be done in hybrid endoscopy suites where ERCP can be performed in the same session if the test is positive. Recent data suggests that the available predictive models for CBD stones (ASGE guidelines—2019) have an

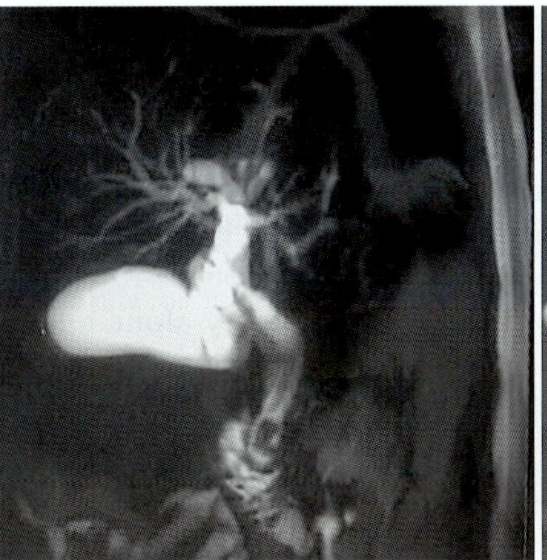
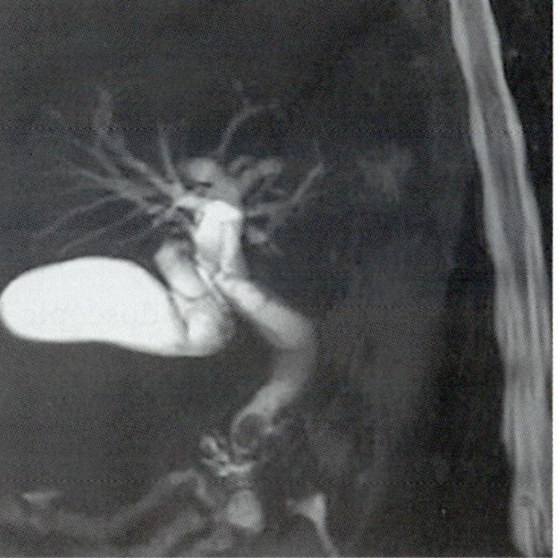

**Fig. 1:** MRCP images showing dilated CBD, filling defect in lower CBD and proximally dilated intrahepatic biliary radicals. (CBD: common bile duct; MRCP: magnetic resonance cholangiopancreatography)

**TABLE 4:** Criteria for difficult stones (ASGE—2019 guidelines).

| *Anatomical factors* | *Stone factors* | *Duct factors* |
|---|---|---|
| An inaccessible papilla:<br>• Aberrant anatomy<br>• Unfavorable duodenal or papillary structures, such as a periampullary diverticulum<br>• Small papilla<br>• Prior surgery, such as Billroth II or Roux-en-Y gastric bypass | • Size (>1.5 cm)<br>• Number: Multiple<br>• Consistency—hard<br>• Shape—square, piston, or faceted<br>• Location of stones—intrahepatic stones | • Contour and diameter at the level of and distal to the stones<br>• Presence of coexisting pathology (e.g., stricture or tumor)<br>• Stones located proximal to a stricture or narrowed distal bile duct<br>• Sigmoid-shaped duct |

accuracy of ~69% even if the clinical factors suggest a high probability. EUS-first approach in such cases, where EUS is performed prior to ERCP has the potential to decrease unnecessary intervention in >40% of the subjects without adding to the adverse effects of missed calculi.[8]

- *Endoscopic retrograde cholangiopancreatography:* ERCP serves as a treatment modality for choledocholithiasis. The success rates vary with characteristics of the CBD stone; ~15% are classified as difficult stones **(Table 4)**. The standard ERCP procedure for uncomplicated stones (<3 in number and <10 mm in size) includes:[9]
  - Successful access to the biliary tree
  - Cholangiogram—for ductal anatomy and stone burden
  - Endoscopic sphincterotomy/balloon dilatation

- Standard pull-type sphincterotomes allow a vertical incision from the papillary orifice in a cephalad direction along the intramural course of the CBD (length: 10–15 mm) depending upon local anatomy, degree of CBD dilation, and size of the stone to be removed
- In case of difficult cannulation, pre-cut papillotomy/access sphincterotomy, needle knife sphincterotomy can be used to gain access into the duct.

*Extraction of stone(s):* Endoscopic biliary sphincterotomy alone allows spontaneous exit of a few stones, while others require various extraction methods. Commonly used devices include balloon or basket catheters. The devices are available in multiple configurations and sizes, and selecting a device is individualized and guided by stone characteristics, bile duct anatomy, and endoscopist preference. A RCT evaluating the benefit of large balloon dilatation demonstrated effective clearance of even >13 mm stones in CBD in 96% cases.[10] For patients with >1 stone, the stone closest to the ampulla is extracted first followed by the rest.

A basket device acts as a mechanical lithotripter and can be used for patients with a nondilated CBD (diameter ≤10 mm) or with multiple stones (>3 stones). When multiple stones are present, each stone is grasped and removed separately to avoid impaction of the basket at the ampulla. The basket is advanced proximal to the stone, it is grasped, closed and can even be used to crush the stones to allow their smooth exit through the papilla. In case, a nonlithotripter basket is used, its size should not be larger than the CBD diameter and it should not be closed tightly as wires get embedded in stone and it becomes difficult to release the stones thereof.

Endoscopic sphincterotomy and stone extraction are effective for clearing the bile duct in 85–90% of patients, with an overall rate of adverse events of approximately 5% and a mortality rate of <1%.[9] Common complications include acute pancreatitis (severe in ~0.5%), bleeding (1%), perforation (0.1–0.6%), basket impaction, and broken handles. Mortality associated with ERCP is 0.2–0.9%.[11]

*Complicated stones:* 10–15% of CBD stones are complicated [stones >1 cm in size, >3 in number, stone location proximal to a biliary stricture, impacted stones, unusual shaped stones, intra-hepatic stones or altered anatomy (Roux-en-Y gastric bypass)]. The extraction of such stones is difficult. Various techniques for stone fragmentation have been described which improve the technical success rates **(Table 5)**.

The success rate for fragmenting stones followed by ductal clearance has ranged from 75 to 90%, and up to 30% of patients require more than one endoscopic session to achieve clearance. Predictors of unsuccessful mechanical lithotripsy include stone impaction, stone size >30 mm, and ratio of stone to bile duct diameter >1. Sphincterotomy combined with balloon

**TABLE 5:** Techniques of lithotripsy for difficult CBD stones.[12-14]

| *Technique* | *Mode of working* | *Success rate* | *Complications* |
|---|---|---|---|
| Electrohydraulic lithotripsy | • Delivers short but rapid electric sparks<br>• Sudden expansion of the surrounding liquid environment generates pressure waves which facilitates stone fragmentation | Done with mother–daughter scope with a success rates of 70–75% | Bleeding or perforation in ~3% |
| Laser lithotripsy | Several lasers have been developed:<br>• Pulsed-dye (coumarin green and rhodamine 6G) and pulsed solid state [neodymium-yttrium aluminum garnet (Nd-YAG)]<br>• Frequency-doubled double-pulse yttrium aluminum garnet (FREDDY)<br>• Alexandrite, and holmium: yttrium aluminum garnet (Ho:YAG)<br>• Short multiple bursts (no more than 5 seconds) under cholangioscopic guidance | 80–85% success rate even with stones up to 2 cm | ~4% adverse events (bleeding and pancreatitis) |
| ESWL (extra-corporeal shock wave lithotripsy) | • It is an alternative to endoscopic technique for difficult CBD stones<br>• Direct contact with the stones is unnecessary<br>• The stones are fragmented using external shock waves under fluoroscopy or ultrasound guidance | • Technical success 55–90%<br>• Advancements in the endoscopic techniques have mitigated the use of ESWL | • Biliary pain<br>• Pancreatitis<br>• Bleeding<br>• Cutaneous petechiae |

dilation is more effective for duct clearance than sphincterotomy alone for large bile duct stones.

Reported rates of adverse events related to ERCP with lithotripsy range from 1 to 14% and include bleeding, pancreatitis, and cholangitis. Events that are unique to mechanical lithotripsy include basket entrapment or fracture of the basket, traction wire, or lithotriptor handle. Entrapped baskets are typically managed nonsurgically by extending the sphincterotomy or using other lithotripsy methods (e.g., cholangioscopy-assisted lithotripsy).

*Extracting the stone fragments:* Following lithotripsy, the stone fragments are removed from the bile duct by grasping them with a basket and pulling the basket through the ampulla and into the duodenum. Stone fragments may also be removed from the bile duct by using an extraction balloon.[13]

Whenever duct clearance is not achieved, establishing drainage by placing a temporary biliary stent is a reasonable option. A biliary stent facilitates drainage and prevents cholangitis until the follow-up ERCP is performed in 2–6 months. Rates of complete ductal clearance after previous ERCP with biliary stenting range from 65 to 93%.

## PERCUTANEOUS TREATMENT OF COMMON BILE DUCT STONES

In the era of endoscopic technical expertise, the role of percutaneous treatment is limited to patients in whom endoscopy is not possible (Roux-en-Y gastrojejunostomy) or is a poor surgical candidate. In percutaneous transhepatic approach, an intrahepatic bile duct is accessed under fluoroscopy and ultrasound guidance. The percutaneous biliary drain (PTBD) is kept in situ for 4–6 weeks. At 6 weeks, a guidewire is passed into the CBD under fluoroscopy and a 7–12 mm angioplasty balloon is used for papillotomy. Stones <1.5 cm can be dealt in a single session by pushing them into the duodenum. The stones are not extracted retrogradely so as to avoid damage to intrahepatic radicals (small diameter) and liver parenchyma. Larger stones (>1.5 cm) can be fragmented with the use of laser lithotripter. Multiple stones usually require multiple sessions. Major complications are subcapsular biloma, cholangitis, and bleeding. Percutaneous intervention is also possible through an access (jejunal) loop fixed in the subcutaneous plane during index hepaticojejunostomy in patients with risk of recurrent (intrahepatic) stones.

In circumstances where the CBD could be cannulated due to anatomic abnormalities (diverticulum at papilla, small papilla), a *rendezvous technique* can be used wherein a percutaneous transhepatic catheter is passed into the duodenum through the CBD and papilla under fluoroscopy guidance and the endoscopist uses it as guide to rail road the papillotome into the CBD. The modern endoscopy suites have all the facilities (fluoroscope, ultrasound, and endoscopes) for such hybrid procedures.

## SURGICAL MANAGEMENT

Management of diagnosed CBD stones include three options:

1. Single stage laparoscopic CBD exploration (CBDE) with cholecystectomy
2. ERCP and CBD clearance followed by laparoscopic/open cholecystectomy
3. Open CBDE with cholecystectomy.

Laparoscopic CBDE with cholecystectomy is a single stage procedure and has a clinical success rate of 85–100%. There are two methods of laparoscopic CBDE:

1. *Trans-cystic CBDE:* After successful dissection of the structures in the hepato-cystic triangle, the cystic duct (should be >4 mm) is isolated and a cholangiogram is performed through an opening in the cystic duct. Stones and their position are noted in the direct cholangiogram. The stones are extracted using a combination of various techniques: forceful flushing, choledochoscopy, and balloon sweep/basket. Complete clearance is ascertained by a check cholangiogram. Cystic duct is finally clipped and the gallbladder is removed.
2. *Choledochotomy and CBDE:* This is useful in a dilated CBD. After clipping the cystic duct, CBD is fully exposed and a longitudinal choledochotomy is made to gain access into the lumen. The stones are cleared using a choledochoscope/nephroscope under vision **(Figs. 2 to 4)**. Later, the CBD is closed primarily or closed over a T-tube. T-tube is a T-shaped silicon catheter with three limbs. Two short limbs are placed in proximal and distal CBD, while the long limb is exteriorized. In the modern era with increasing expertise, T-tubes are seldom used (few indications—recent history of pancreatitis, significant ampullary edema or instrumentation because of an impacted stone).[15]

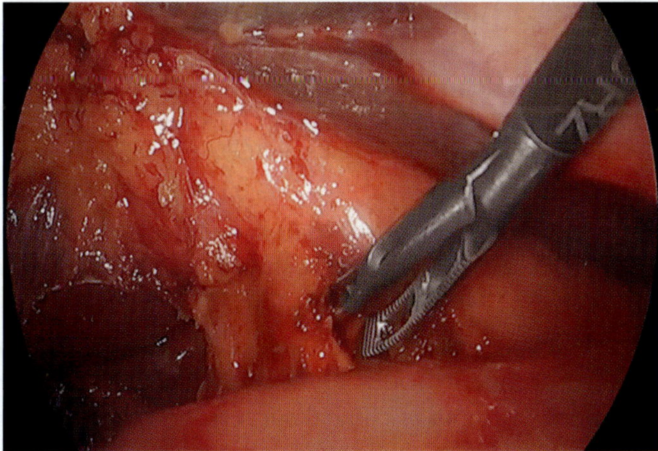

**Fig. 2:** Intraoperative picture showing CBD exploration through a choledochotomy and removal of stones. (CBD: common bile duct)

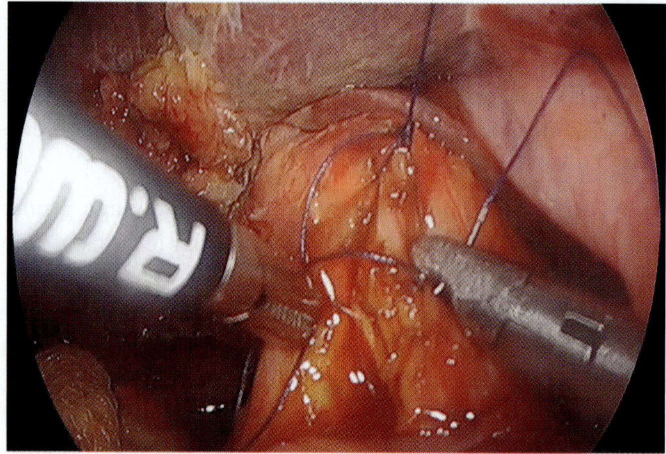

**Fig. 3:** Intraoperative picture showing laparoscopic CBD suturing. (CBD: common bile duct)

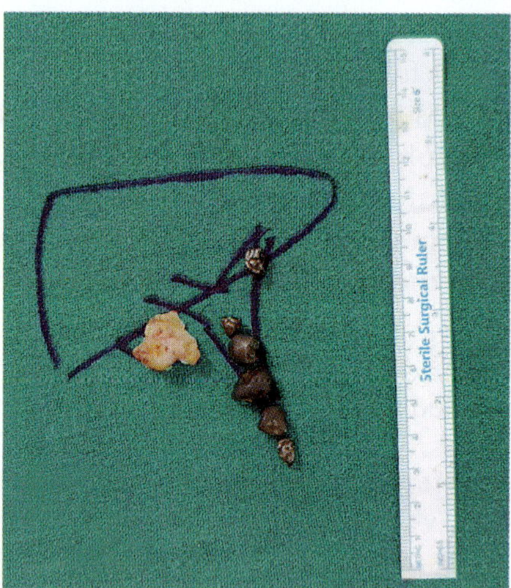


**Fig. 4:** Specimen picture showing retrieved CBD stones after laparoscopic choledochotomy and CBD exploration. (CBD: common bile duct)

The two methods are comparable in outcome; however, the choice depends upon the expertise, condition of the duct, and stone characteristics **(Table 6)**.

*Laparoscopic CBDE versus preoperative ERCP followed by laparoscopic/open cholecystectomy*: Although various RCTs and meta-analyses have shown comparable results in terms of clinical success, morbidity, and mortality with either of the procedure, single stage laparoscopic CBDE is associated with decreased hospital stay and treatment cost.[6] Another meta-analysis including 8 RCTs and 1,130 patients documented better stone clearance

**TABLE 6:** Comparison of laparoscopic CBD exploration options.[16-20]

| *Variables* | *Trans-cystic CBDE* | *Choledochotomy and CBDE* |
|---|---|---|
| Technique | CBD is evaluated through an opening in the cystic duct | Choledochotomy is done and CBD is evaluated |
| Surgical skill | Endoscopic skills are important | Laparoscopic suturing is required |
| Stone characteristics:<br>• Number<br>• Size<br>• Location | <br>• <8<br>• <8 mm<br>• Distal to cystic duct | <br>• Any number<br>• Any size<br>• Entire duct |
| CBD diameter | Possible even in nondilated system | >10 mm |
| Drain placement | Not required | Suggested |
| Contraindications | • Friable cystic duct/medial insertion<br>• Intrahepatic stones<br>• Multiple, large stones | Small-diameter CBD |
| Advantages | • No T-tube, choledochotomy is eliminated, thus mitigating the chances of biliary stricture in future<br>• Shorter hospital stay | • Operating time is less<br>• T-tube if placed—can be used for postoperative access |
| Success rates | 70–95% | 85–100% |
| Hospital stay (in days) | 1–2 | 4–7 |
| Return to work (in days) | 7–10 | 14–30 |

(CBDE: common bile duct exploration)

with single stage procedure.[21] However, new advancements in endoscopic techniques (mechanical and laser lithotripter) have considerably mitigated this difference. The decision to perform ERCP and CBD clearance prior to cholecystectomy is primary institutional preference and is heavily dependent on the availability of equipment and expertise. There are few clinical scenarios where laparoscopic CBDE is superior to two-stage procedure: patients with altered anatomy like in follow-up cases Roux-en-Y gastrojejunostomy or duodenal diverticulae.

## Open Common Bile Duct Exploration

Open CBDE in the modern era is seldom indicated. Few situations which necessitate an open procedure include:

- Mirizzi syndrome type 2 and 3 where there is a fistula between the duct and the gallbladder necessitating bilioenteric bypass

- Failed laparoscopic CBD clearance (if cholecystectomy is possible laparoscopically, then postoperative ERCP for stone clearance is another option)[22]
- Large or impacted CBD stone(s) with failed previous endoscopic interventions in which bilioenteric drainage is indicated
- Anatomic considerations that preclude endoscopic treatment, such as prior gastric resection or duodenal diverticulae
- Open cholecystectomy is indicated as in patients with bilioenteric fistula, severe cholecystitis, or a suspicion for cancer.

*Technique:* The abdomen is accessed through a right upper quadrant subcostal incision, although a midline approach is also acceptable. The liver is retracted superiorly, the duodenum inferiorly, and the stomach is retracted to the left. A generous Kocher maneuver is performed, which allows for manual palpation and manipulation of the distal CBD. The steps of CBD exploration are similar to laparoscopic procedures: dissection of the gallbladder, cholangiogram or choledochoscopy, identification of stones and their position, flushing and extraction under direct vision.

The CBD rent is closed after confirming complete clearance. In patients with dilated CBD (>1.2 cm), impacted ampullary stone, distal impacted stones and distal CBD stricture, recurrent choledocholithiasis or proximal stones (hepatolithiasis), bilioenteric bypass (choledochoduodenostomy—diamond shaped or hepaticojejunostomy—side to side) is indicated.

## Role of Intraoperative Cholangiogram

Approximately 10–15% patients have silent choledocholithiasis at the time of cholecystectomy. Majority of them pass through the papilla without any symptom, hence routine use of IOC during cholecystectomy is debatable.[23] Patients with intermediate risk of CBD stone **(Table 3)** should undergo additional tests (MRCP, EUS) before definitive surgery. In patients where choledocholithiasis is suspected despite a negative MRCP, options include preoperative EUS (sensitivity ~95%) or intraoperative cholangiogram/ultrasound. Data from an European RCT documented similar outcomes with decreased hospital stay, number of bile duct evaluations in favor of intraoperative cholangiograms (IOCs) when compared to endoscopic assessment and clearance.[24] However, the choice of the procedure is largely dependent on institutional protocols and physician's preference.

*Rendezvous technique:* In patients in whom the IOC reveals stones in CBD (not amenable to trans-cystic extraction—small caliber duct or surgeon's preference), the operating team passes a trans-cystic guidewire through the CBD into the duodenum and the endoscopist using his side-view endoscope can gain access into the duct. Thus, this hybrid procedure can take care of the stones in the duct along with cholecystectomy in one go, that too without injuring the CBD (choledochotomy).[25]

## RETAINED AND RECURRENT STONES

Retained CBD stones are those found within 2 years of follow-up after clearance, while recurrent stones are those found in CBD after 2 years of intervention. Common symptoms include recurrent pain in the right upper quadrant of abdomen, fever, jaundice, and sometimes may present with pancreatitis. Index of clinical suspicion and imaging forms the backbone of diagnosis. Often these stones are treated by endoscopy, while a few require surgical intervention.

## FUTURE DIRECTIONS

Emerging artificial intelligence (AI) driven diagnostic tools are poised to improve the diagnostic accuracy and timely intervention. Similar technologies may aid in the surgical planning, thus improving the precision and outcomes. Research can be directed to development of biomarkers for early detection and monitoring of the disease and its complications. Quality improvement strategies and personalized medical treatment approaches can improve the therapeutic success rates. Standardization of care protocols, comprehensive education programs for surgeons and patients and utilization of telemedicine services can ensure specialized care even at peripheral centers.[26,27]

## CONCLUSION

Prevalence of CBD stones is 10–20% along with cholelithiasis. Advances in recent imaging techniques (EUS and MRCP) have replaced ERCP as a diagnostic tool, although it continues to remain the mainstay for the definitive management. Improvements in therapeutic ERCP techniques have been able to achieve high technical success rates (as high as 90–95%), without added morbidity. Endoscopic and laparoscopic treatments of bile duct stones are complementary to each other in terms of definitive management. While endoscopic clearance followed by laparoscopic cholecystectomy is generally followed, upfront surgery with intraoperative IOC/IOUS is a promising approach.

## REFERENCES

1. Rijna H, Kemps WG, Eijsbouts Q, Meuwissen SGM, Cuesta MA. Preoperative ERCP approach to common bile duct stones: results of a selective policy. Dig Surg. 2000;17:229-33.
2. Kiriyama S, Takada T, Strasberg SM, Solomkin JS, Mayumi T, Pitt HA, et al. New diagnostic criteria and severity assessment of acute cholangitis in revised Tokyo Guidelines. J Hepatobiliary Pancreat Sci. 2012;19(5):548-56.

3. Kiriyama S, Kozaka K, Takada T, Strasberg SM, Pitt HA, Gabata T, et al. Tokyo Guidelines 2018: Diagnostic Criteria and Severity Grading of Acute Cholangitis (With videos). J Hepatobiliary Pancreat Sci. 2018;25(1):17-30.
4. Wermke W, Schulz HJ. Sonographische Diagnostik von Gallenwegskonkrementen. Ergebnisse einer prospektiven Studie von 222 Fällen mit Choledocholithiasis [Sonographic diagnosis of bile duct calculi. Results of a prospective study of 222 cases of choledocholithiasis]. Ultraschall Med. 1987;8(3):116-20.
5. Buxbaum JL, Abbas Fehmi SM, Sultan S, Fishman DS, Qumseya BJ, Cortessis VK, et al. ASGE guideline on the role of endoscopy in the evaluation and management of choledocholithiasis. Gastrointest Endosc. 2019;89:1075-105.e15.
6. Dasari BV, Tan CJ, Gurusamy KS, Martin DJ, Kirk G, McKie L, et al. Surgical versus endoscopic treatment of bile duct stones. Cochrane Database Syst Rev. 2013;(9):CD003327.
7. Giljaca V, Gurusamy KS, Takwoingi Y, Higgie D, Poropat G, Štimac D, et al. Endoscopic ultrasound versus magnetic resonance cholangiopancreatography for common bile duct stones. Cochrane Database Syst Rev. 2015;2015(2): CD011549.
8. Maruta A, Iwashita T, Uemura S, Yoshida K, Yasuda I, Shimizu M. Efficacy of the Endoscopic Ultrasound-first Approach in patients with suspected common bile duct stone to avoid unnecessary Endoscopic Retrograde Cholangiopancreatography. Intern Med. 2019;58(12):1673-9.
9. Zhu J, Wang G, Xie B, Jiang Z, Xiao W, Li Y. Minimally invasive management of concomitant gallstones and common bile duct stones: an updated network meta-analysis of randomized controlled trials. Surg Endosc. 2023;37(3):1683-93.
10. Karsenti D, Coron E, Vanbiervliet G, Privat J, Kull E, Bichard P, et al. Complete endoscopic sphincterotomy with vs. without large-balloon dilation for the removal of large bile duct stones: randomized multicenter study. Endoscopy. 2017;49(10):968-76.
11. Orenstein SB, Marks JM, Hardacre JM. Technical aspects of bile duct evaluation and exploration. Surg Clin North Am. 2014;94(2):281-96.
12. Johansson E, Österberg J, Sverdén E, Enochsson L, Sandblom G. Intervention versus surveillance in patients with common bile duct stones detected by intraoperative cholangiography: a population-based registry study. Br J Surg. 2021;108(12):1506-12.
13. Möller M, Gustafsson U, Rasmussen F, Persson G, Thorell A. Natural course vs interventions to clear common bile duct stones: data from the Swedish Registry for Gallstone Surgery and Endoscopic Retrograde Cholangiopancreatography (GallRiks). JAMA Surg. 2014;149(10):1008-13.
14. Kedia P, Tarnasky PR. Endoscopic Management of Complex Biliary Stone Disease. Gastrointest Endosc Clin N Am. 2019;29(2):257-75.
15. Gurusamy KS, Koti R, Davidson BR. T-tube drainage versus primary closure after laparoscopic common bile duct exploration. Cochrane Database Syst Rev. 2013;2013(6):CD005641.
16. Topal B, Aerts R, Penninckx F. Laparoscopic common bile duct stone clearance with flexible choledochoscopy. Surg Endosc. 2007;21(12):2317-21.
17. Zerey M, Haggerty S, Richardson W, Santos B, Fanelli R, Brunt LM, et al. Laparoscopic common bile duct exploration. Surg Endosc. 2018;32(6):2603-12.

18. Lyass S, Phillips EH. Laparoscopic transcystic duct common bile duct exploration. Surg Endosc. 2006;20 Suppl 2:S441-5.
19. Paganini AM, Guerrieri M, Sarnari J, De Sanctis A, D'Ambrosio G, Lezoche G, et al. Thirteen years' experience with laparoscopic transcystic common bile duct exploration for stones. Effectiveness and long-term results. Surg Endosc. 2007;21(1):34-40.
20. Memon MA, Hassaballa H, Memon MI. Laparoscopic common bile duct exploration: the past, the present, and the future. Am J Surg. 2000;179(4):309-15.
21. Zhu HY, Xu M, Shen JH, Yang C, Li F, Li KW, et al. A meta-analysis of single-stage versus two-stage management for concomitant gallstones and common bile duct stones. Clin Res Hepatol Gastroenterol. 2015;39(5):584-93.
22. Grubnik VV, Tkachenko AI, Ilyashenko VV, Vorotyntseva KO. Laparoscopic common bile duct exploration versus open surgery: comparative prospective randomized trial. Surg Endosc. 2012;26(8):2165-71.
23. Sun SX, Kulaylat AN, Hollenbeak CS, Soybel DI. Cost-effective decisions in detecting silent common bile duct gallstones during laparoscopic cholecystectomy. Ann Surg. 2016;263(6):1164-72.
24. Iranmanesh P, Frossard JL, Mugnier-Konrad B, Morel P, Majno P, Nguyen-Tang T, et al. Initial cholecystectomy vs sequential common duct endoscopic assessment and subsequent cholecystectomy for suspected gallstone migration: a randomized clinical trial. JAMA. 2014;312(2):137-44.
25. Tang CN, Tai CK, Ha JP, Tsui KK, Wong DC, Li MK. Antegrade biliary stenting versus T-tube drainage after laparoscopic choledochotomy—a comparative cohort study. Hepatogastroenterology. 2006;53(69):330-4.
26. Johnson KB, Wei WQ, Weeraratne D, Frisse ME, Misulis K, Rhee K, et al. Precision medicine, AI, and the future of personalized health care. Clin Transl Sci. 2021;14:86-93.
27. Liu JC, Cheng CY, Cheng TH, Liu CN, Chen JJ, Hao WR. Unveiling the potential: remote monitoring and telemedicine in shaping the future of heart failure management. Life (Basel). 2024;14:936.

CHAPTER 2

# Gallbladder Cancer: Contemporary Concepts, Challenges, and Evolving Paradigms

*Amir M Parray, Vikram A Chaudhari, Shailesh V Shrikhande*

## INTRODUCTION

Gallbladder cancer (GBC) is the most common biliary tract malignancy and among the most lethal gastrointestinal cancers, carrying the highest mortality of all biliary tumors. Despite representing only 1–2% of gastrointestinal cancers worldwide, nearly half of patients present with advanced, unresectable disease. Long labeled a "silent killer" due to nonspecific symptoms and late diagnosis, advanced GBC is associated with a 5-year survival of <10%.[1-3]

Over the past two decades, advances in imaging, staging laparoscopy, systemic therapy, and surgical technique have begun to reshape management. Precision staging with CT, MRI, PET, and laparoscopy enhances disease mapping and reduces futile resections. Neoadjuvant chemotherapy increasingly acts as a biological filter, while pivotal trials such as BILCAP and ABC-02 have established capecitabine and gemcitabine–cisplatin as systemic backbone.[2,3]

Few cancers illustrate the intersection of geography and oncological uncertainty as starkly as GBC. This marked epidemiologic disparity creates profound inconsistencies in surgical expertise, staging protocols, and systemic therapy pathways. In regions of high incidence, resource constraints often collide with complex decision-making, producing wide variation in the extent of surgical resection, nodal clearance, and the use of neoadjuvant or adjuvant therapies. This chapter reviews the contemporary landscape of GBC—covering epidemiology, staging, surgical standards, systemic therapies, the paradigm of futility, and emerging precision oncology—emphasizing biology-driven, multidisciplinary care beyond surgical radicality.

## GLOBAL EPIDEMIOLOGY AND RISK FACTORS

Gallbladder cancer shows striking geographic clustering, with the highest incidence in South America—particularly Chile and Bolivia (21–27 per 100,000 women)—followed by northern India, Pakistan, and Korea. Indigenous South American women bear the greatest global burden, while the Indo-Gangetic belt of India (Uttar Pradesh, Bihar, Assam) remains a hotspot with rates exceeding 10 per 100,000. In contrast, Japanese and Korean cohorts often present earlier, reflecting better healthcare access and incidental detection at cholecystectomy.[1-5]

A strong female predominance (3:1–6:1) peaks in the sixth and seventh decades, linked to estrogen exposure, parity-related biliary stasis, and higher gallstone prevalence. Gallstones are the dominant risk factor, present in 70–90% of patients, with stone size >3 cm conferring a tenfold risk increase. Other inflammatory and premalignant conditions include xanthogranulomatous cholecystitis, porcelain gallbladder, anomalous pancreaticobiliary duct junction, and choledochal cysts (lifetime risk >10%). Chronic *Salmonella typhi* carriage contributes in South Asia, while environmental exposures such as aflatoxin, pesticides, and heavy metals exacerbate incidence in endemic regions.[4,5]

Molecularly, TP53 mutations dominate (50–70%), while KRAS and PIK3CA mutations drive proliferative signaling. ERBB2 (HER2) amplification (10–15%) confers an aggressive phenotype but provides a therapeutic target. FGFR2 fusions (~3%) and microsatellite instability (MSI-H/dMMR, ~2–3%) offer opportunities for precision and immunotherapy.[6,7]

## ADVANCES IN DIAGNOSTIC EVALUATION AND STAGING

Accurate staging is central to GBC management, as up to 15% of upfront resections prove futile due to early recurrence or rapid postoperative mortality. Modern advances in cross-sectional imaging, PET-CT, endoscopic ultrasound (EUS), and staging laparoscopy have transformed preoperative evaluation.

Most patients present with vague, gallstone-like symptoms, while in endemic regions incidental GBC is detected in 0.7–2% of cholecystectomy specimens. Elevated CA19-9 (>100 U/mL) predicts nodal metastasis and unresectability. Multidetector CT with triphasic acquisition remains the first-line modality, achieving 85–90% accuracy in advanced (T3–T4) disease but limited sensitivity for early or micrometastatic disease. MRI with hepatobiliary contrast improves detection of subtle hepatic infiltration and sub-centimeter metastases and distinguishes peritoneal-side T2a from hepatic-side T2b disease.[8-10]

The EUS offers high-resolution evaluation with 89% accuracy for T staging and 77% for nodal staging, enabling precise distinction of T1a (mucosal) from T1b (muscular) invasion, fine-needle aspiration (FNA) of pericholedochal nodes, and staging of incidental cancers. 18F-FDG PET/CT detects occult metastases in 15–20% of radiologically resectable patients, outperforming CT for nodal and distant disease. Beyond staging, >50% reduction in SUVmax after neoadjuvant chemotherapy correlates with pathological response and improved survival, while novel tracers such as ^68Ga-FAPI PET show superior tumor-to-background contrast.[2,3,11-14]

Staging laparoscopy remains indispensable, identifying occult peritoneal or hepatic metastases in 25–35% of radiologically resectable T2–T4 cases. Its yield is highest in T3/T4 disease, nodal involvement, or CA19-9 elevation, sparing nearly one-third of patient's unnecessary laparotomy.[15,16] Current guidelines recommend an integrated algorithm: high-quality CT/MRI as baseline, PET-CT for systemic staging in ≥T2 tumors, EUS with FNA in equivocal cases, and routine staging laparoscopy for T2–T4 or node-positive disease.[2,3,15,16]

## SURGICAL MANAGEMENT: OMEGA INSIGHTS, INSTITUTIONAL LESSONS, FUTILITY, AND GLOBAL CONSENSUS

Surgery remains the only curative option for GBC, but outcomes are dictated more by tumor biology than surgical radicality. The OMEGA study, the largest international collaborative dataset (>3,600 patients, 133 centers), revealed profound heterogeneity in surgical practice, reflecting institutional philosophy more than evidence-based consensus. The extent of hepatic resection ranged from wedge excision to right hepatectomy, yet outcomes in node-positive or margin-positive disease did not improve with greater radicality. Over 40% of patients undergoing major hepatectomy for T3 tumors recurred systemically within a year, underscoring the futility of aggressive surgery in biologically advanced disease.[17,18]

High-volume institutional series reinforces these lessons. At Tata Memorial Centre (>1,300 resections), neoadjuvant chemotherapy (NACT) improved R0 rates and disease-free survival in borderline resectable and node-positive tumors, with >90% R0 achieved in responders compared with poor outcomes after upfront surgery. Japanese and Korean registries confirmed extended cholecystectomy with segment IVb/V resection and lymphadenectomy as the standard for T2 disease, but also highlighted that anatomically radical surgery cannot overcome adverse biology in node-positive or advanced disease.[19-21]

The recognition of futility represents a major conceptual advance. Multicenter analyses show that 10–15% of upfront resections are futile, defined by early recurrence or perioperative death. Predictors include R1 margins, N2 nodal burden, jaundice, and major vascular invasion—features reflecting systemic spread rather than surgical inadequacy. Increasingly, staging laparoscopy, PET, EUS, and NACT response serve as filters to avoid futile laparotomy, while emerging AI-based radiomics and biomarker models are being developed to refine resectability prediction.[22,23]

To address global heterogeneity, expert consensus guidelines from IHPBA and NCCN recommend a tiered, biology-driven approach. Simple cholecystectomy suffices for T1a, while extended cholecystectomy is generally favored for T1b. For T2 disease, IVb/V resection with lymphadenectomy is standard, with T2b (hepatic-side) tumors carrying worse prognosis than T2a (peritoneal-side). In T3–T4 disease, major hepatectomy or multivisceral resection is justified only in carefully selected patients with favorable biology, given the predominance of systemic recurrence. Mandatory nodal clearance includes stations 8, 12, and 13, while para-aortic dissection remains investigational. Global guidelines also emphasize routine PET and laparoscopy before radical surgery in all ≥T2 cases.[2,3]

Collectively, OMEGA, institutional lessons, and international consensus converge on a single principle: GBC surgery must be biology-driven, guideline-aligned, and globally standardized. Radicality cannot offset systemic disease; meaningful survival requires rigorous staging, systemic therapy, and careful patient selection.

## NEOADJUVANT TREATMENT: BIOLOGY-DRIVEN SELECTION

Neoadjuvant chemotherapy (NACT) is emerging as a rational strategy in GBC, addressing the disease's systemic propensity and functioning as a biological filter for surgical decision-making. Even after curative-intent resection, 50–60% of patients relapse within 2 years, predominantly with systemic recurrence. NACT offers multiple advantages: downstaging borderline resectable tumors, treating micrometastatic disease early, enabling biological selection by sparing non-responders futile laparotomy, and providing dynamic prognostic information through radiological or PET-based regression.[24-28]

Institutional data from endemic regions have been pivotal. At Tata Memorial Centre (Mumbai, India), which pioneered NACT in GBC, node-positive or borderline resectable patients achieved R0 resections in >90% of responders, with superior disease-free survival versus upfront surgery. Korean multicenter registry data similarly showed improved outcomes with preoperative gemcitabine–cisplatin. Systematic reviews reinforce these findings, reporting higher resectability and survival in T3/T4 or node-positive disease.[24-28]

Ongoing randomized trials aim to define standard practice. The GAIN trial (AIO-HEP-0116) compares neoadjuvant gemcitabine–cisplatin with upfront surgery in resectable GBC, focusing on survival and R0 rates. Indian multicenter efforts led by Tata Memorial are testing perioperative chemotherapy ± radiotherapy, incorporating PET-based response stratification.[29,30] Early-phase global studies are evaluating chemo-immunotherapy combinations, targeting subsets such as MSI-high and PD-L1-positive tumors.[31]

While not yet universally incorporated into guidelines, converging evidence supports NACT for borderline resectable, node-positive, and locally advanced GBC, particularly in endemic regions where systemic relapse dominates. With results from ongoing trials, NACT is poised to become the global standard for biologically advanced but technically resectable disease.

## STAGE-SPECIFIC SURGICAL MANAGEMENT

Surgery remains the cornerstone of treatment in resectable GBC, but the extent of radicality must be balanced against biological aggressiveness. Large studies and high-volume centers consistently demonstrate that while anatomical clearance is essential for cure, escalation of surgery beyond biological limits does not improve outcomes and may increase morbidity. Stage-specific strategies have therefore been refined to maximize oncologic benefit while minimizing futile radicality.[2,3,32]

For *T1a disease,* confined to the lamina propria, simple cholecystectomy is sufficient and curative, with 5-year survival exceeding 95%. Historically, port-site excision was performed after laparoscopic cholecystectomy due to concerns about implantation, but modern data demonstrate negligible risk with current retrieval techniques, making further excision unnecessary.[2,3,33]

In *T1b disease,* invasion of the muscularis layer carries a 15–20% risk of nodal metastasis. Extended cholecystectomy with hepatic resection and lymphadenectomy has been standard. Current evidence suggests that high-risk features—poor differentiation, lymphovascular or perineural invasion, tumor size >2 cm, or positive cystic duct margin—justify radical surgery. Selected low-risk T1b tumors, especially well-differentiated lesions without adverse features, may be managed with simple cholecystectomy, though this remains controversial.[2,3,34]

*T2 disease,* involving the perimuscular connective tissue, is pivotal. Consensus recommends extended cholecystectomy with wedge or segment IVb/V hepatic resection and regional lymphadenectomy. The distinction between T2a (peritoneal) and T2b (hepatic) tumors is critical: T2a lesions may be adequately treated with wedge excision, while T2b lesions more often require formal IVb/V segmentectomy. Extended resection improves 5-year survival to 65% compared with 54% for simple cholecystectomy.[2,3,35-37]

*T3 disease,* with serosal invasion or adjacent organ involvement, is more complex. Major hepatectomy or en bloc resection of contiguous organs (colon, duodenum, and pancreas) may be considered in anatomically resectable, node-negative patients, but systemic recurrence remains the dominant failure pattern, and survival benefit is limited to carefully selected cases. *T4 disease,* defined by main portal vein/hepatic artery involvement or multi-organ invasion, is rarely resectable. In select centers in Japan and India, hepatopancreaticoduodenectomy (HPD) has been attempted, but with 10–15% perioperative mortality and limited long-term benefit. Such surgery should only be undertaken in expert centers and in highly selected patients with favorable biology.[2-5,34-37]

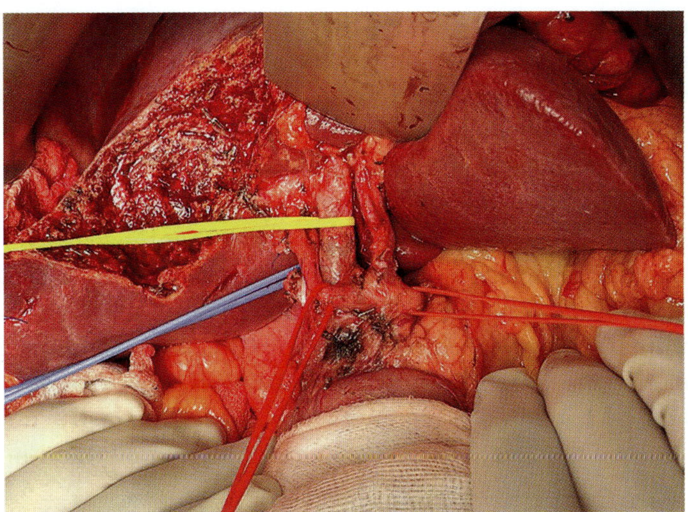

**Fig. 1:** Portal lymphadenectomy and liver wedge resection.

The surgical technique of portal lymphadenectomy and liver wedge resection is illustrated in **Figure 1**.

*Vascular resection*, a mainstay in perihilar cholangiocarcinoma and borderline pancreatic cancer, remains controversial in GBC. Portal vein or hepatic artery resection may theoretically achieve R0 margins when hilar structures are abutted, but high-level evidence for survival benefit is lacking. Existing reports are limited to small series with high recurrence risk, and most expert groups agree vascular resection should be confined to rare, technically feasible cases in high-volume HPB centers with advanced reconstruction capability.[2-5,34-37]

*Lymphadenectomy* is indispensable for staging and prognosis. Retrieval of at least six lymph nodes is required for accurate AJCC staging. Standard dissection includes stations 12 (hepatoduodenal ligament), 8 (hepatic artery), and 13 (posterior pancreaticoduodenal). Para-aortic dissection (station 16) has not shown consistent survival benefit and remains investigational. Meta-analyses of >27,000 patients confirm that systematic lymphadenectomy improves staging accuracy and is independently associated with better survival in T1b–T3 disease. In incidental GBC after index cholecystectomy, timely re-resection with radical cholecystectomy and nodal dissection restores survival outcomes to those seen with planned radical surgery. High-volume centers consistently achieve higher nodal yields, underscoring the need for centralization of care.[2,3,38]

*Minimally invasive and robotic approaches* have reshaped surgical practice, especially in early or incidental GBC. While historically avoided due to concerns over port-site metastasis, contemporary multicenter series and meta-analyses confirm that laparoscopic and robotic radical cholecystectomy can achieve comparable R0 rates, nodal yields, and long-term survival to open surgery, with reduced blood loss, shorter hospital stay, and faster recovery. Outcomes depend on meticulous oncologic technique—avoidance of gallbladder perforation, port-site protection, and adherence to open principles. Network meta-analyses show no difference in oncologic endpoints between open and minimally invasive approaches, but locally advanced and hilar-involved tumors still mandate open surgery to facilitate vascular control and complex reconstruction.[39]

In summary, stage-specific surgery for GBC is guided by a unifying principle: *anatomical radicality improves survival only when aligned with tumor biology.* Extended resections and vascular reconstructions must be judiciously employed, nodal staging must be rigorous, and minimally invasive approaches are safe only in expert hands.

## SYSTEMIC THERAPY: ADJUVANT, PALLIATIVE, AND PRECISION MEDICINE

High systemic relapse rates after R0 resection make systemic therapy integral to GBC management, spanning adjuvant, palliative, and precision oncology settings. In the adjuvant space, the *BILCAP trial* established capecitabine as standard of care, demonstrating improved survival in resected biliary cancers, particularly node- and margin-positive GBC. Other regimens, including gemcitabine–cisplatin and S-1 (used in Japan), have not surpassed capecitabine, which remains the global benchmark.[40,41]

For advanced disease, the *ABC-02 trial* defined gemcitabine–cisplatin as the first-line standard, extending median survival to 11.7 months versus 8.1 with gemcitabine alone. Intensification with nab-paclitaxel plus gemcitabine–cisplatin has shown encouraging phase II responses, with phase III validation ongoing. On progression, the *ABC-06 trial* established FOLFOX as standard second-line therapy, conferring a modest survival benefit (6.2 vs. 5.3 months).[40-43]

Molecular profiling now guides treatment in defined subsets. *HER2 amplification/overexpression* (~10–15%) predicts benefit from trastuzumab, pertuzumab, and antibody–drug conjugates such as trastuzumab deruxtecan. *FGFR2 fusions* (~2–3%) respond to FGFR inhibitors including pemigatinib and futibatinib, while IDH1 mutations, rare in GBC, are under study with IDH inhibitors.[31,44]

Immunotherapy is reshaping practice. The *TOPAZ-1 trial* showed that adding durvalumab to gemcitabine–cisplatin significantly improved survival in advanced biliary tract cancers, establishing chemo-immunotherapy as a new frontline standard. In biomarker-selected disease, MSI-H/dMMR

(~2–3% of GBC) predicts dramatic responses to PD-1 inhibitors such as pembrolizumab.[31,44,45]

Together, these advances mark a decisive shift: systemic therapy in GBC has evolved from empiric cytotoxics to a tiered, biology-driven paradigm integrating adjuvant capecitabine, frontline chemo-immunotherapy, rational second-line chemotherapy, and targeted or immunotherapy in molecularly defined subsets.

## FUTURE DIRECTIONS: CTDNA, RADIOMICS, AI, AND GLOBAL COLLABORATION

The future of GBC management lies in biology-driven personalization. Circulating tumor DNA (ctDNA), radiomics, and artificial intelligence (AI) are poised to transform risk stratification and treatment selection, while international registries and consensus frameworks remain critical to reducing disparities and translating innovation into global practice.

### Circulating Tumor DNA and Molecular Response

Given GBC's systemic biology, ctDNA-based minimal residual disease (MRD) monitoring is highly attractive. In biliary cancers, postoperative ctDNA positivity predicts early recurrence and inferior survival, often preceding imaging by months. Serial ctDNA kinetics track clonal evolution (e.g., TP53, PIK3CA), guiding therapy escalation in persistent disease or de-escalation when MRD remains negative. Composite definitions integrating PET and pathology are promising, though GBC-specific trials remain essential.[46,47]

### Radiomics and Quantitative Imaging Biomarkers

Radiomics extracts quantitative features from CT/MRI, capturing tumor phenotype beyond visual assessment. In biliary cancers, models predict microvascular invasion, nodal spread, peritoneal disease, and survival. For GBC, early models suggest predictive value for hepatic-side T2b invasion, nodal risk, and systemic relapse—key triggers for NACT versus upfront surgery. Integration with PET metrics (MTV, ΔSUVmax) and serum markers may enhance futility prediction.[48]

### Artificial Intelligence for Decision Support

AI platforms are advancing staging from descriptive imaging to predictive modeling. Early tools predict resectability and futility using integrated imaging and clinical data. Future multiomic systems will combine radiomics, histopathology, ctDNA, and genomics to individualize NACT selection and trial matching. Validation through prospective and randomized AI-enabled trials is needed.[46-48]

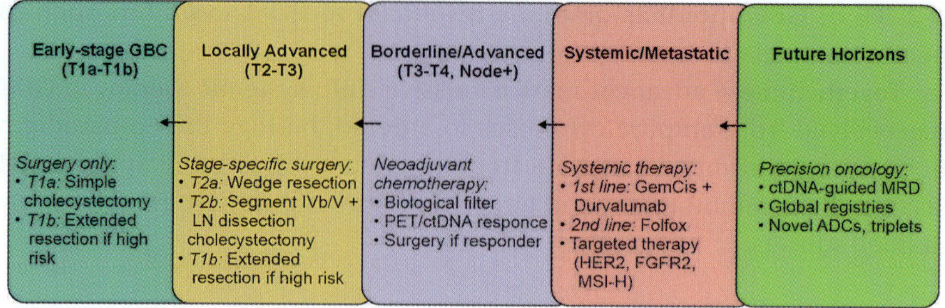


**Fig. 2:** Roadmap for modern treatment of gallbladder cancer.

## Global Collaboration, Registries, and Implementation Science

OMEGA underscored wide disparities. Registries such as China Registry for Gallbladder Cancer (CRGGC) benchmark quality indicators including staging laparoscopy, nodal yield, and PET use.[49] Embedding guideline-aligned checklists from IHPBA/NCCN and pragmatic trials such as GAIN and OPT-IN will standardize biology-first sequencing. Tele-MDTs and surgical mentoring remain vital for capacity building.[2,3,50]

## Translational Horizons

Emerging innovations include FAP-targeted PET with theranostic potential, HER2- and TROP2-directed ADCs, and rational triplets combining chemotherapy, immunotherapy, and targeted agents guided by PD-L1, TMB, MSI-H, and myeloid signatures. In summary, ctDNA-guided MRD, radiomics- and AI-enabled prediction, and international collaboration promise to embed biology-driven precision into real-world GBC care.

A roadmap for modern treatment of GBC is summarized in **Figure 2**.

## CONCLUSION

Gallbladder cancer management is shifting from radical resections toward biology-driven personalization. Rigorous staging, selective use of neoadjuvant chemotherapy, stage-specific surgery, and biomarker-directed systemic therapy represent the pillars of modern care. The future lies in integrating ctDNA, radiomics, AI, and global registries to reduce disparities and standardize outcomes. Multidisciplinary, biology-first approaches will define the next era of GBC management.

## REFERENCES

1. Bao W, Qiao L, Li M, Shi G, Liu L. Trends and cross-country inequalities in the global, regional, and national burden of gallbladder and biliary tract cancer from 1990 to 2021, along with the predictions for 2035. Cancer Epidemiol. 2025;96:102802.

2. Palepu J, Endo I, Chaudhari VA, Murthy GVS, Chaudhuri S, Adam R, et al. IHPBA-APHPBA International Study Group of Gallbladder Cancer; 'IHPBA-APHPBA clinical practice guidelines': international Delphi consensus recommendations for gallbladder cancer. HPB (Oxford). 2024;26(11):1311-26.
3. Benson AB 3rd, D'Angelica MI, Abrams T, Ahmed A, Akce M, Anaya DA, et al. Biliary Tract Cancers, Version 2. 2025, NCCN Clinical Practice Guidelines in Oncology. J Natl Compr Canc Netw. 2025;23(9):403-18.
4. Waller GC, Sarpel U. Gallbladder Cancer. Surg Clin North Am. 2024;104(6): 1263-80.
5. Qiu S, Zeng W, Zhang J, Xie J, Chen X. The Global and Regional Burden of Gallbladder and Biliary Tract Cancer and Attributable Risk Factors: Trends and Predictions. Liver Int. 2025;45(4):e70025.
6. Giraldo NA, Drill E, Satravada BA, Dika IE, Brannon AR, Dermawan J, et al. Comprehensive Molecular Characterization of Gallbladder Carcinoma and Potential Targets for Intervention. Clin Cancer Res. 2022;28(24):5359-67.
7. Ebata N, Fujita M, Sasagawa S, Maejima K, Okawa Y, Hatanaka Y, et al. Molecular Classification and Tumor Microenvironment Characterization of Gallbladder Cancer by Comprehensive Genomic and Transcriptomic Analysis. Cancers (Basel). 2021;13(4):733.
8. Rana P, Kalage D, Soundararajan R, Gupta P. Update on the Role of Imaging in the Diagnosis, Staging, and Prognostication of Gallbladder Cancer. Indian J Radiol Imaging. 2024;35(2):218-33.
9. Cassese G, Han HS, Yoon YS, Lee JS, Cho JY, Lee HW, et al. Preoperative Assessment and Perioperative Management of Resectable Gallbladder Cancer in the Era of Precision Medicine and Novel Technologies: State of the Art and Future Perspectives. Diagnostics (Basel). 2022;12(7):1630.
10. Kim HJ, Park MS, Lee J, Kim KW, Yu JS, Chung JJ, et al. Role of gadoxetic acid-enhanced MRI in gallbladder carcinoma. Eur Radiol. 2013;23(12):3294-303.
11. El Chafic AH, Dewitt J, Leblanc JK, Sherman S, McHenry L, Al-Haddad MA. Role of EUS-FNA in incidental gallbladder cancer. Endosc Ultrasound. 2017;6(5):324-30.
12. Kim YJ, Yun M, Lee WJ, Kim KS, Lee JD. Clinical value of FDG PET/CT in gallbladder cancer. Eur J Nucl Med Mol Imaging. 2010;37(2):335-42.
13. Shukla PJ, Barreto SG, Arya S, Shrikhande SV, Hawaldar R, Purandare N, et al. Does PET-CT scan have a role prior to radical re-resection for incidental gallbladder cancer? HPB (Oxford). 2008;10(6):439-45.
14. Zhao L, Chen S, Lin Y, Chen X, Li X, Xu H, et al. Fibroblast activation protein-targeted PET for biliary cancers. Clin Cancer Res. 2021;27(2):479-88.
15. Goel M, Agarwal AK, Kumar V, Shukla NK, Verma AK, Saxena R, et al. Staging laparoscopy in gallbladder cancer: predictive yield and impact. Ann Surg Oncol. 2013;20(9):3102-9.
16. Agarwal AK, Mandal S, Singh S, Tandon P, Verma A, Sakhuja P. Predictors of positive yield of staging laparoscopy in gallbladder cancer. Ann Surg. 2013;258(3):519-25.
17. Balakrishnan A, Barmpounakis P, Demiris N, Prassas D, Notas G, Macheras A, et al. Surgical outcomes of gallbladder cancer: the OMEGA retrospective, multicentre, international cohort study. EClinicalMedicine. 2023;59:101951.

18. Balakrishnan A, Barmpounakis P, Demiris N, Andersson B, Brañes A, de Aretxabala X, et al. OMEGA Study Investigators. Assessment of nodal staging and risk factors for nodal involvement in gallbladder cancer. BJS Open. 2025;9(3):zraf056.
19. Patkar S, Patel S, Gupta A, Ramaswamy A, Ostwal V, Goel M, et al. Lessons learnt from 1300 consecutive gallbladder cancer surgeries: evolving role of peri-operative chemotherapy. Eur J Surg Oncol. 2023;49(9):107035.
20. Lee SE, Choi YS, Kim YH, Heo JS, Jeong CY, Lee WJ, et al. Prognostic Significance of Tumor Location in T2 Gallbladder Cancer: A Korea Tumor Registry System Biliary Pancreas (KOTUS-BP) Database Analysis. J Clin Med. 2020;9(10):3268.
21. Kato H, Horiguchi A, Ohtsuka T, Nanashima A, Unno M, Wakai T, et al. Annual report of Japanese biliary tract cancer registry from 2021: Focus on the rate of R0 resection, postoperative complications, and site of lymph node metastasis. J Hepatobiliary Pancreat Sci. 2025;32(5):339-49.
22. Dutta U, Goel M, Shukla PJ, Shrikhande SV. Futility in gallbladder cancer surgery: lessons from India. Indian J Gastroenterol. 2018;37(3):248-55.
23. Serenari M, Berti D, Rivera B, Newhook TE, Kristjanpoller W, Ruzzenente A, et al. Optimizing Outcomes in Gallbladder Cancer: Identifying Predictors of Futile Up-Front Surgery in a Global Multi-center Study. Ann Surg Oncol. 2025; 32(6):4374-82.
24. Varshney P, Baghmar S, Sirohi B, Abou-Alfa GK, Cao HT, Sharma LM, et al. Neoadjuvant treatment for incidental gallbladder cancer: A systematic review. Ann Hepatobiliary Pancreat Surg. 2025;29(2):113-20.
25. Chaudhari VA, Ostwal V, Engineer R, Chopra S, Ramaswamy A, Goel M, et al. Neoadjuvant chemotherapy in node-positive gallbladder cancer: institutional experience. HPB (Oxford). 2018;20(5):416-24.
26. Goel M, Singh RK, Kapoor VK, Agarwal AK, Tandon R, Mohan N, et al. Neoadjuvant chemotherapy in locally advanced gallbladder cancer: Tata Memorial Centre experience. Ann Surg Oncol. 2019;26(5):1340-7.
27. Xiong Y, Yang Z, Gong A, Lin Y, Yan J, Zhang Y, et al. Prognostic impact of neoadjuvant chemotherapy in localized or locoregionally advanced gallbladder cancer: a SEER-based population analysis. Cancer Control. 2024; 31:1-11.
28. Patkar S, Gundavda K, Polusany K, Yelamanchi R, Varty GP, Shah N, et al. Predicting clinical benefit response after neoadjuvant chemotherapy in locally advanced gallbladder cancer: retrospective analysis. BJS Open. 2025; 9(4):zraf077.
29. Goetze TO, Bechstein WO, Bankstahl US, Keck T, Königsrainer A, Lang SA, et al. Neoadjuvant gemcitabine and cisplatin followed by radical surgery versus immediate surgery in locally advanced gallbladder cancer (GAIN): a multicentre, randomized, phase 3 trial protocol. BMC Cancer. 2020;20(1):122.
30. Engineer R, Patkar S, Lewis SC, Sharma AD, Shetty N, Ostwal V, et al. A phase III randomised clinical trial of perioperative therapy (neoadjuvant chemotherapy versus chemoradiotherapy) in locally advanced gallbladder cancers (POLCAGB): study protocol. BMJ Open. 2019;9(6):e028147.
31. Oh DY, He AR, Qin S, Chen LT, Okusaka T, Vogel A, et al. Durvalumab plus gemcitabine–cisplatin in advanced biliary tract cancer (TOPAZ-1). N Engl J Med. 2022;386(9):898-910.

32. Barreto SG, Dutt A, Sirohi B, Shrikhande SV. Gallbladder cancer: a journey of a thousand steps. Future Oncol. 2018;14(13):1299-306.
33. Lee SE, Jang JY, Lim CS, Kang MJ, Kim SW, Kim YH, et al. Surgical treatment for T1 gallbladder cancer: a Korean multicenter analysis. World J Gastroenterol. 2011;17(2):174-80.
34. Vega EA, Mellado S, Chirban AM, de la Fuente HA, Ferrero A, Giuliante F, et al. Extent of liver resection for incidental gallbladder cancer: how much is too much? Ann Surg Oncol. 2023;30(11):6594-600.
35. Shirai Y, Tsukada K, Ohtani T, Hatakeyama K. Radical surgery for gallbladder carcinoma: long-term results. World J Surg. 2002;26(9):1011-7.
36. Kondo S, Nimura Y, Kamiya J, Nagino M, Kanai M, Uesaka K. Radical surgery for advanced gallbladder cancer. Br J Surg. 2002;89(2):165-71.
37. D'Angelica M, Dalal KM, DeMatteo RP, Fong Y, Blumgart LH, Jarnagin WR. Analysis of the extent of resection for adenocarcinoma of the gallbladder. Ann Surg Oncol. 2009;16(4):806-16.
38. Papageorge MV, de Geus SWL, Woods AP, Ng SC, Drake FT, Merrill A, et al. Lymphadenectomy in gallbladder adenocarcinoma: Are we doing enough? Am J Surg. 2022;224(1 Pt B):423-8.
39. Chee MYM, Wu AGR, Fong KY, Yew A, Koh YX, Goh BKP. Robotic, laparoscopic and open surgery for gallbladder cancer: a systematic review and network meta-analysis. Surg Endosc. 2024;38(9):4846-57.
40. Primrose JN, Fox R, Palmer DH, Malik HZ, Prasad R, Mirza D, et al. Capecitabine as adjuvant therapy for biliary tract cancer (BILCAP): a phase 3 trial. Lancet Oncol. 2019;20(5):663-73.
41. Li Y, Zhou Y, Hong Y, He M, Wei S, Yang C, et al. The Efficacy of Different Chemotherapy Regimens for Advanced Biliary Tract Cancer: A Systematic Review and Network Meta-Analysis. Front Oncol. 2019;9:441.
42. Shroff RT, Javle M, Xiao L, Kaseb AO, Varadhachary GR, Wolff RA, et al. Gemcitabine, cisplatin, and nab-paclitaxel for advanced biliary tract cancers: a phase 2 trial. JAMA Oncol. 2019;5(6):824-30.
43. Lamarca A, Palmer DH, Wasan HS, Ross PJ, Ma YT, Arora A, et al. Advanced Biliary Cancer Working Group. Second-line FOLFOX chemotherapy versus active symptom control for advanced biliary tract cancer (ABC-06): a phase 3, open-label, randomised, controlled trial. Lancet Oncol. 2021;22(5):690-701.
44. Marabelle A, Le DT, Ascierto PA, Di Giacomo AM, De Jesus-Acosta A, Delord JP, et al. Efficacy of pembrolizumab in MSI-H/dMMR cancers. J Clin Oncol. 2020;38(1):1-10.
45. Kassab J, Saba L, Gebrael G, Kais S, Kassab R, Kourie HR. Update on immunotherapy in the management of gallbladder cancer. Immunotherapy. 2023;15(1):35-42.
46. Okamura Y, Yamashita YI, Imai K, Nakagawa S, Hashimoto D, Chikamoto A, et al. Circulating tumor DNA in biliary tract cancers: opportunities and challenges. J Hepatobiliary Pancreat Sci. 2021;28(5):383-91.
47. Parikh AR, Van Seventer EE, Siravegna G, Hartwig AV, Jaimovich A, He Y, et al. Minimal residual disease detection using ctDNA in gastrointestinal cancers. Nat Rev Clin Oncol. 2021;18(12):760-73.

48. Lambin P, Leijenaar RTH, Deist TM, Peerlings J, De Jong EEC, Van Timmeren J, et al. Radiomics: the bridge between medical imaging and personalized medicine. Nat Rev Clin Oncol. 2017;14(12):749-62.
49. Ren T, Li Y, Zhang X, Geng Y, Shao Z, Li M, et al. China Registry for Gallbladder Cancer (CRGGC): study protocol. BMJ Open. 2021;11(2): e038634.
50. Shishir K Maithel, Sung Chul Hong, Cecilia Grace Ethun, Cristina R Ferrone, Flavio G Rocha, Charles A Staley, et al. Optimal perioperative therapy for incidental gallbladder cancer (OPT-IN): A randomized phase II/III trial—ECOG-ACRIN EA2197. J Clin Oncol 41, TPS620-TPS620(2023). DOI:10.1200/JCO.2023.41.4_suppl.TPS620

CHAPTER 3

# Large Bowel Obstruction

*Yajnadatta Sarangi, Sanjay K, Rahul*

## INTRODUCTION

Large bowel obstruction (LBO), defined as obstruction distal to the ileocecal valve, accounts for approximately 20–25% of all intestinal obstructions and is more frequently encountered in elderly patients. It carries significant morbidity and mortality, particularly when complicated by ischemia or perforation, where mortality rates may reach 10–20%.[1]

The causes of LBO are diverse and may be malignant or benign. Malignancy, particularly colorectal cancer (CRC), is the most common etiology. Approximately 8–13% of CRCs present with obstruction at the time of diagnosis, and up to 25% develop obstruction during the disease course. Obstruction is often the first clinical presentation in left-sided tumors. The sigmoid colon is the most common site of obstruction, with nearly 75% of obstructing tumors occurring distal to the splenic flexure.[2] Benign causes of LBO, although less common, remain clinically important. These include diverticular disease with stricture, volvulus (particularly of the sigmoid colon), inflammatory bowel disease (IBD), ischemic colitis, radiation-induced strictures, and postsurgical or anastomotic strictures.

In recent years, the management of malignant LBO has evolved considerably. Traditionally, emergency surgery was the mainstay of treatment. With the advent of self-expanding metal stents (SEMS), treatment paradigms have shifted. These recent advances, along with improved imaging and endoscopic techniques, highlight the importance of individualized, evidence-based decision-making in the management of LBO.

## ETIOLOGY

The causes of LBO can be broadly categorized as functional (adynamic) or mechanical **(Table 1)**. Based on etiology, it can be either malignant or benign. Based on the site of obstruction, it can be categorized as right-sided (proximal to the splenic flexure), left-sided (distal to the splenic flexure), or rectal obstruction, with left-sided disease being the most common. Based on the duration of symptoms, obstruction may be acute (lasting hours to days), subacute (lasting days to weeks), or chronic/recurrent (lasting weeks to months). Pathophysiologically, it may be further distinguished as

**TABLE 1:** Various causes of large bowel obstruction.[3]

| *Obstruction type* | *Causes of large bowel obstruction* |
|---|---|
| Mechanical | Neoplastic |
| | Volvulus (sigmoid/cecal/transverse colon) |
| | Diverticular disease |
| | Intussusception |
| | Incarcerated hernia |
| | Abscess/inflammation/inflammatory bowel disease |
| | Adhesions |
| | Foreign body (rare) |
| | Fecal impaction (rare) |
| Functional | Toxic megacolon |
| | Pseudo-obstruction |

simple obstruction, where vascular supply and viability remain intact, or complicated obstruction, where ischemia, necrosis, or perforation has set in. Such classifications are clinically important as they guide both the urgency and type of intervention.

One of the common benign causes of LBO (after malignancy and diverticulitis) is volvulus of the sigmoid colon, followed by volvulus of the cecum. Transverse colon and splenic flexure volvulus are rare. Benign LBO can result from a wide spectrum of intrinsic, extrinsic, and functional pathologies. Intrinsic causes include luminal narrowing from diverticular disease, IBD, ischemic colitis, radiation-induced injury, tuberculosis, traumatic injury, or anastomotic strictures. Uncommon causes include intraluminal factors such as foreign bodies, food bolus impaction (particularly in the elderly), or drug packets. Extrinsic compression may arise from gynecologic neoplasms, peritoneal carcinomatosis, lymphadenopathy, or inflammatory conditions like pancreatitis. Endometriosis is notable for its ability to cause obstruction by both intrinsic and extrinsic involvement. Retroperitoneal fibrosis, although rare, can also lead to obstruction through fibrotic encasement of bowel loops and adjacent structures, often secondary to infections, malignancy, medications, or prior radiotherapy. Additional unusual causes include congenital adhesive bands, migration of medical devices (e.g., intrauterine devices), and pharmacobezoars in patients with chronic constipation and redundant colon.[3]

Acute colonic pseudo-obstruction (*Ogilvie's syndrome*) is characterized by colonic dilatation in the absence of a mechanical obstruction. It typically affects the cecum and ascending colon, though it can involve the entire colon. The exact mechanism is unclear, but it is believed to result from dysregulation of the autonomic control of colonic motility, resulting in ineffective

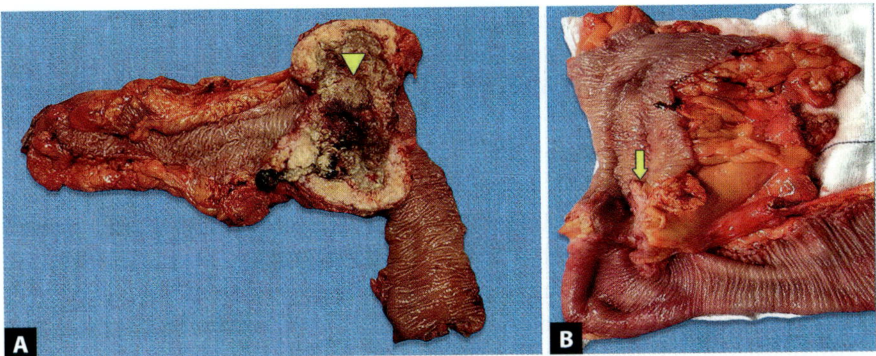


**Figs. 1A and B:** (A) Cicatrizing growth at the splenic flexure of the colon (arrowhead); (B) Proliferative growth in the cecum (arrow).

smooth muscle contraction. Risk factors include advanced age, electrolyte disturbances (hypomagnesemia, hypercalcemia, and hypothyroidism), medications (opioids, calcium-channel blockers, antidepressants, and anticholinergics), severe systemic illness, postoperative states, trauma, and neurological disorders (e.g., Parkinson's disease, multiple sclerosis, spinal cord injury).

The descending and sigmoid colon are the most common sites of malignant obstruction. Left-sided CRCs are typically annular and constricting ("cicatrizing"), in contrast to right-sided tumors, which are often ulcero-proliferative **(Figs. 1A and B)**. In addition, stool in the left colon is more solid and lumen is narrower, thus further predisposing it to mechanical obstruction.

## PATHOPHYSIOLOGY

In LBO, as the bowel distends (due to accumulation of gas and fluid), intraluminal pressure starts to increase. The gas (primarily of bacterial origin) consists largely of nitrogen (~90%) and hydrogen sulfide. Progressive distension is exacerbated by impaired propulsion and ongoing bacterial fermentation. Increased intraluminal pressure initially compromises the venous drainage, thus resulting in wall congestion, edema, and mucosal injury. Persistent obstruction and sustained intraluminal pressure later impairs the capillary inflow, culminating in ischemia. If left untreated, it evolves into transmural necrosis and eventually perforation. Bacterial overgrowth and mucosal breakdown facilitate translocation of organisms and toxins, contributing to systemic sepsis.

The degree and rapidity of distension are influenced by the competence of the ileocecal valve.

- *Competent valve:* A closed-loop obstruction is created. The colon—especially the cecum, being the most distensible segment—undergoes rapid distension. Once the diameter exceeds 12 cm, the risk of ischemia and perforation rises sharply. Mucosa becomes ischemic in 3–4 hours, and transmural infarction followed by perforation occurs within 6 hours.

- *Incompetent valve:* The obstruction decompresses retrogradely into the small bowel. Although this reduces the colonic pressure, progressive dilatation of small bowel ensues, often with fecalization and bacterial overgrowth.

Fluid and electrolyte disturbances result from reduced oral intake, impaired absorption, repeated vomiting, sequestration of fluid within the obstructed bowel, and transudation into the peritoneal cavity. These changes can cause hypovolemia, metabolic derangements, and systemic toxicity, particularly when ischemia or perforation supervenes.

## HISTORY AND PHYSICAL EXAMINATION

The clinical presentation of LBO varies with the level of block. Common features include abdominal pain, progressive distension, nausea, vomiting, and obstipation. When the ileocecal valve is incompetent, colonic contents decompress into the small intestine, often resulting in feculent vomiting. In contrast, a competent ileocecal valve prevents decompression, leading to progressive colonic dilatation and marked right iliac fossa pain. Digital rectal examination may reveal an empty rectum, mass in rectum or finger smeared with fresh blood. Long-standing obstruction complicated by ischemia or perforation may present with fecal peritonitis, characterized by generalized abdominal pain, guarding or rigidity, and systemic features of sepsis. In a study of 150 consecutive cases of acute mechanical bowel obstruction, 24% involved the large bowel. The most frequent presenting features were inability to pass flatus (90%) or stool (80.6%), along with abdominal distension (65.3%).[4]

## CLINICAL FEATURES OF COLORECTAL MALIGNANCY-ASSOCIATED OBSTRUCTION

Obstruction due to left-sided CRC typically presents with alternating constipation and diarrhea, rectal bleeding, and weight loss. These symptoms may persist for weeks or months before frank obstruction ensues. A family history of CRC is positive in some.

## CLINICAL FEATURES OF BENIGN CAUSES OF LARGE BOWEL OBSTRUCTION

Sigmoid volvulus occurs most often in patients with chronic constipation and reduced mobility, particularly in those who are bedridden or are living in long-term care facilities. It usually presents abruptly with abdominal pain, constipation, and marked distension. On examination, the abdomen may reveal significant distension and tympany. Cecal volvulus often mimics small bowel obstruction.

Pseudo-obstruction can closely resemble a true mechanical obstruction; however, pain is an uncommon feature. These patients may continue to pass gas, present with either constipation or diarrhea, and abdominal distension.

## CLINICAL FEATURES OF OTHER ETIOLOGY-ASSOCIATED OBSTRUCTION

Large bowel obstruction may also result from less common causes. Diverticular disease typically presents with pain, fever, a palpable mass, and proximal colonic distension. Hernia-related obstruction manifests as an irreducible mass with overlying skin changes, most often at inguinal, spigelian, or lumbar sites. Endometriosis and other pelvic pathologies, such as uterine fibroids or malignancy, may present with pelvic pain, dysmenorrhea, rectal pain, or altered bowel habits. Fecal impaction, frequently seen in chronically ill, debilitated, or constipated patients, is characterized by abdominal pain, distension, fecal incontinence, and hard pellet like stool in the rectum; complications include stercoral ulceration and perforation. Retroperitoneal fibrosis is associated with back or flank pain, fever, weight loss, and fatigue. Intussusception may cause nonspecific symptoms such as abdominal pain, nausea, vomiting, altered bowel habit, or hematochezia. In cases of perforation, patients often exhibit signs of peritonitis with diffuse guarding, accompanied by signs of systemic instability (tachycardia and hypotension).

## COMPLICATIONS OF LARGE BOWEL OBSTRUCTION

Patients with LBO may present with complications that influence clinical course and management:

- *Bowel ischemia:* Severe pain disproportionate to clinical findings, fever, and tachycardia.
- *Perforation with peritonitis:* Acute severe pain, abdominal distension, fever, and guarding/rigidity.
- *Contained perforation with abscess:* Localized pain, fever, and/or phlegmon.
- *Sepsis and multiorgan dysfunction:* Systemic inflammatory response with shock and organ failure(s).
- *Fluid and electrolyte disturbances:* Irritability, confusion, arrhythmias, nausea, and fatigue.
- *Aspiration pneumonia:* Cough, fever, dyspnea in patients with persistent vomiting.

## EVALUATION

Obtaining a detailed history, a thorough physical examination, and imaging are crucial in evaluating a suspected LBO. Laboratory tests for anemia, infection, renal function, and electrolytes are initiated to drive resuscitation and focused treatment. Leukocytosis and acidosis may indicate tissue ischemia.

## IMAGING

The evaluation usually begins with *plain radiography*, which is widely available, quick, and inexpensive. Supine and upright abdominal X-rays demonstrate a dilated colon proximal to the site of obstruction, absence of rectal gas, and characteristic air-fluid levels **(Figs. 2A to D)**. In advanced cases, plain radiographs can also reveal complications such as pneumoperitoneum, pneumatosis intestinalis, or portal venous gas, which signal necrosis or perforation. Sensitivity for plain radiographs is ~80–90%, with specificity ranging from 65–75%, though diagnostic accuracy varies with the underlying pathology and interpreter's expertise. Plain films are especially

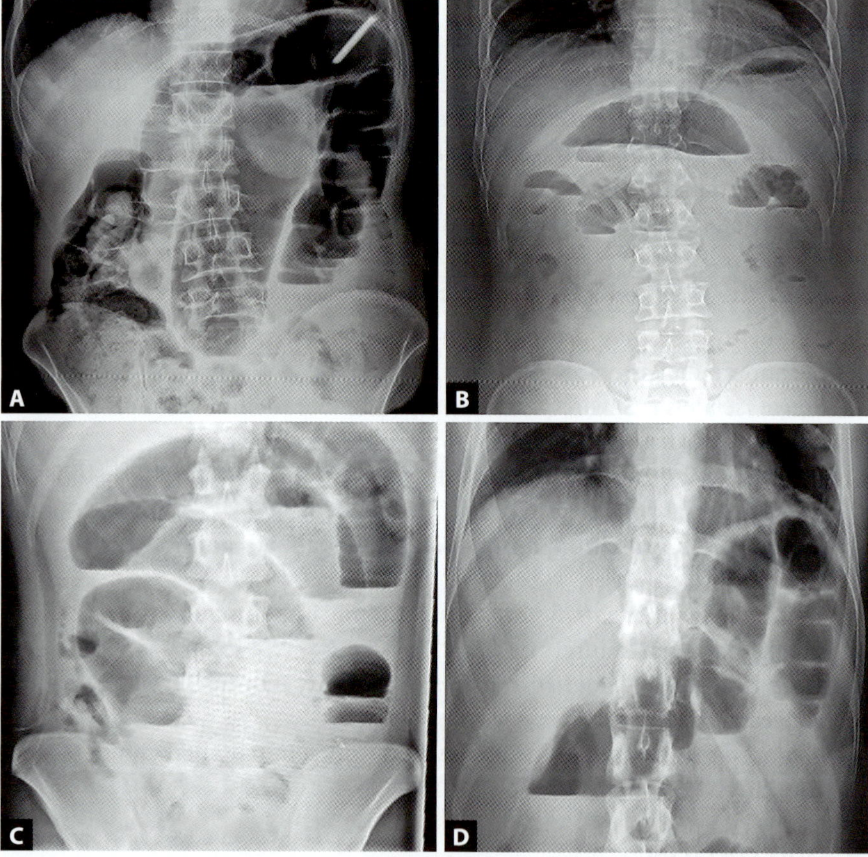

**Figs. 2A to D:** X-ray images of large bowel obstruction. (A) Dilated transverse colon and descending colon in a case of sigmoid colon growth; (B) Dilated colon with air fluid level; (C) Air fluid level with the absence of rectal gas; (D) Dilated transverse colon in a case of descending colon malignancy.

valuable in volvulus (classic signs—*coffee bean or bird beak* configurations) **(Figs. 3A to C)**. A sigmoid volvulus may extend into the right upper quadrant in a large U-shaped loop, while a cecal volvulus may remain in the right lower quadrant or migrate into the left upper quadrant, sometimes displacing the appendix alongside the distended cecum. Additional features on X-rays include: loss of haustrations in advanced IBD or ischemic conditions, *lead-pipe appearance* in ulcerative colitis (smooth, featureless colonic walls) **(Fig. 4)**. Radiography is also important in identifying toxic megacolon: massive colonic dilatation (transverse colon >6 cm) accompanied by loss of haustrations in addition to systemic signs of toxicity. Early recognition and prompt medical or surgical intervention are often lifesaving.

X-ray helps in distinguishing pseudo-obstruction (*Ogilvie's syndrome*) from mechanical LBO. Pseudo-obstruction shows diffuse dilatation of colon

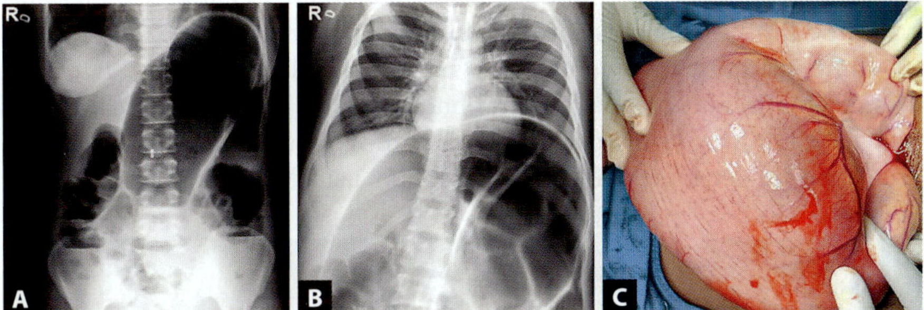


**Figs. 3A to C:** (A and B) Coffee bean sign sigmoid volvulus on abdominal X-ray; (C) Intraoperative photograph of dilated sigmoid colon.

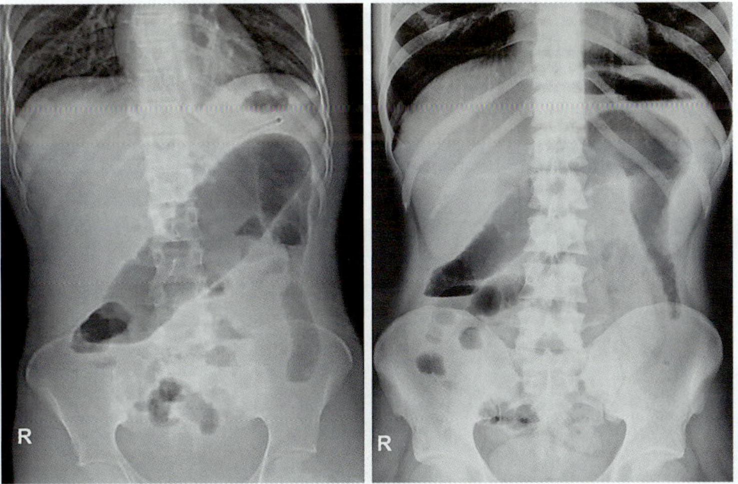


**Fig. 4:** Acute severe ulcerative colitis. Loss of haustration of colon with lead pipe appearance.

without a clear transition point, reaching up to the pelvis; unlike mechanical obstruction. Air-fluid levels are often absent. In equivocal cases, a water-soluble contrast enema can help differentiate pseudo-obstruction from true obstruction by outlining the transition point in mechanical cases. On the other hand, diffuse passage of contrast suggests functional dilatation. However, radiographs alone cannot determine the precise site, cause, or severity of obstruction, which highlights the importance of cross-sectional imaging.

*Multidetector computed tomography (MDCT)* is the gold standard in evaluating suspected LBO, with sensitivity and specificity ~90%. It not only clinches the diagnosis of obstruction but also localizes the transition point, identifies the underlying etiology, and complications. In volvulus, CT demonstrates the *Whirl sign* of twisted mesenteric vessels and the site of torsion. In diverticular disease, CT typically shows segmental symmetric wall thickening, pericolic fat stranding, and inflammatory changes, sometimes with free fluid or abscess formation. Malignancy is often characterized by short segment involvement, asymmetric wall thickening, irregular enhancement, and associated lymphadenopathy **(Figs. 5 and 6)**. It also helps in identifying synchronous lesions in the colon **(Fig. 7)**. CT also plays a crucial role in detecting adult intussusception, usually caused by a malignant

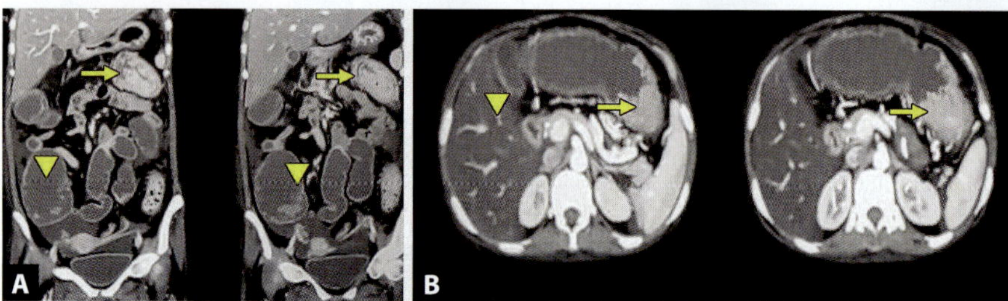


**Figs. 5A and B:** Computed tomographic scan in cases of colonic malignant obstruction. (A) Growth in the splenic flexure of the colon (small arrow), dilated proximal colon (arrowhead); (B) Growth in distal transverse colon (small arrow), fatty liver, indicating malnutrition (arrowhead) can be appreciated.

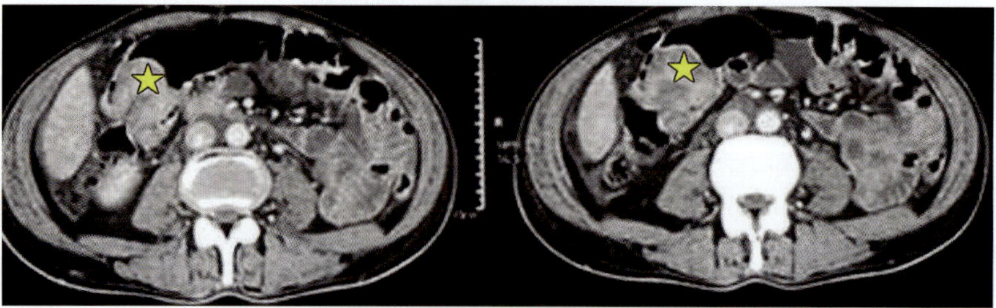

**Fig. 6:** Computed tomographic scan showing malignant growth in hepatic flexure of colon (yellow star).

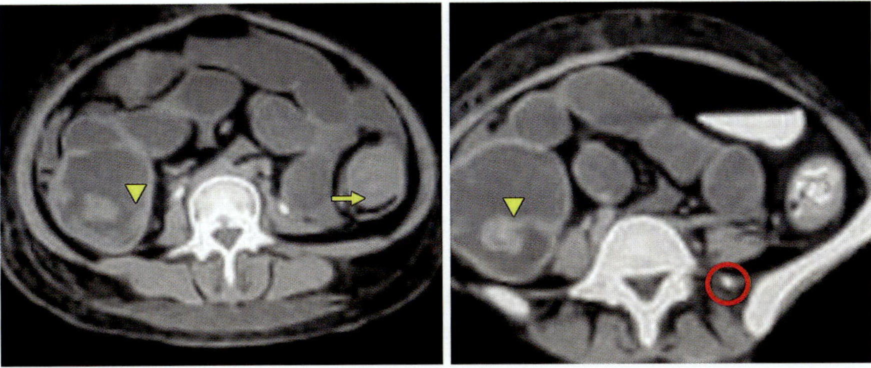

**Fig. 7:** Computed tomographic scan showing (small arrow) malignant obstructing growth in descending colon with polypoidal lesion in cecum (arrowhead) a paracolic node (red circle).

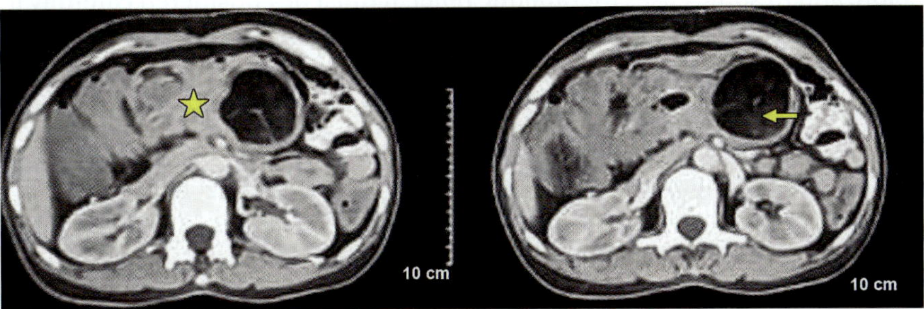


**Fig. 8:** Computed tomographic scan showing colonic intussusception (star) with the mesocolic vessel (yellow arrow) which can be appreciated inside lumen (target sign).

lead point, where the *"Target sign"* with telescoped bowel loops and mesenteric fat within the lumen can be appreciated **(Fig. 8)**. In inflammatory bowel disease, CT can demonstrate strictures, wall thickening, mucosal hyperenhancement, fistulae, or abscesses, at times mimicking malignancy. Importantly, CT can also identify toxic megacolon with precision, revealing massive colonic dilatation, wall thinning, pericolonic inflammation, and sometimes pneumatosis or free air (in presence of ischemia). CT is invaluable in differentiating true mechanical obstruction from pseudo-obstruction. In pseudo-obstruction, colonic dilatation extends up to the rectum without a discrete transition point.

CT can provide critical staging information in obstruction due to malignancy: local invasion, regional nodal involvement, and distant metastases, thereby guiding decisions regarding resection, diversion, or palliative stenting. Recent literature emphasizes the impact of timely CT scans in acute setting: early imaging correlates with reduced morbidity and mortality by enabling rapid diagnosis and intervention.[5] Post-processing techniques, including multiplanar reconstructions, further enhance diagnostic accuracy by clearly depicting tortuous or redundant colonic segments and provide a surgical "roadmap". Pneumatosis within the cecum or colon often indicates ischemia and possibly imminent perforation.

Water-soluble contrast enema is valuable when CT findings are equivocal. In suspected sigmoid volvulus, in addition to clinching the diagnosis, it can achieve therapeutic decompression in a few cases. In pseudo-obstruction, instillation of contrast helps exclude a mechanical cause and may stimulate colonic motility. However, the routine use of contrast enemas has declined with the widespread availability of high-quality CT.

## Role of Colonoscopy in Large Bowel Obstruction

Colonoscopy may play a selective but valuable role in the management of LBO, particularly for diagnosis, decompression, assessment of the proximal colon, and in some cases therapeutic relief. It must be considered carefully in the context of patient's condition, etiology, and therapeutic goals. In a 20-year retrospective study of non-conservatively managed LBO, colonoscopy was used in about 24% of cases as monotherapy and in ~7% as combination therapy (with surgery).[6] Safety remains a major concern: colonoscopy in mechanical obstruction carries the risk of perforation, especially if ischemia is suspected.

When safe, colonoscopy may be used in obstructed CRC—if the cancer is resectable—to evaluate the proximal colon for synchronous lesions or decompress the bowel. SEMS can be used to relieve obstruction. In one study, including patients with resectable malignant colorectal obstruction after effective stent placement, complete colonoscopy to the cecum was possible in ~93%; synchronous cancer was identified in nearly 10%, which changed the surgical approach plan.[7] If the mass is unresectable, the role of colonoscopy remains limited to providing tissue diagnosis and possible palliative stenting.

## Techniques

Insufflation must be done cautiously (minimal insufflation with gentle decompression) in the presence of LBO. Typically, carbon-dioxide rather than air insufflation is preferred as it is rapidly absorbed, decreasing the risk of overdistension. If a stent is in place, scope passage through SEMS must be gentle to avoid stent migration or injury. Bowel preparation is often minimal or modified in obstruction. Rectal enemas or lavage, are preferred over full oral preparation.

In volvulus, particularly sigmoid volvulus, flexible sigmoidoscopy has a therapeutic role: initial endoscopic detorsion/decompression is recommended in uncomplicated cases without signs of bowel ischemia or perforation. American Society of Colorectal Surgeons (ASCRS) and ASGE guidelines recommend endoscopic untwisting as first-line management for sigmoid volvulus, reserving surgery for failures or when there is evidence of gangrene or perforation.[8] Colonoscopy may also allow assessment of mucosal viability in volvulus. In cecal volvulus, colonoscopic detorsion is generally not recommended: surgery is the standard of care.

## MANAGEMENT

Management of benign conditions is rather straightforward **(Table 2)**, whereas management of malignant LBO requires detailed evaluation for optimal outcome.

**TABLE 2:** Management of benign causes of large bowel obstruction.

| *Cause* | *Acute phase management* | *Definitive management* |
|---|---|---|
| Sigmoid volvulus | • Resuscitation (IV fluids, correction of electrolytes)<br>• Nasogastric decompression<br>• Endoscopic detorsion/ decompression with flexible sigmoidoscopy or colonoscopy if no peritonitis/ ischemia<br>• Avoid aggressive insufflation; prefer $CO_2$ | • Elective sigmoid colectomy after stabilization (recommended due to high recurrence rates)<br>• If patient unfit: consider percutaneous endoscopic colostomy (PEC) in selected cases<br>• Hartmann's procedure<br>• Sigmoidopexy (extraperitonealization of sigmoid colon) |
| Cecal volvulus | • Resuscitation and stabilization<br>• Colonoscopic decompression not recommended | • Right hemicolectomy (preferred)<br>• Cecopexy or tube cecostomy in frail/unfit patients |
| Diverticular stricture | • Stabilize, IV fluids, broad-spectrum antibiotics<br>• Bowel rest, NG decompression | • Elective sigmoidectomy (laparoscopy if feasible)<br>• Resection and anastomosis or Hartmann's procedure depending on patient status and contamination |
| Inflammatory bowel disease (IBD) stricture—e.g., Crohn's, ulcerative colitis (UC) | • Stabilization, steroids, or biologics if acute flare<br>• Avoid endoscopic dilation in toxic megacolon or acute inflammation<br>• Short-term decompression if needed | • Elective resection of affected segment (Crohn's)<br>• Sub-total colectomy in UC with refractory disease/ strictures<br>• Endoscopic balloon dilation for short, accessible strictures in Crohn's |

*Contd...*

*Contd...*

| *Cause* | *Acute phase management* | *Definitive management* |
|---|---|---|
| Post-surgical or anastomotic stricture | • Initial stabilization<br>• Exclude ischemia or recurrence with imaging | • Endoscopic balloon dilation (first-line)<br>• Surgical revision if dilation fails |
| Radiation-induced stricture | • Stabilization<br>• Exclude perforation/ischemia<br>• Bowel rest | • Segmental resection or bypass if severe<br>• Endoscopic dilation may be attempted but recurrence common |
| Fecal impaction | • Manual disimpaction, enemas, osmotic laxatives<br>• NG decompression if vomiting: Exclude stercoral perforation | • Long-term bowel regimen (laxatives, dietary modification)<br>• Treat underlying causes (neurologic, immobility, medications) |
| Endometriosis involving colon | • Stabilization<br>• Imaging (CT/MRI) to assess extent | • Elective resection of involved segment<br>• Medical therapy (hormonal suppression) in selected cases |
| Adhesions (possible after colorectal surgery) | • Conservative: fluids, nasogastric decompression, correction of electrolytes<br>• Oral neat contrast | Surgical adhesiolysis if recurrent or complicated |
| Intussusception (benign lead point, e.g., lipoma, polyp) | • Stabilize<br>• Imaging confirmation<br>• Gentle colonoscopic reduction in adults sometimes attempted | Segmental resection (since malignancy must always be excluded in adults) |
| Toxic megacolon (complication of UC, Crohn's, or infectious colitis) | • Intensive supportive care (fluids, electrolytes)<br>• High-dose IV steroids in UC/ Crohn's<br>• Broad-spectrum antibiotics<br>• NG/rectal tube decompression<br>• Avoid colonoscopy due to perforation risk | Subtotal colectomy with end ileostomy if medical therapy fails or perforation occurs |

(NG: nasogastric)

## Initial Management

Targeted fluid resuscitation and metabolic corrections should be started as soon as a patient of LBO lands in the emergency. Nasogastric tube decompression relieves abdominal distention, especially in patients with an incompetent ileocecal valve. Serial imaging may be required to monitor the distension in pseudo-obstructions. Patients with increasing cecal distension are at increased risk of perforation and should be considered for early intervention.

For patients with perforation, source control is the primary objective. A perforation proximal to the tumor typically leads to widespread fecal contamination and sepsis. Damage control measures should be initiated within hours of initial resuscitation. It is important to achieve a central venous pressure of 8–12 mm Hg, a mean arterial pressure >65 mm Hg, and a central venous oxygen saturation of ≥70%. Vasopressors (norepinephrine and epinephrine), broad-spectrum antibiotics covering anaerobes, and Gram-negative organisms are tailored according to needs. In hemodynamically unstable patients, image-guided drainage of associated abscess is vital for source control.

## Etiology-guided Interventions

### *Benign Large Bowel Obstruction*

Principles of management of LBO remain the same and often require a multidisciplinary approach.

### *Malignant Large Bowel Obstruction*

*Management of left-sided obstructing CRC:* Left-sided malignant LBO is a surgical emergency. Management strategy depends on patient stability, tumor stage, surgical expertise, and institutional resources. Treatment options include: proximal loop colostomy, Hartmann's procedure (HP), and resection with primary anastomosis (RPA) as well as endoscopic intervention—SEMS and transanal decompression tubes (TDT) as bridge therapy.

## Surgical Management

### *Resection and Primary Anastomosis*

Resection and primary anastomosis is the preferred option for resectable, uncomplicated obstructions in physiologically stable patients without high-risk features (e.g., hemodynamic instability, frailty, co-morbidities). Anastomotic leak (AL) rates range between 2.2 and 12%, comparable to the 2–8% rate after elective surgery. Its main advantage is avoiding a second major operation. Risk stratification (age, co-morbidities, and tumor stage) and assessment of anastomotic blood supply (including indocyanine green angiography) are critical before performing RPA. Outcomes improve when surgery is performed by colorectal specialists. A protective stoma does not reduce the rate of AL, but decreases the probability of re-exploration.

### *Hartmann's Procedure*

Hartmann's procedure (HP) is generally indicated in high-risk patients or in emergency where surgical expertise is limited. It includes resection of

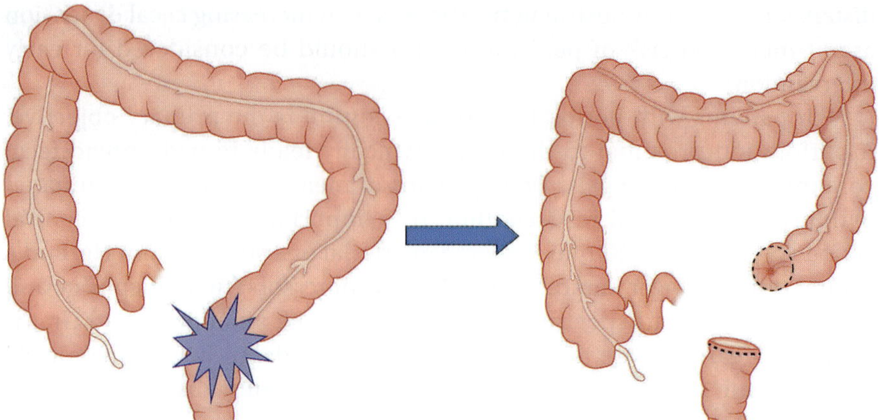

**Fig. 9:** Hartmann's procedure for sigmoid colon growth. Distal stump is closed and proximal end is fashioned as end colostomy.

the diseased segment (usually descending colon, sigmoid colon, or upper rectum), closure of the distal stump and proximal colostomy. **(Fig. 9)**. While HP avoids the risk of AL, it may end up in a permanent stoma (~60–70%) due to chemotherapy complications or disease progression. Evidence suggests no significant survival advantage of HP over RPA.

### *Loop Colostomy*

A diverting loop colostomy is primarily reserved for unresectable tumors or severely ill patients unfit for major surgery, and when SEMS is not feasible or available. It provides rapid decompression with minimal surgical trauma and facilitates patient stabilization and staging. Randomized studies have demonstrated no significant survival advantage for colostomy compared with resection, limiting its role to palliation or as a temporary measure rather than a definitive treatment. Therefore, in patients with resectable disease, either RPA or a HP should be the primary intent.

Traditionally, LBO has been considered an absolute contraindication to laparoscopy because of the high-risk patient profile and the level of operative technical difficulties due to dilated and vulnerable bowel. With the wider adoption of colorectal laparoscopy and growing surgical expertise, several small series have reported encouraging outcomes, but no randomized trials are available.

## Endoscopic Management

### *Transanal Decompression Tube*

Transanal decompression tube is an endoscopic technique to relieve colonic obstruction and optimize the patients for elective resection. Reported technical success rates are between 80 and 100%, while clinical success

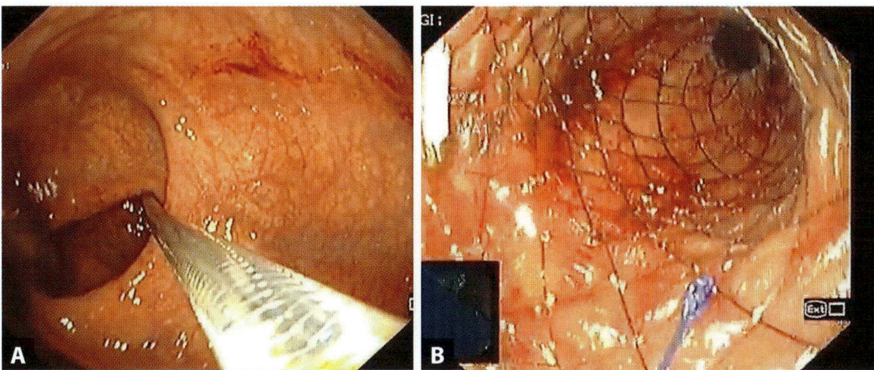

**Figs. 10A and B:** (A) Self-expanding metallic stent placement through the scope; (B) Deployed stent in descending colon.

ranges from 72 to 100%.[9] Most studies employed the Dennis colorectal tube (Covidien, Mansfield, MA, USA), which is inserted over a guidewire to facilitate placement. Complications such as perforation are uncommon (<10%). Advantages over SEMS include lower cost and reduced tumor handling. Nonetheless, strong comparative evidence is lacking, and its application largely depends on institutional preference.

### *Self-expandable Metallic Stents*

The introduction of SEMS, which can be deployed via colonoscopy, has broadened their role in the management of LBO. Beyond their use as a palliation tool to avoid a stoma, SEMS are now also employed to convert emergency surgery into an elective procedure, thus reducing morbidity, mortality, and the need for permanent stomas **(Figs. 10A and B)**.

A few randomized controlled trials (RCTs) have compared SEMS placement with a diverting stoma, concluding that SEMS is a suitable alternative to colostomy **(Table 3)**. It offers improved quality of life and avoids the psychological repercussions associated with a stoma, in addition to being cost-effective. In one study, patients and their family members found an ostomy unacceptable.[10] On the contrary, none of the patients with stents reported any inconvenience related to the procedure.

The SEMS can be used in two situations:

1. *Palliation:* The World Society of Emergency Surgery (WSES) recommends SEMS over colostomy for palliation, as it avoids a permanent stoma, improves quality of life, and shortens hospital stay. Several RCTs and meta-analyses confirm comparable survival and morbidity to colostomy. In patients with unresectable disease, there is a growing consensus that SEMS are associated with superior outcomes compared to diversion stoma for palliation.

**TABLE 3:** RCTs and meta-analysis exploring the role of SEMS in obstructing left-sided colon cancers.

| *S. N.* | *Authors* | *Type of study* | *Sample size* | *Results* | *References* |
|---|---|---|---|---|---|
| ***Palliation (SEMS vs. loop colostomy):*** | | | | | |
| 1. | Fiori et al., 2012 | RCT | SEMS (11) vs. Loop colostomy (11) | SEMS associated with less early morbidity, less length of hospital stay, early oral intake and improved QOL. Similar OS | 10 |
| 2. | Liang et al., 2014 | Meta-analysis | | • *Hospital stay:* Significantly shorter with SEMS<br>• *Early complications and 30-day mortality:* Lower with SEMS<br>• *Late complications (e.g., stent re-obstruction, migration):* Higher with SEMS compared to surgery<br>• *OS:* No significant difference between SEMS and surgery | 15 |
| 3. | Van Hooft et al., 2011 | RCT | SEMS (10) vs. Loop colostomy (11) | High number of stent related perforation lead to early termination of trial | 16 |
| 4. | Takahashi et al., 2015 | Meta-analysis | | • SEMS associated with less complications, mortality and stoma creation but associated with significantly higher risk of perforation of large bowel and late complication<br>• SEMS associated with improved long-term survival | 17 |
| 5. | Young et al. (2015) | RCT | SEMS (26) vs. surgical management (26) | SEMS insertion provided better short-term QOL and fewer complications compared to stoma surgery | 13 |

*Contd...*

*Contd…*

| *S. N.* | *Authors* | *Type of study* | *Sample size* | *Results* | *References* |
|---|---|---|---|---|---|
| ***BTS: SEMS and planned surgery versus ES*** | | | | | |
| 1. | Cheung et al., 2009 | RCT | BTS (24) vs. ES (24) | BTS lower morbidity and stoma rates, faster recovery, and equivalent oncologic outcomes compared with conventional emergency open surgery | 18 |
| 2. | Alcántara et al., 2011 | RCT | BTS (15) vs. ES (15) | • *Stoma rate:* Significantly lower in stent group (0% vs. 27%)<br>• *Morbidity:* Lower in stent group (13% vs. 40%)<br>• *Mortality:* No significant difference<br>• *Hospital stay:* Shorter in stent group<br>• *Anastomotic leak:* None in either group<br>• *Oncologic outcomes:* Similar between groups (R0 resection and lymph node yield) | 19 |
| 3. | Pirlet et al., 2011 | RCT | BTS (30) vs. ES (30) | • *Technical success of stent:* 46% (low, with multiple failures)<br>• *Complications:* Higher in the stent group (including perforations), leading to early trial termination<br>• *Mortality:* Similar between groups<br>• *Stoma rates and oncologic clearance:* No clear benefit due to high stent failure | 14 |
| 4. | Ghazal et al., 2013 | | BTS (11) vs. ES (11) | • *Morbidity:* Lower in stent group (9% vs. 45%)<br>• *Mortality:* None in either group.<br>• *Stoma rate:* Much lower in stent group (0% vs. 36%)<br>• *Hospital stay:* Shorter in stent group<br>• *Oncologic outcomes:* Similar between groups (R0 resection, lymph node yield) | 20 |

(BTS: bridge to surgery; ES: emergency surgery; OS: overall survival; QOL: quality of life; RCT: randomized controlled trial; SEMS: self-expanding metallic stent)

2. *Bridge to surgery (BTS):* SEMS as BTS allows conversion of emergency to elective resection, enabling bowel preparation, better staging, and laparoscopic surgery. Short-term outcomes are favorable with lower stoma rates and reduced hospital stay. In one recent meta-analysis by McHugh et al.,[11] colonic stenting for malignant left-sided colorectal obstruction was associated with a significantly lower permanent stoma rate, reduced overall complications, lower surgical site infection rates and thus decreased morbidity. The author also found that SEMS placement frequently facilitated minimally invasive surgery and improved the likelihood of primary anastomosis. Long-term oncologic outcomes remain debated, with some studies reporting higher local recurrence. Therefore, SEMS as a BTS should be best considered in selected cases at tertiary centers. Studies comparing emergency surgery with BTS using SEMS have shown that BTS is associated with comparable short-term outcomes (including postoperative morbidity, mortality, and length of hospital stay), however increases the likelihood of laparoscopic surgery.

Complications include perforation (up to 13%), migration, and risk of chemotherapy interruption, especially with bevacizumab. Guidelines (e.g., ESGE) caution against SEMS in patients planned for antiangiogenic therapy. SEMS carry inherent risks; the Dutch Stent-in I RCT reported four stent-related perforations among 10 patients, leading to three deaths and premature trial termination.[12] Furthermore, studies suggest that palliative SEMS may reduce overall survival by increasing local complications, forcing discontinuation.[13] RCTs comparing long-term outcomes have not demonstrated significant differences in overall survival with SEMS. However, some studies have reported a trend toward reduced disease-free survival (DFS) and higher rates of tumor ulceration, perineural invasion, and lymph node involvement in the SEMS group compared with surgery-only patients **(Table 3)**. The key concern is the potential increased risk of recurrence due to stent-related perforation, which has been reported in up to 13% of cases.[14]

### *Technical Considerations for Stent Placement*

Self-expanding metal stent is most commonly made of *nitinol* (an alloy of nickel and titanium). It has the ability to generate strong radial force while maintaining flexibility. Deployment can be performed under endoscopic guidance with fluoroscopic assistance or radiological guidance with selective endoscopy inputs **(Figs. 10A and B)**. Two delivery techniques are commonly used: through-the-scope (TTS), in which a stent preloaded into a 10-Fr catheter is passed through the endoscope's working channel, and over-the-wire (OTW), in which the stent is advanced across the stricture over a guidewire.

Self-expanding metal stents are further classified as uncovered or covered. The multicenter HASID study involving 469 patients recommended uncovered stents for higher clinical success and lower complication rates.[21] Similarly, a systematic review and meta-analysis confirmed the advantages of uncovered stents: fewer complications, lower rates of stent migration, longer duration of patency, and a reduced need for stent reinsertion.[22]

In some cases, advanced intra-abdominal malignancies and peritoneal carcinomatosis can cause extrinsic compression of the colon, more often affecting the transverse and descending segments. A meta-analysis of retrospective studies found that SEMS placement in such extra-colonic malignancies is associated with higher technical and clinical failure compared with intraluminal obstructing lesions.[23] This is thought to result from factors such as prior abdominal surgery, chemotherapy, radiotherapy, or multifocal disease. Technical difficulties with stent deployment are also observed in cases of very tight or long strictures, multifocal obstruction, and angulation or kinking of the bowel, which may prevent guidewire passage. The literature rarely stratifies obstruction severity or correlates it with technical success in acutely angulated strictures, though a pre-intervention Colorectal Obstruction Scoring System (CROSS) score of 0 has been associated with difficult stent placement **(Table 4)**.[24]

Accurate stent placement generally requires fluoroscopy guidance during the procedure, while post-procedural abdominal radiographs or CT scans are used to confirm stent expansion and positioning. Clinical success is defined as relief of obstructive symptoms with colonic decompression, usually achieved within 72 hours of deployment. Full bowel preparation is not essential; however, gentle carbon dioxide insufflation is preferred to minimize the risk of perforation. The use of prophylactic antibiotics may be appropriate in cases with a high risk of perforation or when bacterial translocation is suspected.

Overall, SEMS placement is a technically demanding but highly effective procedure when performed by experienced gastroenterologists, with success rates exceeding 90% in appropriately selected patients. Careful patient selection, recognition of technical pitfalls, and optimal device choice remain critical to maximize safety and outcomes.

**TABLE 4:** CROSS (Colorectal Obstruction Scoring System) scoring system based on level of oral intake.[24]

| *Level of oral intake* | *Score* |
|---|---|
| Requiring continuous decompression | 0 |
| No oral intake | 1 |
| Tolerates liquid or enteral tube feeding | 2 |
| Tolerates soft solids, low-residue, or full diet with symptoms of stricture* | 3 |
| Tolerates full diet without symptoms of stricture* | 4 |

*Note*: *Symptoms of stricture include abdominal pain/cramps, abdominal distension, nausea, vomiting, constipation, and diarrhea

## Endoscopic Ultrasound-guided Entero-colostomy with Lumen-apposing Metal Stent

Recently, a novel application of EUS-guided lumen-apposing metal stent (LAMS) placement to create an entero-colonic bypass in patients with MBO has shown promising results. Under EUS guidance, the dilated small bowel loop proximal to the obstruction is identified. A LAMS is then deployed to create a direct anastomosis between the small intestine and the colon, allowing intestinal contents to bypass the obstructed segment. The saddle-shaped design of LAMS provides strong anchorage, reduces the risk of leakage, and maintains luminal patency. This approach offers rapid decompression, avoids emergency surgery, and may be particularly useful in patients who are poor surgical candidates. However, it remains an emerging technique with scarce data on long-term outcomes.

The reported technical success (defined as the correct deployment of the LAMS between the colon and the small bowel) in a study was 80% ($n$ = 8), while clinical success (defined as the resolution of the obstruction for at least 14 days after the procedure) was 70% ($n$ = 7), with only one major adverse event (10%), which was aspiration.[25] A schematic representation of the management strategy for left-sided obstruction is shown in **Flowchart 1**.

**Flowchart 1:** Management of obstructed left sided colon cancer.

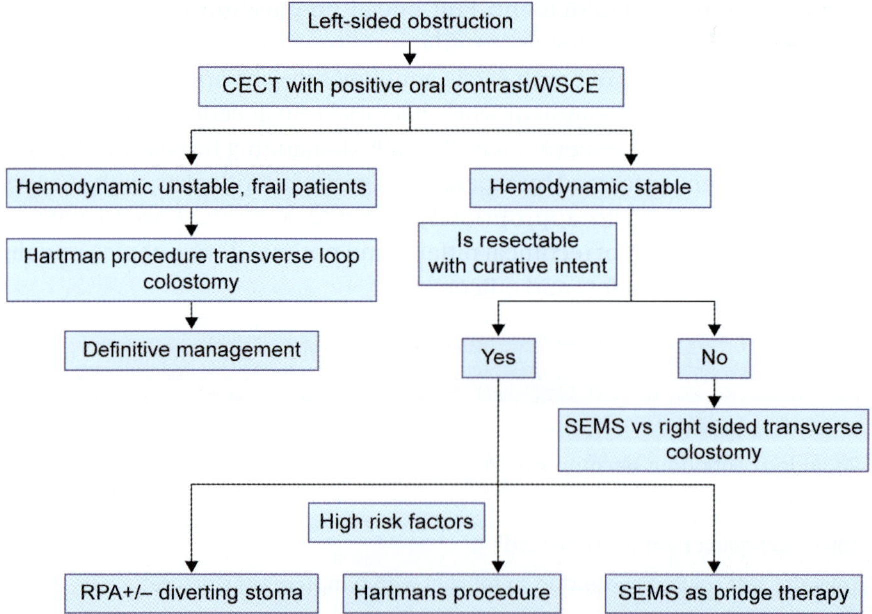


(CECT: contrast-enhanced CT scan; RPA: resection and primary anastomosis; SEMS: self-expanding metallic stent; WSCE: water-soluble contrast enema; High risk factors: Anemia, low albumin, hemodynamic instability, frail patients)

## OBSTRUCTED RECTAL CANCER GROWTH

Obstructed rectal cancer usually signifies locally advanced disease. Highest chance of survival is with elective surgery following neoadjuvant therapy. Therefore, the approach in obstruction should be limited to relieve obstruction, thus opening the possibility of subsequent multimodal treatment. Direct comparative trials between endoscopic stenting and fecal diversion are lacking. However, the use of SEMS in low rectal cancers has been linked to chronic pain and tenesmus, resulting in reduced quality of life. In addition, tumor necrosis after chemoradiation can predispose to stent migration or perforation. Since many patients with low rectal cancer ultimately require a stoma—either a permanent stoma after abdominoperineal resection or a temporary stoma following low anterior resection, a diverting stoma is generally preferred over SEMS for acute rectal obstruction. The choice of stoma, type, and site should be made in anticipation of the planned definitive surgery.

### Loop Ileostomy Versus Loop Colostomy Versus End Colostomy

The decision regarding type (end vs. loop) and site (sigmoid vs. transverse) should be tailored to the patient's condition and the definitive surgical strategy. In emergency rectal obstruction where a future anastomosis is planned, a loop ileostomy is suitable only if the obstruction is partial or the ileocecal valve is incompetent. When the obstruction is complete and the ileocecal valve remains competent, a colostomy is preferred. In high-risk patients unfit for general anesthesia, a left-sided loop colostomy can be fashioned under local anesthesia using a trephine approach. In routine practice, however, a right-sided loop transverse colostomy is most frequently performed, as it provides effective decompression, can later function as a protective stoma following definitive resection, is technically straightforward due to the mobility of the transverse colon, reduces the risk of marginal artery injury, and preserves the left iliac fossa for a potential permanent sigmoid colostomy. When abdominoperineal resection is anticipated, an end sigmoid colostomy is a reliable alternative.

## OBSTRUCTING RIGHT COLON CANCER

In cases of acute obstruction due to right-sided colon cancer, right hemicolectomy with primary anastomosis is the treatment of choice, despite the fact that these patients are often elderly and present with more advanced locoregional disease compared with those harboring left-sided lesions. When a primary anastomosis is deemed unsafe, a terminal ileostomy with a colonic mucous fistula serves as a reasonable alternative. Anatomical considerations favor surgery in this region: the hepatic flexure is easier to mobilize than the splenic flexure, mobility of small bowel facilitates ileocolic anastomosis without the need for additional maneuvers, and the blood supply to the ileocolic segment is typically robust, unlike "watershed" areas of the left colon and rectum that rely heavily on the marginal arcade and hypogastric vessels. Nonetheless, the creation of an ileostomy should be judiciously considered, given the risk of significant fluid and electrolyte disturbances. Nonsurgical options are limited, as stenting or tube decompression of the right colon is technically challenging. Reported AL rates following emergency right colectomy range from 0.5–4.6% in perforated cases, compared with 0.5–1.4% following elective procedures.

For unresectable right-sided cancers, a side-to-side internal bypass between the terminal ileum and transverse colon may be undertaken, or a loop ileostomy be fashioned. Cecostomy is no longer recommended because of its high rates of malfunction and complications. The use of SEMS as a BTS in right colon obstruction is generally discouraged. Right-sided stenting is technically demanding and supported by limited evidence. Nonetheless, meta-analyses have shown encouraging results, with high technical success rates.[26] Compared to emergency resection, SEMS in right-sided malignant obstruction has also been linked to reduced postoperative complications. However, the absence of RCTs highlights the need for further research.

A schematic representation of the management strategy for right-sided obstruction is shown in **Flowchart 2**.

**Flowchart 2:** Management of obstructed right sided colon cancer.

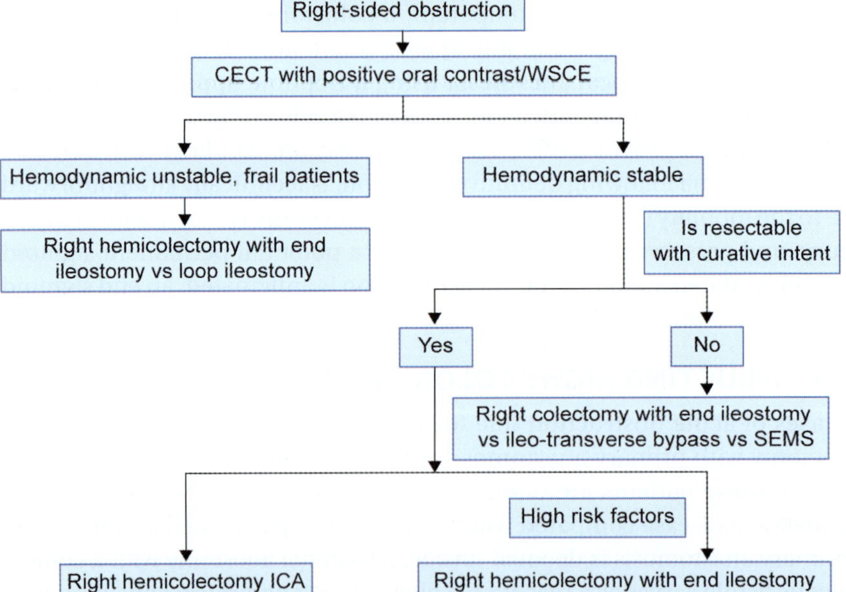


(CECT: contrast-enhanced CT scan; ICA: ileo-colic anastomosis; SEMS: self-expanding metallic stent; WSCE: water-soluble contrast enema; High risk factors: Anemia, low albumin, hemodynamic instability, frail patients)

## CONCLUSION

Management of LBO depends on the underlying cause, tumor location, and hemodynamic condition of the patient. In benign causes, management is relatively straightforward with resection or decompression, often resulting in favorable outcomes. Right-sided malignant obstruction is often treated with hemicolectomy and primary anastomosis; if unsafe, a terminal ileostomy with colonic fistula. Stenting as a BTS is rarely used. Left-sided obstruction offers multiple options: RPA is preferred in stable patients, whereas HP is reserved for high-risk or unstable patients. Diverting stomas serve mainly as temporary or palliative measures. Endoscopic techniques, including TDT and SEMS, can be used either as a BTS or for palliation, facilitating bowel decompression and minimally invasive surgery. For low rectal obstruction, diverting stomas are generally preferred over SEMS due to pain, stent migration, and oncologic considerations. EUS-guided entero-colostomy with lumen-apposing metal stents are promising but remain limited to specialized centers.

## ACKNOWLEDGMENT

We sincerely acknowledge Professor Samir Mohindra (Department of Gastroenterology, SGPGI, Lucknow) and Professor Shashi Prakash Mishra (Department of General Surgery, BHU, Varanasi) for their invaluable contribution to the chapter (in form of clinically relevant photographs and inputs).

## REFERENCES

1. Pavlidis ET, Galanis IN, Pavlidis TE. Management of obstructed colorectal carcinoma in an emergency setting: An update. World J Gastrointest Oncol. 2024;16:598-613.
2. Neri B, Citterio N, Schiavone SC, Biasutto D, Rea R, Martino M, et al. Malignant Bowel Occlusion: An Update on Current Available Treatments. Cancers (Basel). 2025;17(9):1522.
3. Quinn K, Davis ME, Carter L, Shortell CK, Sommer C. Emergency General Surgery-A Misnomer? Am Surg. 2018;84:1214-6.
4. Markogiannakis H, Messaris E, Dardamanis D, Pararas N, Tzertzemelis D, Giannopoulos P, et al. Acute mechanical bowel obstruction: clinical presentation, etiology, management and outcome. World J Gastroenterol. 2007;13:432-7.
5. Imuta M, Awai K, Nakayama Y, Murata Y, Asao C, Matsukawa T, et al. Multidetector CT findings suggesting a perforation site in the gastrointestinal tract: analysis in surgically confirmed 155 patients. Radiat Med. 2007;25:113-8.
6. Jun L, ChangYi S. Diagnostic Value of Plain and Contrast Radiography, and Multi-slice Computed Tomography in Diagnosing Intestinal Obstruction in Different Locations. Indian J Surg. 2015;77:1248-51.
7. Vitale MA, Villotti G, d'Alba L, Frontespezi S, Iacopini F, Iacopini G. Preoperative colonoscopy after self-expandable metallic stent placement in patients with acute neoplastic colon obstruction. Gastrointest Endosc. 2006;63:814-9.

8. Naveed M, Jamil LH, Fujii-Lau LL, Al-Haddad M, Buxbaum JL, Fishman DS, et al. American Society for Gastrointestinal Endoscopy guideline on the role of endoscopy in the management of acute colonic pseudo-obstruction and colonic volvulus. Gastrointest Endosc. 2020;91:228-35.
9. Li C-Y, Guo S-B, Wang N-F. Decompression of acute left-sided malignant colorectal obstruction: comparing transanal drainage tube with metallic stent. J Clin Gastroenterol. 2014;48:e37-42.
10. Fiori E, Lamazza A, Schillaci A, Femia S, Demasi E, Decesare A, et al. Palliative management for patients with subacute obstruction and stage IV unresectable rectosigmoid cancer: colostomy versus endoscopic stenting: final results of a prospective randomized trial. Am J Surg. 2012;204:321-6.
11. McHugh FT, Ryan ÉJ, Ryan OK, Tan J, Boland PA, Whelan MC, et al. Management Strategies for Malignant Left-Sided Colonic Obstruction: A Systematic Review and Network Meta-analysis of Randomized Controlled Trials and Propensity Score Matching Studies. Dis Colon Rectum. 2024;67:878-94.
12. Repici A, De Caro G, Luigiano C, Fabbri C, Pagano N, Preatoni P, et al. WallFlex colonic stent placement for management of malignant colonic obstruction: a prospective study at two centers. Gastrointest Endosc. 2008;67:77-84.
13. Young CJ, De-Loyde KJ, Young JM, Solomon MJ, Chew EH, Byrne CM, et al. Improving Quality of Life for People with Incurable Large-Bowel Obstruction: Randomized Control Trial of Colonic Stent Insertion. Dis Colon Rectum. 2015;58:838-49.
14. Pirlet IA, Slim K, Kwiatkowski F, Michot F, Millat BL. Emergency preoperative stenting versus surgery for acute left-sided malignant colonic obstruction: a multicenter randomized controlled trial. Surg Endosc. 2011;25:1814-21.
15. Liang T, Sun Y, Wei Y, Yang DX. Palliative treatment of malignant colorectal obstruction caused by advanced malignancy: a self-expanding metallic stent or surgery? A system review and meta-analysis. Surg Today. 2014;44:22-33.
16. van Hooft JE, Veld JV, Arnold D, Beets-Tan RGH, Everett S, Götz M, et al. Self-expandable metal stents for obstructing colonic and extracolonic cancer: European Society of Gastrointestinal Endoscopy (ESGE) Guideline – Update 2020. Endoscopy. 2020;52:389-407.
17. Takahashi H, Okabayashi K, Tsuruta M, Hasegawa H, Yahagi M, Kitagawa Y. Self-Expanding Metallic Stents Versus Surgical Intervention as Palliative Therapy for Obstructive Colorectal Cancer: A Meta-analysis. World J Surg. 2015;39:2037-44.
18. Tung KLM, Cheung HYS, Ng LWC, Chung CC, Li MK. Endo-laparoscopic approach versus conventional open surgery in the treatment of obstructing left-sided colon cancer: long-term follow-up of a randomized trial. Asian J Endosc Surg. 2013;6:78-81.
19. Alcántara M, Serra-Aracil X, Falcó J, Mora L, Bombardó J, Navarro S. Prospective, controlled, randomized study of intraoperative colonic lavage versus stent placement in obstructive left-sided colonic cancer. World J Surg. 2011;35:1904-10.
20. Ghazal A-HA, El-Shazly WG, Bessa SS, El-Riwini MT, Hussein AM. Colonic endolumenal stenting devices and elective surgery versus emergency subtotal/total colectomy in the management of malignant obstructed left colon carcinoma. J Gastrointest Surg. 2013;17:1123-9.
21. Oh H-H, Cho S-B, Hong J-Y, Kim DH, Yang HC, Kim SW, et al. Clinical outcomes of palliative self-expandable metal stent placement in right- and left-sided

malignant colon obstruction: A Honam Association for the Study of Intestinal Disease (HASID) multicenter study. Medicine. 2022;101:e30156.
22. Mashar M, Mashar R, Hajibandeh S. Uncovered versus covered stent in management of large bowel obstruction due to colorectal malignancy: a systematic review and meta-analysis. Int J Colorectal Dis. 2019;34:773-85.
23. Ali FS, Gandam MR, Hussain MR, Mualla N, Khuwaja S, Sundararajan N, et al. Self-expanding metal stents for the treatment of malignant colon obstruction from extra-colonic malignancy versus intra-colonic malignancy: a systematic review and meta-analysis. Surg Endosc. 2023;37:4179-92.
24. Ohki T, Yoshida S, Yamamoto M, Isayama H, Yamada T, Matsuzawa T, et al. Determining the difference in the efficacy and safety of self-expandable metallic stents as a bridge to surgery for obstructive colon cancer among patients in the CROSS 0 group and those in the CROSS 1 or 2 group: a pooled analysis of data from two Japanese prospective multicenter trials. Surg Today. 2020;50:984-94.
25. Neri B, Stigliano S, Biasutto D, Citterio N, Lisotti A, Fusaroli P, et al. Endoscopic ultrasound-guided entero-colostomy with lumen-apposing metal stent as a rescue treatment for malignant intestinal occlusion: a multicenter study. Endoscopy. 2025;57:77-82.
26. Kanaka S, Matsuda A, Yamada T, Ohta R, Sonoda H, Shinji S, et al. Colonic stent as a bridge to surgery versus emergency resection for right-sided malignant large bowel obstruction: a meta-analysis. Surg Endosc. 2022;36:2760-70.

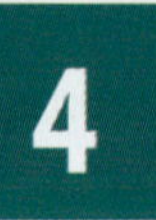

CHAPTER 4

# Nonvariceal Upper Gastrointestinal Bleeding

*Vikram Kate, Deeksha Kapoor, Anandhi Amaranathan*

## INTRODUCTION

Upper gastrointestinal bleeding (UGIB) is defined when the source of the bleeding is proximal to the ligament of Treitz, such as the esophagus, stomach, and duodenum. Clinically, UGIB presents as hematemesis, coffee-ground vomiting, or melena, and less commonly as hematochezia when it is a brisk and copious bleeding. UGIB is broadly classified into two distinct categories based on the etiology and pathophysiology as variceal and nonvariceal bleeding. Variceal bleeding arises primarily from dilated, tortuous, and submucosal veins, typically in the distal esophagus or gastric fundus, secondary to portal hypertension due to chronic liver disease or extrahepatic portal venous obstruction (EHPVO). Nonvariceal upper gastrointestinal bleeding (NVUGIB), the focus of this chapter, comprises all other sources of bleeding in the upper gastrointestinal tract not related to varices or portal hypertension.

The NVUGIB accounts for 70–80% of all cases of UGIB, making it the more prevalent subtype in both community and hospital settings.[1] Peptic ulcer disease remains the leading cause globally; however, the incidence has declined in some high-income countries due to efforts to eradicate *Helicobacter pylori* (*H. pylori*) and the widespread use of PPIs. The other causes of NVUGIB include non-steroidal anti-inflammatory drugs (NSAID)-induced gastropathy, erosive gastritis, Mallory–Weiss syndrome, Dieulafoy's lesion, and vascular ectasias. These have shown variable prevalence depending on demographic, environmental, and healthcare access factors.

## EPIDEMIOLOGICAL BURDEN

The global incidence of UGIB ranges between 48 and 160 cases per 100,000 population per year, with hospital admission rates for NVUGIB reported between 30 and 70 per 100,000 persons/year.[2,3] In India, hospital-based data suggest a disproportionately high burden of NVUGIB due to a combination of over-the-counter use of NSAIDs, high prevalence of *H. pylori* infection, and delayed presentation.[4,5] Despite advances in endoscopic and pharmacological therapies, in-hospital mortality for NVUGIB remains at 3–10%, with significantly higher rates in the elderly and patients with comorbidities. In the event of rebleeding, the mortality rate can increase by up to 14–20%.[1,6,7]

Early and accurate identification of the underlying etiology of NVUGIB is critical, as it guides immediate management decisions, including endoscopic interventions, pharmacologic therapy, and secondary prevention. For instance, the approach to an actively bleeding duodenal ulcer differs significantly from that of a Dieulafoy lesion or a hemorrhage related to malignancy. Furthermore, risk stratification tools such as the Glasgow-Blatchford Score (GBS) and Rockall Score rely partly on etiologic understanding for optimal use.[7]

This chapter reviews the etiological spectrum of NVUGIB, emphasizing both common and rare causes, their pathophysiological mechanisms, diagnostic features, and clinical implications. The goal is to equip clinicians, surgeons, and trainees with a detailed understanding of NVUGIB, thereby supporting prompt, evidence-based decision-making and ultimately improving patient outcomes.

## CLINICAL PRESENTATION AND SYMPTOMATOLOGY

The key symptoms of NVUGIB include hematemesis and melena. Hematemesis, which can present as vomiting of fresh blood, or in an altered form described as a coffee-ground vomitus, occurs in about 30–50% of cases. It indicates active or recent bleeding from an upper gastrointestinal source, more often from the esophagus or stomach. This can be due to peptic ulcer disease, Mallory-Weiss tears, or erosive mucosal disease.[8,9] Melena, or the passage of black, tarry stools, indicates the presence of bleeding which is slow and occurs over a period. NVUGIB more commonly presents with melena than hematemesis, occurring in 70–80% of cases. It usually requires a blood loss of at least 50–100 mL and a source usually proximal to the colon. It involves exposure of blood to gastric acid and intestinal enzymes for at least 8–14 hours which impart the black color. Hematochezia, characterized by the passage of bright red blood per rectum, is uncommon in NVUGIB but may occur with brisk upper gastrointestinal (GI) bleeding when intestinal transit is rapid. This presentation is more often in patients with massive UGIB and has been associated with hemodynamic instability and a higher mortality rate. Associated postural dizziness, syncope, or lightheadedness indicates acute blood loss leading to hypoperfusion, especially in elderly or volume-depleted patients. Association of epigastric pain is common with peptic ulcer disease, especially in bleeding gastric or duodenal ulcers, which remain the leading causes of NVUGIB.[5] In case of subacute or chronic blood loss commonly due to occult GI bleeding, presentation is with iron deficiency anemia, fatigue, and pallor. A clinical history of drug use, such as NSAIDs, aspirin, and corticosteroids, is imperative. These drugs are strongly associated with gastroduodenal ulceration and erosion. The risk is higher in elderly patients and those with *H. pylori* infection. The use of antiplatelet agents such as clopidogrel, ticagrelor, and anticoagulants such as warfarin or other direct oral anticoagulants can be associated with NVUGIB. The chance of an associated GI bleed significantly increases if the patient has pre-existing mucosal bleeding. Ischemic heart disease or heart failure may amplify the morbidity from blood loss.[5]

## CLINICAL ASSESSMENT, EXAMINATION, AND RISK STRATIFICATION

Clinical assessment in a patient with NVUGIB aims at three immediate goals: assessing and stabilizing the patient's hemodynamic status, establishing the cause of bleeding, and assessing the severity to identify associated comorbidities and high-risk features that may determine prognosis and management. All patients with a suspected upper GI bleed should undergo immediate assessment of airway, breathing, and circulation to detect the risk of aspiration, hypoxia, or hemodynamic instability. The presence of tachycardia, hypotension, tachypnea, and altered mental status are critical indicators of significant blood loss. After stabilization, a physical examination should assess for jaundice, ascites, or hepatosplenomegaly, which may suggest underlying liver disease. An abdominal examination should evaluate for abdominal masses, hepatosplenomegaly, and ascites. A per rectal examination is performed to look for melena and/or hematochezia. Risk stratification is crucial for facilitating informed decision-making regarding urgent interventions. Clinical tools, such as the GBS and Rockall scores, utilize signs like hypotension, tachycardia, and the presence of comorbidities to inform decisions regarding the timing of endoscopy, the need for intensive care, and the requirement for blood transfusions and/or interventions.[2] Regardless of the hemoglobin level at admission, patients presenting with syncope, tachycardia, hypotension, and massive hematemesis should be considered high-risk and managed in the intensive care unit.

## DIFFERENTIAL DIAGNOSIS AND CAUSES OF NONVARICEAL UPPER GASTROINTESTINAL BLEEDING

Peptic ulcer disease remains the most common cause of NVUGIB, responsible for about 50–70% of cases globally. The principal causes of peptic ulcer disease are *H. pylori* infection and NSAID use, with additional factors such as burns, head injuries, smoking, and alcohol abuse also contributing.[10] Duodenal ulcers situated on the posterior wall of the duodenum tend to bleed more significantly, often due to the erosion of the gastroduodenal or rarely left gastric artery. NSAIDs and antiplatelet agents, which can cause gastritis and duodenitis, are also well-known causes of NVUGIB, especially in elderly patients and those with cardiovascular conditions. With a widespread use of endoscopic evaluation and standardized *H. pylori* eradication protocols, the proportion of ulcer-related NVUGIB due to *H. pylori* has markedly declined.[11,12]

However, drug-induced mucosal injury—particularly from NSAIDs and antiplatelets—has become a more prominent cause of bleeding.[9] This primarily occurs through the inhibition of cyclooxygenase-1 (COX-1), an enzyme always present in the gastric mucosa that produces prostaglandins crucial for protecting the mucosa. The suppression of COX-1 reduces mucus and bicarbonate secretion, hampers mucosal blood flow, and impairs epithelial repair, creating an environment vulnerable to acid-related damage, especially in the gastric antrum and duodenum. Antiplatelet drugs aspirin and P2Y12 inhibitors such as clopidogrel and ticagrelor increase bleeding risk further by impairing primary hemostasis. When these drugs are combined with dual antiplatelet therapy (DAPT), the risk of major gastrointestinal bleeding can be 2–3 times higher than with monotherapy following percutaneous coronary interventions. Low-dose aspirin alone, particularly in elderly patients, is a common cause of occult or overt gastrointestinal blood loss.[2,9,11,13] Risk stratification tools, such as the HAS-BLED and ATRIA scores, are utilized in clinical practice to assess bleeding risk for patients on long-term antithrombotic therapy; however, they are primarily validated for intracranial and systemic bleeding. The HEMORR 2 HAGES and ORBIT scores are also employed in the gastrointestinal context.[2,9,11,13] The concurrent use of corticosteroids, selective serotonin reuptake inhibitors, or anticoagulants significantly heightens the likelihood of gastrointestinal complications when patients are taking NSAIDs or antiplatelet agents. Additionally, *H. pylori*-associated peptic ulcer disease tends to have lower rates of rebleeding. Endoscopic classification using the Forrest system categorizes ulcers based on signs of recent hemorrhage, guiding the urgency and type of endoscopic treatment. High-risk lesions (Forrest Ia: spurting, Ib: oozing, IIa: visible vessel) are associated with rebleeding rates exceeding 20% if left untreated.

Mallory–Weiss syndrome (MWS) accounts for approximately 5–10% of NVUGIB cases and is characterized by longitudinal mucosal lacerations at the gastroesophageal junction, typically on the gastric side of the cardia. A sudden increase in intra-abdominal or intragastric pressure, usually triggered by forceful retching, vomiting, coughing, or straining, causes shearing stress at the gastroesophageal junction. Predisposing factors include alcohol use, hiatal hernia, recurrent vomiting due to gastroparesis, pregnancy, bulimia, and conditions that impair esophageal compliance or mucosal integrity.[14]

Dieulafoy's lesions are a caliber-persistent artery although, rare can cause severe UGIB, representing about 1–2% of NVUGIB cases.[15] A large, abnormal submucosal artery protrudes through a small mucosal defect, usually without associated ulceration, erosion, or inflammation.

These lesions most commonly occur in the proximal stomach, within 6 cm of the gastroesophageal junction, along the lesser curvature.[15] Bleeding is typically intermittent, and patients may present with hematemesis, melaena, or hematochezia, often accompanied by hemodynamic instability. An urgent upper GI endoscopy is often required; however, detection can be challenging due to the lesion's small size and lack of surrounding ulceration. Features suggestive of a Dieulafoy's lesion include active arterial spurting from a pinpoint defect, a visible vessel with minimal mucosal damage, or an adherent clot without an ulcer base.

*Uncommon causes:* Angiodysplasia of the upper GI tract is an uncommon cause of nonvariceal upper GI bleeding (2–6% of cases), typically affecting elderly patients and those with comorbidities such as chronic kidney disease or aortic stenosis. Age-related degeneration of vascular integrity is often implicated, explaining its higher prevalence in the elderly (>60 years). It is often associated with systemic comorbidities such as chronic kidney disease, aortic stenosis (Heyde's syndrome), and von Willebrand disease.[16] Gastric antral vascular ectasia (GAVE) causes NVUGIB in approximately 4% of cases but may be underdiagnosed due to its often occult and insidious presentation. It is characterized by ectatic, dilated mucosal capillaries and venules in the gastric antrum that are prone to spontaneous bleeding. GAVE, also known as "watermelon stomach" is frequently associated with systemic conditions, particularly cirrhosis, chronic kidney disease, systemic sclerosis, and autoimmune connective tissue disorders. GAVE is distinct from portal hypertensive gastropathy which is associated with cirrhosis and portal hypertension. Diagnosis of GAVE is primarily by upper GI endoscopy, where GAVE appears as longitudinal red stripes of ectatic vessels radiating from the pylorus across the antrum, resembling the stripes of a watermelon, hence the term. A biopsy may be used for confirmation or to rule out other pathologies.[16]

Neoplasms, such as gastric adenocarcinoma, gastrointestinal stromal tumors, and primary gastric lymphomas, account for approximately 1–5% of cases. Gastric adenocarcinoma is the most common malignancy associated with GI bleeding.[17] Other rare conditions include primary and secondary aortoenteric fistulae, hemobilia, hemosuccus pancreaticus, and pseudoaneurysms, especially in the setting of chronic pancreatitis.[14,18] **Table 1** describes the clinical variability of presentation based on the etiology of NVUGIB.

## MANAGEMENT OF NONVARICEAL UPPER GASTROINTESTINAL BLEEDING

### Initial Management, Resuscitation, and Risk Stratification

Initial management of nonvariceal UGIB involves prompt hemodynamic assessment with large-bore IV access and volume resuscitation, aiming for

**TABLE 1:** Clinical variability based on etiology.

| *Etiology* | *Typical presentation* |
|---|---|
| Peptic ulcer disease (PUD) | Most common cause of NVUGIB. Often presents with melena or hematemesis. Epigastric pain may precede or follow bleeding. History of NSAID use or *H. pylori* is common |
| Erosive gastritis or duodenitis | Often presents with low-grade bleeding, sometimes asymptomatic except for melena. May follow alcohol use, stress, and NSAIDs |
| Mallory–Weiss tear | Sudden-onset hematemesis following retching or vomiting, often in alcoholics or pregnant women. Usually self-limited |
| Dieulafoy's lesion | Massive, painless hematemesis or melena, with intermittent bleeding. No associated ulcer or inflammation |
| Gastric antral vascular ectasia (GAVE) | Also known as "watermelon stomach." Typically presents with chronic occult bleeding and iron deficiency anemia. Often seen in cirrhotics and autoimmune disease |
| Angiodysplasia | Presents with intermittent melena or occult blood loss. More common in elderly patients. May be associated with aortic stenosis (Heyde's syndrome) |
| Neoplastic bleeding | Typically indolent with chronic blood loss symptoms; overt hematemesis or melena is less common. May be associated with weight loss, early satiety, or dysphagia |
| Postinterventional bleeding | Iatrogenic bleeding post-endoscopic therapy, stenting, biopsy, or surgery. Presentation is variable based on timing and intervention site. |

(NVUGIB: nonvariceal upper gastrointestinal bleeding; NSAIDs: nonsteroidal anti-inflammatory drugs; *H. pylori: Helicobacter pylori*)

a restrictive transfusion threshold such as hemoglobin <7 g/dL, increased to <8 g/dL for patients with cardiovascular comorbidities to reduce rebleeding and mortality. Risk stratification using validated composite scores, such as the GBS, AIMS65, and Rockall, enables the early identification of low-risk patients suitable for outpatient management and high-risk individuals requiring urgent intervention.[7,19] The GBS is useful, as a score of 0–1 has high sensitivity (≥99%) for ruling out the need for hospital-based interventions, and scores ≥7 strongly predict the need for transfusion or endoscopic therapy. By combining clinical stabilization, careful transfusion strategies, and early risk stratification, particularly by GBS, clinicians can effectively prioritize patients, optimize resource allocation, and improve outcomes in NVUGIB.[11,19,20]

### Pre-endoscopy Management

In cases of NVUGIB, stabilizing hemodynamics takes priority before endoscopy, and a restrictive transfusion strategy is supported by systematic reviews and meta-analyses showing lower all-cause mortality and rebleeding rates without increasing ischemic risk compared to liberal transfusion.[21,22] Restrictive thresholds do not increase in-hospital or 30-day mortality or rebleeding rates, while decreasing transfusion reactions and interventions.[21] High-dose PPI therapy, administered as an initial 80 mg IV bolus followed by continuous infusion or intermittent dosing, has been shown in this report to significantly reduce rebleeding and the need for surgery or repeat endoscopy.[21] However, it does not affect mortality. Subgroup analysis of the data suggested that intermittent versus continuous PPI infusion provides similar effectiveness in reducing early rebleeding rates, offering flexibility in clinical practice.[5] However, it is emphasized that PPIs are no substitute for endoscopic interventions, which remain the primary modality for definitive hemostasis in NVUGIB, and the delivery of PPIs should not delay endoscopy. While adjunctive prokinetic therapy such as with erythromycin may enhance endoscopic visualization, a recent meta-analysis does not support the routine use of other agents such as tranexamic acid or octreotide in NVUGIB.[23] However, octreotide may be considered as an adjunct to endoscopic management for variceal bleed in patients with portal hypertension. Overall, evidence-based pre-endoscopy management, which combines restrictive transfusion and targeted PPI use, promotes better preparation for endoscopic intervention and improves patient outcomes.

## ENDOSCOPY AND INTERVENTIONS

### Timing of Endoscopy

Current international guidelines recommend performing upper GI endoscopy within 24 hours after hemodynamic resuscitation and medical optimization, since timely endoscopy identifies the bleeding source and enables endoscopic hemostasis when feasible and indicated.[23] Randomized trials show that in high-risk patients, an urgent endoscopy within 6 hours did not reduce 30-day mortality compared with endoscopy at 6–24 hours, despite detecting more active bleeding and prompting more immediate therapy.[24] Extensive territory-wide cohort analyses and aggregated observational data suggest that outcomes such as mortality, repeat endoscopy, intensive care unit (ICU) admission are generally better when therapeutic endoscopy is performed within the 6–24 hour window versus either ultra-urgent (<6 h) or delayed (>24 h) procedures, likely reflecting the benefit of prior resuscitation and optimization.[25] Systematic reviews and meta-analyses similarly report no clear mortality advantage for routine endoscopy earlier than 24 hours. However, early endoscopy may shorten the length of stay and has been shown to reduce transfusion requirements.[25] Consequently, the timing of endoscopy should be individualized as an early or urgent endoscopy is appropriate for persistent hemodynamic instability or ongoing massive bleeding despite resuscitation **(Flowchart 1)**. At the same time, stable high-risk patients are usually best served by endoscopy performed promptly within the first 24 hours after hemodynamic optimization.[23,25]

## METHODS OF ENDOSCOPIC INTERVENTION

There are three preferred modalities of endoscopic therapy for the management of NVUGIB. These include injection therapy, thermal coagulation, and mechanical clipping of the bleeding vessel.[2] Injection therapy, usually with dilute epinephrine (1:10,000) at or near the base of the bleeding ulcer, leads to control of the bleeding through vasoconstrictive effect of epinephrine and a rapid tamponade effect on the bleeding vessel through the tissue compression by the volume injected. However, it is associated with higher rebleeding rates when used alone; hence, guidelines recommend combining it with a second modality for a complete hemostasis.[26] Thermal coagulation with heater probe and bipolar electrocoagulation achieves hemostasis by coagulating bleeding vessels and remains effective for spurting or oozing ulcers when applied directly with firm pressure.[2] Monopolar hemostatic forceps achieve a higher rate of initial hemostasis, at 98%, compared to hemostatic clips, which achieve initial hemostasis in approximately 80% of cases.[27] Hemostatic clips used with the endoscope provide immediate mechanical vessel closure. They are beneficial for focal bleeding points with a visible vessel or adherent clot, although their success is reduced in fibrotic ulcer bases or difficult anatomical locations.[28] Evidence shows that all three methods, when used judiciously in a combination therapy, achieve initial hemostasis rates above 90% reducing rebleeding compared to monotherapy.[26] These techniques form the core of modern endoscopic hemostasis and remain first-line interventions despite the availability of newer devices.

## ADVANCED ENDOSCOPIC THERAPEUTIC TECHNIQUES

Recent advances in endoscopic hemostasis broaden effective options for refractory or high-risk nonvariceal bleeding beyond traditional injection, thermal, and clip techniques. Over-the-scope clips (OTSC), used as first-line or salvage therapy, have been linked in meta-analyses with significantly lower 30-day rebleeding rates (pooled RR ~0.58, 95% CI 0.41–0.82) and higher clinical success compared to standard endoscopic treatments, though without a consistent mortality benefit.[29] This supports their role, especially in large (more than 2 cm), fibrotic, or refractory ulcers. Hemostatic powders (TC-325/Hemospray) achieve very high immediate hemostasis rates, and multiple recent randomized controlled trials (RCTs) and meta-analyses

**Flowchart 1:** Algorithmic approach for the management of bleeding due to peptic ulcer disease.

Patient with suspected nonvariceal upper GI bleed

- Evaluate hemodynamic stability
- Glasgow Blatchford Score (GBS)

- Start a high dose of proton pump inhibitors (PPI) (8 mg/hr., after an 80 mg bolus dose)
- Consider erythromycin or metoclopramide
- Stop antiplatelets/ anticoagulants until stabilization and evaluation

- Hemodynamically
- Unstable

→ • Intensive care unit admission • Restrictive blood transfusion

→ Persistent instability, need of multiple transfusions → Urgent endoscopic therapy/surgery

→ Stabilized → Endoscopy within 24 hours and endoscopic risk stratification of the ulcer by Forrest Classification

- Hemodynamically
- Stable, GBS >1

→ Hospitalization and evaluation

- Hemodynamically
- Stable, GBS<1

→ Evaluation on out-patient basis

Forrest Classification:

- F1a (active spurting)
- F1b (active oozing)
- F2a (nonbleeding visible vessel)
- F2b (adherent clot)

→

- Needs endoscopic hemostasis
- Consider combination or dual therapy
- In F2b, consider clot removal to assess high-risk stigmata

→

*Endoscopic hemostasis-successful:*
- PPI x 72 hrs
- Resume antiplatelets in 72 hours
- *H. pylori* eradication if tested positive

*Second look endoscopy:*
- If monotherapy was used initially
- Doubtful hemostasis
- Clinical evidence of re-bleed

*Refractory bleeding:*
- Consider hemospray
- Consider thermocoagulation
- Transarterial embolization
- Surgery

- F2c (flat pigmented spot)
- F3 (clean base)

→

- No endoscopic hemostasis needed
- Start oral PPI +/- *H. pylori* eradication
- Re-start antiplatelets

(PPI: proton pump inhibitors)

indicate reduced short-term (7–30 day) rebleeding when utilized as primary or salvage therapy—particularly as a temporary "bridge" to definitive treatment in malignant or diffuse bleeding—although durability beyond 30 days varies.[30] Endoscopic suturing and cap-mounted devices offer durable mechanical closure for selected lesions such as large mucosal defects, tumor bleeding, or hemorrhage postendoscopic mucosal resection or endoscopic submucosal dissection and are increasingly employed when clipping proves technically challenging.[31] The present data demonstrate high technical success but variable rebleeding depending on lesion type and operator experience.

## TRANSCATHETER ARTERIAL EMBOLIZATION

In refractory NVUGIB, transcatheter arterial embolization (TAE) achieves immediate hemostasis in 80–95% of cases, with technical success rates exceeding 90% in recent series.[28] Indications include persistent or recurrent bleeding after endoscopic therapy, inability to treat due to anatomical constraints, and high surgical risk. Modern microcatheter systems, coils, liquid embolics such as n-butyl cyanoacrylate, and calibrated microspheres have all contributed to improved patient outcomes. A meta-analysis shows comparable mortality to surgery but with fewer complications and shorter recovery times, despite higher rebleeding rates (15–30%).[32] Complications occur in <5% of cases and include access-site hematomas, contrast nephropathy, and rare bowel ischemia.[32] Early referral after failed endoscopy improves hemostatic success and reduces transfusion needs. Current guidelines recommend TAE as the preferred salvage treatment over surgery in most high-risk patients.[28,32]

## MANAGEMENT OF REBLEEDING FOLLOWING ENDOSCOPIC THERAPY

Rebleeding is defined as new onset of hematemesis, coffee-ground vomitus or melena, with an increasing pulse rate over 110 per minute and decreasing blood pressure below 90 mm of Hg after a 24-h period of stable vital signs following endoscopic treatment.[33] Rebleeding occurs in 15–25% of NVUGIB cases after initially successful endoscopic hemostasis, with risk strongly linked to the Forrest classification: Ia (spurting) ~55%, IIa (visible vessel) ~43%, IIb (adherent clot) ~22%, IIc (flat pigmented spot) ~10%.[13] A recent retrospective cohort study on 386 patients demonstrated that, in addition to Forrest stigmata, hypoalbuminemia ≤30 g/L, presentation with shock and hematemesis, and prolonged prothrombin time independently predicted rebleeding within 72 hours, yielding a C-index of 0.854 for a new multivariable risk model.[34]

A meta-analysis of routine second-look endoscopy on 9 RCTs ($n$ = 1,452) has shown no significant reduction in rebleeding (RR 0.79; 95% CI: 0.51–1.23), surgery, mortality, or transfusion requirements compared with single endoscopy, supporting selective use in high-risk cases only.[35] When rebleeding occurs, repeat endoscopic therapy achieves hemostasis in ~75–85% of cases, with combination strategies of thermal and mechanical approaches demonstrating higher success rates than monotherapy.[23] If endoscopy fails, transcatheter arterial embolization (TAE) is preferred over immediate surgery, achieving primary hemostasis in ~90% of cases and avoiding laparotomy, although with rebleeding rates of 10–20%.[36] Surgery is now reserved mainly for cases where both endoscopic and interventional radiology (IR) interventions fail, or in unstable patients with ongoing massive bleeding.

## SURGICAL INTERVENTION

Surgical intervention for NVUGIB has sharply declined over recent decades from approximately 10–13% in the 1990s to ≤2% by 2021–2024, due to the rise of effective endoscopic and IR techniques.[37] Surgery remains indispensable in <5% of refractory cases particularly when endoscopic and TAE options fail or are contraindicated. Outcomes data show that surgical hemostasis, typically by oversewing of bleeding ulcers with and acid reducing surgery or ulcer resection, carries a 30-day mortality of up to 29%, primarily driven by patient comorbidity and hemodynamic instability at presentation.[38] In comparative retrospective studies and meta-analyses involving 427 patients undergoing TAE and 650 patients undergoing surgery = 650, TAE demonstrated no significant mortality benefit over surgery, despite a higher incidence of rebleeding post-TAE. However, significant heterogeneity was found among these studies.[38] More recent systematic reviews on TAE report technical success at ~84%, clinical success at around 67%, a rebleeding rate of ~27%, complications in 6%, and 30-day mortality at around 8%.[39] This evidence supports a modern algorithm where surgery is reserved for cases where IR is unavailable, fails, or pathological factors such as perforated ulcer or malignancy necessitate operative management. Hence, a multidisciplinary approach with endoscopic therapy, IR, and surgery ensures optimal selection with individualized management of the patients with NVUGIB.

In patients requiring operative control of peptic ulcer hemorrhage after failure of endoscopic and/or IR therapy, the standard open approach is a longitudinal pyloroduodenotomy with identification and ligation of the bleeding vessel which is often the gastroduodenal artery followed by transverse closure as a Heineke–Mikulicz pyloroplasty. Historically, adjunctive acid-reducing procedures such as truncal vagotomy or antrectomy were added, but in the modern era their routine use has declined because *H. pylori* eradication and proton pump inhibitors (PPIs) lower recurrence risk. Bleeding gastric ulcers are treated with a surgical procedure of distal gastrectomy or wedge resection depending on ulcer type with stable patients, whereas omental patch with ulcer edge biopsy serves as a damage-control option in unstable patients.[40]

## OTHER ETIOLOGY FOR NONVARICEAL UPPER GASTROINTESTINAL BLEEDING

### Mallory–Weiss Syndrome

Mallory–Weiss syndrome is managed supportively in most cases, as ~80–90% of bleeds cease spontaneously with hemodynamic stabilization alone. Endoscopic intervention is indicated for active bleeding, a visible vessel, or an adherent clot, with epinephrine injection achieving initial hemostasis in >90% of cases, often followed by thermal coagulation or hemoclipping to reduce the rebleeding risk to <10%.[41] Mechanical clipping provides slightly higher definitive hemostasis rates compared to injection alone, especially in spurting lesions. Proton pump inhibitors are routinely administered post-endoscopy to promote mucosal healing, though no RCTs specifically address their efficacy in Mallory–Weiss syndrome. Transcatheter arterial embolization or surgery is rarely required and is reserved for cases unresponsive to endoscopic therapy, occurring in less than 1–2% of modern series.[42]

### Dieulafoy's Lesion

Dieulafoy's lesion is best managed with prompt endoscopic therapy, which achieves primary hemostasis in 85–95% of cases.[15] Considering the need for diffuse coagulation, cauterization by thermal energy is usually not recommended for Dieulafoy's lesion. Rebleeding, which occurs in up to 15% of patients, is managed with repeat endoscopy. Transcatheter arterial embolization is effective in >90% of refractory cases, while surgery is rarely required.[32] PPIs are given post-procedure to support mucosal healing, although their role in Dieulafoy's lesion-specific outcomes is not well defined.

### Nonvariceal Upper Gastrointestinal Bleeding due to Malignant Lesions

The NVUGIB from malignant lesions accounts for 5–10% of upper GI bleeds and is associated with high 3-day mortality of 20–40% due to advanced disease and comorbidities.[17] Endoscopic therapy provides temporary hemostasis, with pooled success rates of 68–85% but rebleeding rates of 30–40% within 7–14 days. Mechanical clipping is often limited by tumor friability. In contrast, thermal modalities such as heater probe, argon plasma coagulation (APC) achieve initial control in ~80% of cases, but efficacy is reduced in large, ulcerated masses. Hemostatic powders, such as TC-325, have shown immediate hemostasis in 85–95% of cases in recent meta-analyses, with lower early rebleeding rates at 20–25% compared to standard therapy in tumor bleed.[43] Combination strategies such as epinephrine injection plus APC or clips modestly improve durability but remain palliative. For refractory cases, transcatheter arterial embolization achieves hemostasis in 70–90% of cases with a complication rate of 5–8%, although tumor neovascularity predicts earlier recurrence. Definitive control depends on tumor-directed therapy like surgical resection, palliative radiotherapy, or systemic chemotherapy, tailored to oncologic stage and patient performance status.

## Post-interventional Bleeding

Rarely, iatrogenic bleeding can happen following procedures such as postendoscopic therapy, stenting, biopsy, or surgery. It may be commonly self-limiting, however, sometimes it may be alarming and may need intervention or surgery to control it. Presentation is variable based on timing and intervention site. The algorithmic approach for the management is depicted in **Flowcharts 1 and 2**.

**Flowchart 2:** Algorithmic approach for other etiology management of nonvariceal non-ulcer upper gastrointestinal bleeding.

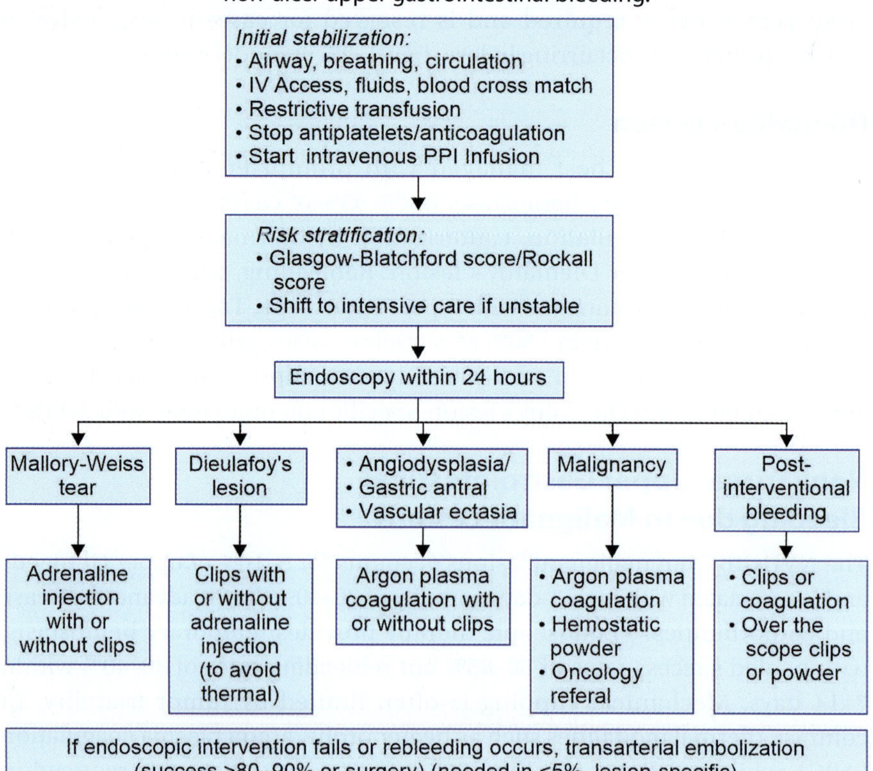


(PPI: proton pump inhibitors)

## FUTURE DIRECTIONS AND RESEARCH GAPS

The field is rapidly embracing device-driven hemostasis and precision-guided therapy, but important questions remain about durability, comparative effectiveness, and cost-effectiveness. Randomized data and pooled analyses increasingly support hemostatic powders, such as TC-325, as effective immediate control agents and as a bridge to definitive therapy. However, longer-term durability and head-to-head comparisons versus combination mechanical/thermal therapy are still limited and under active investigation.[43] Over-the-scope clips and advanced endoscopic suturing demonstrate higher technical and clinical success in treating large, fibrotic, or refractory lesions. However, there is a need for larger randomized trials comparing OTSC/suturing to standard combination therapy, as well as cost-utility analyses in different healthcare settings.[29] Doppler endoscopic probe (DEP) guidance has demonstrated promising reductions in early rebleeding by objectively confirming arterial flow obliteration. Ongoing studies are evaluating DEP-directed algorithms to determine who truly benefits from additional therapy.[44] Emerging topical sealants and next-generation powders/gels such as UI-EWD, Nexpowder™ (UI-EWD, Nextbiomedical, Incheon, South Korea) are in late-phase clinical testing, including several randomized trials assessing noninferiority or superiority to standard care, which should clarify their role for malignant and diffuse bleeding.[31] Artificial intelligence and machine-learning risk models are being developed to enhance early triage, predict the need for intervention, and facilitate intra-procedural lesion detection; however, prospective multicenter validation and integration into clinical pathways remain a significant research gap.[45] Finally, there is an urgent need for pragmatic, multicenter randomized comparisons that evaluate patient-centered outcomes—rebleeding at 30/90 days, need for interventional radiology/surgery, quality of life, transfusion burden, and costs—rather than just immediate hemostasis, to determine which new technologies should be widely adopted versus reserved as salvage tools.

## CONCLUSION

Nonvariceal upper gastrointestinal bleeding accounts for three-fourths of all cases of upper gastrointestinal bleeding and peptic ulcer remains the leading cause, however, its incidence has declined due to eradication of *H. pylori* and the widespread use of PPIs. The key symptoms include hematemesis and melena. Clinical assessment aims at three immediate goals: stabilizing the patient's hemodynamic status, establishing the cause of bleeding, and assessing the severity to identify associated comorbidities and high-risk features that may determine prognosis and management. Clinical tools, such as the GBS and Rockall scores, utilize signs such as hypotension, tachycardia, and the presence of comorbidities to determine the timing of endoscopy, the need for intensive care, and the requirement for blood transfusions and/or interventions. Apart from peptic ulcer, other causes include Mallory–Weiss syndrome, Dieulafoy's lesions, angiodysplasia of the upper GI tract, gastric antral vascular ectasia (GAVE), neoplasms, such as gastric adenocarcinoma and gastrointestinal stromal tumors. Initial management of nonvariceal upper gastrointestinal bleeding involves prompt hemodynamic stabilization and performing upper GI endoscopy within 24 hours to identify the bleeding source and endoscopic hemostasis when feasible and indicated. The preferred modalities of endoscopic therapy include injection therapy, thermal coagulation, and mechanical clipping of the bleeding vessel. Over-the-scope clips and transcatheter arterial embolization are used in refractory bleeding. When rebleeding occurs, repeat endoscopic therapy achieves hemostasis in ~75–85% of cases, with combination strategies of thermal and mechanical approaches demonstrating higher success rates than monotherapy. Surgery is now rarely needed and is reserved primarily when both endoscopic and interventional radiology interventions fail, or in unstable patients with ongoing massive bleeding. Artificial intelligence and machine-learning risk models are being developed to improvise the management of the NVUGIB.

## REFERENCES

1. Bai Y, Li ZS. Guidelines for the diagnosis and treatment of acute non-variceal upper gastrointestinal bleeding (2015, Nanchang, China). J of Digest Diseases. 2016;17(2):79-87.
2. Barkun AN, Almadi M, Kuipers EJ, Laine L, Sung J, Tse F, et al. Management of Nonvariceal Upper Gastrointestinal Bleeding: Guideline Recommendations From the International Consensus Group. Ann Intern Med. 2019;171(11):805-22.
3. Hearnshaw SA, Logan RFA, Lowe D, Travis SPL, Murphy MF, Palmer KR. Acute upper gastrointestinal bleeding in the UK: patient characteristics, diagnoses and outcomes in the 2007 UK audit. Gut. 2011;60(10):1327-35.
4. Raj A, Kaeley N, Prasad H, Patnaik I, Bahurupi Y, Joshi S, et al. Prospective observational study on clinical and epidemiological profile of adult patients presenting to the emergency department with suspected upper gastrointestinal bleed. BMC Emerg Med. 2023;23(1):107.
5. Kate V, Sureshkumar S, Gurushankari B, Kalayarasan R. Acute Upper Non-variceal and Lower Gastrointestinal Bleeding. J Gastrointest Surg. 2022;26(4):932-49.
6. Kurien M, Lobo AJ. Acute upper gastrointestinal bleeding. Clin Med (Lond). 2015;15(5):481-5.
7. Anchu AC, Mohsina S, Sureshkumar S, Mahalakshmy T, Kate V. External validation of scoring systems in risk stratification of upper gastrointestinal bleeding. Indian J Gastroenterol. 2017;36(2):105-12.
8. Sung JJ, Chiu PW, Chan FKL, Lau JY, Goh K lee, Ho LH, et al. Asia-Pacific working group consensus on non-variceal upper gastrointestinal bleeding: an update 2018. Gut. 2018;67(10):1757-68.
9. Kamboj AK, Hoversten P, Leggett CL. Upper Gastrointestinal Bleeding: Etiologies and Management. Mayo Clin Proc. 2019;94(4):697-703.

10. Mittal S, Trakroo S, Kate V, Jagdish S. Evaluation of the effect of presence of blood in the stomach on endoscopic diagnostic tests for *Helicobacter pylori* infection. Indian J Med Microbiol. 2011;29(4):379-82.
11. Malfertheiner P, Megraud F, O'Morain CA, Gisbert JP, Kuipers EJ, Axon AT, et al. Management of *Helicobacter pylori* infection-the Maastricht V/Florence Consensus Report. Gut. 2017;66(1):6-30.
12. Singh SP, Ahuja V, Ghoshal UC, Makharia G, Dutta U, Zargar SA, et al. Management of *Helicobacter pylori* infection: The Bhubaneswar Consensus Report of the Indian Society of Gastroenterology. Indian J Gastroenterol. 2021;40(4):420-44.
13. Laine L, Jensen DM. Management of patients with ulcer bleeding. Am J Gastroenterol. 2012;107(3):345-60; quiz 361.
14. Kate V, Ananthakrishnan N, Siva Ram G. Non-variceal upper gastrointestinal bleeding: Current concept in management. In: Recent Advances in Surgery, 1 edition. New Delhi: Jaypee Brothers Medical Publisher; 2009. pp. 262-77.
15. Baxter M, Aly E. Dieulafoy's lesion: current trends in diagnosis and management. annals. 2010;92(7):548-54.
16. Sami SS, Al-Araji SA, Ragunath K. Review article: gastrointestinal angiodysplasia - pathogenesis, diagnosis and management. Aliment Pharmacol Ther. 2014;39(1):15-34.
17. Ofosu A, Ramai D, Latson W, Adler DG. Endoscopic management of bleeding gastrointestinal tumors. Ann Gastroenterol. 2019;32(4):346-51.
18. Cui HY, Jiang CH, Dong J, Wen Y, Chen YW. Hemosuccus pancreaticus caused by gastroduodenal artery pseudoaneurysm associated with chronic pancreatitis: A case report and review of literature. World J Clin Cases. 2021;9(1):236-44.
19. Stanley AJ, Laine L, Dalton HR, Ngu JH, Schultz M, Abazi R, et al. Comparison of risk scoring systems for patients presenting with upper gastrointestinal bleeding: international multicentre prospective study. BMJ. 2017;356: i6432.
20. Saltzman JR, Tabak YP, Hyett BH, Sun X, Travis AC, Johannes RS. A simple risk score accurately predicts in-hospital mortality, length of stay, and cost in acute upper GI bleeding. Gastrointest Endosc. 2011;74(6):1215-24.
21. Teutsch B, Veres DS, Pálinkás D, Simon OA, Hegyi P, Erőss B. Potential benefits of restrictive transfusion in upper gastrointestinal bleeding: a systematic review and meta-analysis of randomised controlled trials. Sci Rep. 2023;13(1):17301.
22. Kola G, Sureshkumar S, Mohsina S, Sreenath G, Kate V. Restrictive versus liberal transfusion strategy in upper gastrointestinal bleeding: A randomized controlled trial. Saudi J Gastroenterol. 2021;27(1):13-9.
23. Gralnek IM, Stanley AJ, Morris AJ, Camus M, Lau J, Lanas A, et al. Endoscopic diagnosis and management of nonvariceal upper gastrointestinal hemorrhage (NVUGIH): European Society of Gastrointestinal Endoscopy (ESGE) Guideline – Update 2021. Endoscopy. 2021;53(03):300-32.
24. Lau JYW, Yu Y, Tang RSY, Chan HCH, Yip HC, Chan SM, et al. Timing of Endoscopy for Acute Upper Gastrointestinal Bleeding. N Engl J Med. 2020;382(14):1299-308.
25. Bai L, Jiang W, Cheng R, Dang Y, Min L, Zhang S. Does Early Endoscopy Affect the Clinical Outcomes of Patients with Acute Nonvariceal Upper Gastrointestinal Bleeding? A Systematic Review and Meta-Analysis. Gut Liver. 2023;17(4):566-80.
26. Vergara M, Bennett C, Calvet X, Gisbert JP. Epinephrine injection versus epinephrine injection and a second endoscopic method in high-risk bleeding ulcers. Cochrane Database Syst Rev. 2014;2014(10):CD005584.

27. Toka B, Eminler AT, Karacaer C, Uslan MI, Koksal AS, Parlak E. Comparison of monopolar hemostatic forceps with soft coagulation versus hemoclip for peptic ulcer bleeding: a randomized trial (with video). Gastrointest Endosc. 2019;89(4):792-802.
28. Loffroy R, Rao P, Ota S, De Lin M, Kwak BK, Geschwind JF. Embolization of acute nonvariceal upper gastrointestinal hemorrhage resistant to endoscopic treatment: results and predictors of recurrent bleeding. Cardiovasc Intervent Radiol. 2010;33(6):1088-100.
29. Faggen AE, Kamal F, Lee-Smith W, Khan MA, Sharma S, Acharya A, et al. Over-the-Scope Clips Versus Standard Endoscopic Treatment for First Line Therapy of Non-variceal Upper Gastrointestinal Bleeding: Systematic Review and Meta-Analysis. Dig Dis Sci. 2023;68(6):2518-30.
30. Deliwala SS, Chandan S, Mohan BP, Khan S, Reddy N, Ramai D, et al. Hemostatic spray (TC-325) vs. standard endoscopic therapy for non-variceal gastrointestinal bleeding: A meta-analysis of randomized controlled trials. Endosc Int Open. 2023;11(3):E288-95.
31. Li XJ, Fung BM. Advancements in endoscopic hemostasis for non-variceal upper gastrointestinal bleeding. World J Gastrointest Endosc. 2024;16(7):376-84.
32. Beggs AD, Dilworth MP, Powell SL, Atherton H, Griffiths EA. A systematic review of transarterial embolization versus emergency surgery in treatment of major nonvariceal upper gastrointestinal bleeding. Clin Exp Gastroenterol. 2014;7:93-104.
33. Agarwal A, Kumar SS, Sadasivan J, Kate V. Antibiotic prophylaxis in the prevention of rebleeding in acute variceal hemorrhage: A randomized trial. J Pharmacol Pharmacotherap. 2015;6(1):24-9.
34. Lai Y, Xu Y, Zhu Z, Pan X, Long S, Liao W, et al. Development and validation of a model to predict rebleeding within three days after endoscopic hemostasis for high-risk peptic ulcer bleeding. BMC Gastroenterol. 2022;22:64.
35. Kamal F, Khan MA, Lee-Smith W, Sharma S, Imam Z, Henry C, et al. Role of routine second-look endoscopy in patients with acute peptic ulcer bleeding: meta-analysis of randomized controlled trials. Gastrointest Endosc. 2021;93(6):1228-37.
36. Wong TCL, Wong KT, Chiu PWY, Teoh AYB, Yu SCH, Au KWL, et al. A comparison of angiographic embolization with surgery after failed endoscopic hemostasis to bleeding peptic ulcers. Gastrointest Endosc. 2011;73(5):900-8.
37. Du RC, Ling LX, Hu YX, Xiao YT, Zhou YA, Hu Y. Research trends on endoscopic therapy for non-variceal upper gastrointestinal bleeding: a bibliometric analysis from 1991 to 2024. Int J Surg. 2024;111(1):1473-6.
38. Tarasconi A, Baiocchi GL, Pattonieri V, Perrone G, Abongwa HK, Molfino S, et al. Transcatheter arterial embolization versus surgery for refractory non-variceal upper gastrointestinal bleeding: a meta-analysis. World J Emerg Surg. 2019;14:3.
39. Matsumoto T, Yoshimatsu R, Shibata J, Osaki M, Maeda H, Miyatake K, et al. Transcatheter arterial embolization of nonvariceal gastrointestinal bleeding with n-butyl cyanoacrylate or coils: a systematic review and meta-analysis. Sci Rep. 2024;14(1):27377.
40. Kate V, Kalayarasan R, Elamurugan T, Ananthakrishnan N. Surgery for peptic ulcer disease. In: Textbook of Surgical Gastroenterology. New Delhi: Jaypee Brothers Medical Publisher; 2016. pp. 283-99.

41. Lee JY, Park HW, Choi JY, Lee JS, Koo JE, Chung EJ, et al. *Helicobacter pylori* Infection with Atrophic Gastritis Is an Independent Risk Factor for Advanced Colonic Neoplasm. Gut Liver. 2016;10(6):902-9.
42. Lee S, Ahn JY, Jung HY, Jung KW, Lee JH, Kim DH, et al. Effective endoscopic treatment of Mallory-Weiss syndrome using Glasgow-Blatchford score and Forrest classification. J Dig Dis. 2016;17(10):676-84.
43. Hussein M, Alzoubaidi D, O'Donnell M, de la Serna A, Bassett P, Varbobitis I, et al. Hemostatic powder TC-325 treatment of malignancy-related upper gastrointestinal bleeds: International registry outcomes. J Gastroenterol Hepatol. 2021;36(11):3027-32.
44. Jensen DM, Kovacs TOG, Ohning GV, Ghassemi K, Machicado GA, Dulai GS, et al. Doppler Endoscopic Probe Monitoring of Blood Flow Improves Risk Stratification and Outcomes of Patients With Severe Nonvariceal Upper Gastrointestinal Hemorrhage. Gastroenterology. 2017;152(6):1310-1318.e1.
45. Luo D, Kuang F, Du J, Zhou M, Liu X, Luo X, et al. Artificial Intelligence-Assisted Endoscopic Diagnosis of Early Upper Gastrointestinal Cancer: A Systematic Review and Meta-Analysis. Front Oncol. 2022;12:855175.

CHAPTER 5

# The Role of Intraoperative Ultrasound in Hepato-Pancreato-Biliary Surgery

*Somaiah Aroori, Venakt Vineeth Amavasya, Poornima Aiswarya Munagala, Vasileios K Mavroeidis*

## INTRODUCTION

Hepato-pancreato-biliary (HPB) operations are highly complex and technically challenging procedures. There is a wide variety of indications for surgery, ranging from stone disease to malignant tumors. Due to the complexity of HPB surgery, pre- and intraoperative planning is essential in minimizing intra- and postoperative complications. Currently, surgeons plan surgery based on preoperative ultrasound (US), computed tomography (CT), and magnetic resonance imaging (MRI), as well as intraoperative examination. Although the currently available cross-sectional imaging is highly sensitive and specific, these investigations have shortcomings, including the inability to provide real-time updates once the operation begins. After the liver is mobilized, CT and MRI cannot assist with anatomical orientation or reveal subtle intrahepatic anatomical variations that may become apparent during surgery. Their accuracy in predicting resectability is not absolute, and their sensitivity and specificity, while high, still fall short of 100%. Small tumors—particularly those adjacent to major vessels or within cirrhotic livers—may be missed. They also cannot guide margin marking, assess blood flow to the remnant liver, and reliably detect vascular patency. Furthermore, they offer no support for intraoperative interventions such as planning ablation, performing targeted biopsies, or guiding intrahepatic indocyanine green (ICG) injections—all of which require real-time, direct imaging capabilities.

In addition to preoperative planning, surgeons also rely on visual inspection and palpation before planning the type of liver resection. However, in 20–40% of patients, surgeons may not be able to see and feel the deeply located and small tumors; therefore, surgeons require an intraoperative tool that complements preoperative imaging and intraoperative examination, providing additional information that can be repeated as many times as necessary without causing any morbidity, and that tool is intraoperative ultrasound (IOUS).

Intraoperative ultrasound has slowly grown to become one of the most trusted tools in HPB surgery. The idea of bringing ultrasound into the operating theatre started to take shape in the late 1960s and early 1970s, with the first experimental use reported in neurosurgery in the United States. Soon after, surgeons in Japan and Europe began applying the technique to abdominal procedures. The significant advancement came in the mid-1970s with the invention of real-time two-dimensional B-mode ultrasonography.[1] By the 1980s, the actual value of IOUS in liver surgery became clear. Pioneers such as Makuuchi in Japan and Bismuth in France showed that ultrasound performed during the operation could detect tiny hepatocellular carcinomas (HCC) and hidden colorectal metastases (CRLM) that were not visible on standard imaging.[2,3]

Through the 1990s, IOUS became part of routine practice in complex resections and liver transplantation. It provided surgeons with a method to map out vessels within the liver, plan reconstructions, and minimize injuries. The technology then kept pace with the rise of minimally invasive surgery. Smaller laparoscopic probes became available in the 2000s, enabling the same level of precision to be applied to laparoscopic and later robotic liver resections. Over the past decade, contrast-enhanced ultrasound (CE-US) using microbubbles and liver-specific agents, such as Sonazoid, has significantly enhanced sensitivity, particularly for lesions in patients with cirrhosis or those who have undergone chemotherapy. Today, it is often combined with ICG fluorescence, 3D planning, and fusion imaging to support parenchyma-sparing, anatomical liver resections and ablations. This chapter discusses the role of IOUS in liver, pancreas, and biliary surgery.

## WHAT IS INTRAOPERATIVE ULTRASOUND?

Intraoperative ultrasound, compared to percutaneous US, is a real-time investigative tool that is placed directly on the organ of interest, thereby bypassing the barriers that can limit standard ultrasound, such as the skin, abdominal wall, or bowel gas. The probes, typically operating at frequencies between 7 and 15 MHz, and the direct approach provide superior image quality and sensitivity. The additional advantage of IOUS is that it can be repeated as many times as possible and can be performed by a surgeon.

## WHAT DOES A LIVER SURGEON NEED TO KNOW BEFORE SURGERY?

Before we describe the role of IOUS in liver surgery, it is essential to understand the information surgeons need to know before planning liver surgery. Unlike the planning of other intra-abdominal surgeries, planning liver surgery is significantly more complex due to the highly intricate intra- and extrahepatic anatomy, associated anatomical variations, dual blood supply, variable pathology, the nature of the liver parenchyma, as well as the size and function of the remnant liver. Surgeons also need to consider whether they should aim for R0 or R1 resection, as well as the location and number of tumors/segments involved, and signs of portal hypertension. Based on the above information, as well as the patient's performance status, liver function, and the presence/absence of extrahepatic disease, surgeons will determine the type, extent, and approach to liver surgery.

## THE ROLE OF INTRAOPERATIVE ULTRASOUND IN LIVER SURGERY

Intraoperative ultrasound serves as an invaluable extension of preoperative imaging, confirming what has already been identified while also uncovering lesions that may have been missed on earlier scans. Its real-time capability allows surgeons to pinpoint the exact location and size of lesions, determine segmental involvement, and assess their relationship to key inflow and outflow vessels. IOUS allows for the three-dimensional reconstruction of the relationship between tumors and intrahepatic vasculature, which is essential for surgical planning and individualizing the type and extent of resection.

## CHARACTERIZATION OF LIVER TUMORS

Intraoperative ultrasound also helps to characterize the various liver lesions/ tumors, which is essential for obtaining a correct diagnosis before deciding on the need for liver resection. However, it is not uncommon to encounter benign and malignant liver pathologies in the same patient. This information can help surgeons ensure that they only remove the tumors that require resection. Hemangioma and liver cysts are the most commonly encountered benign lesions. Hemangiomas are well-circumscribed, hyperechoic (echo-bright) lesions with slightly irregular walls. Simple liver cysts are anechoic, well-circumscribed, with posterior acoustic enhancement and lack color on Doppler. Adenomas are premalignant tumors, which are either hypoechoic (20–30%) or hyperechoic (<30%), discrete lesions with a hypoechoic halo due to fat sparing. Focal nodular hyperplasia is a benign tumor that is well-demarcated, mostly isoechoic, with a hyperechoic central scar. HCC is also a well-circumscribed hypoechoic tumor often with increased vascularity on color doppler. However, large HCCs often have a mixed echogenic pattern **(Figs. 1A and B)**. Colorectal liver metastases (CRLM) are the most common metastases, typically appearing as discrete, mixed-echogenic lesions with a hypoechoic halo surrounding them **(Fig. 2)**. Focal fatty sparing is a hypoechoic area that is usually close to the falciform ligament junction with segment 4B/3.

## ASSESSMENT OF THE BACKGROUND LIVER PARENCHYMA

Intraoperative ultrasound is a highly sensitive investigation tool in assessing the status of liver parenchyma. Typically, a preoperative MRI provides

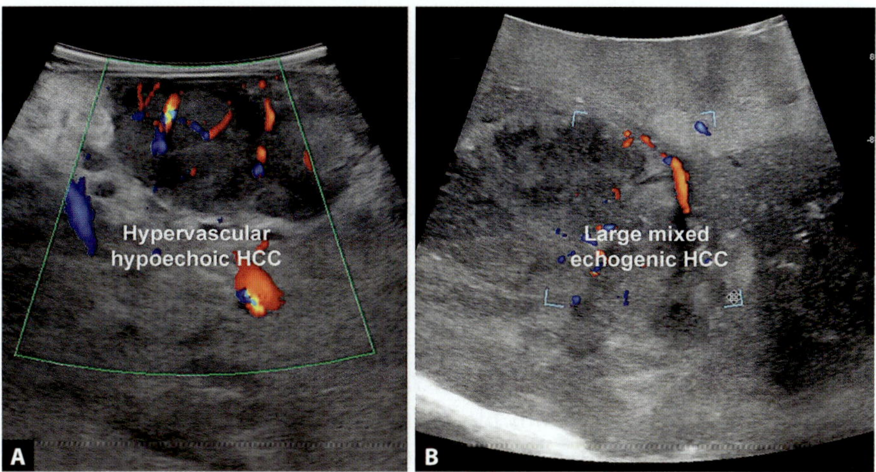


**Figs. 1A and B:** (A) An ultrasound image of a liver demonstrating a hypoechoic hypervascular HCC within a cirrhotic liver; (B) Demonstrates a large mixed echogenic hypervascular HCC. (HCC: hepatocellular carcinoma)

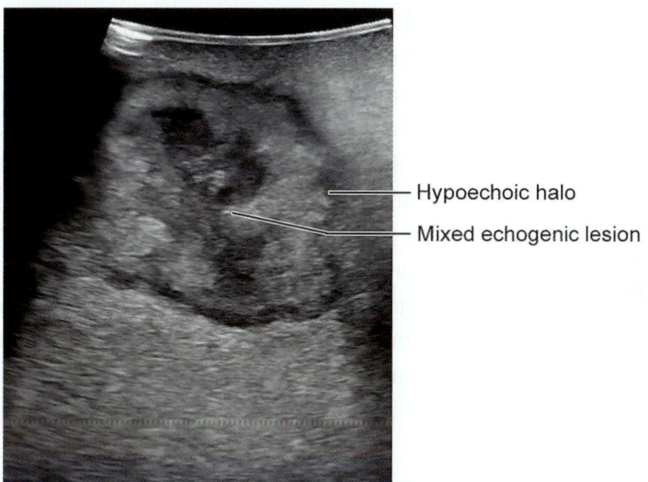


**Fig. 2:** An ultrasound image of a liver demonstrating a well-defined mixed echogenic lesion with a hypoechoic halo around it—typical of a colorectal metastasis.

information about the liver's background status; however, if proton density fat fractionation is not calculated, the MRI may underestimate the extent of steatosis. A steatotic liver has an echo-bright appearance compared to a normal liver. Surgeons can use this information before deciding whether or not to carry out major hepatectomies, especially in patients with borderline future remnant liver. A cirrhotic liver will have a moth-eaten appearance, with regenerative nodules appearing as echo-bright areas, and the normal liver in-between appears as hypoechoic areas.

## VASCULAR ASSESSMENT

Intraoperative ultrasound will help identify intrahepatic vascular anatomy, as well as anatomical variations and vascular involvement. The portal vein, hepatic artery, and hepatic veins all have an anechoic appearance (black tubular structures) with a color signal on Doppler assessment. The type of color depends on the direction of blood flow to the ultrasound probe. The following features will help one to differentiate the portal vein, hepatic artery, and hepatic vein **(Table 1)**. The most important feature that helps differentiate between the three vascular structures is the pulse wave pattern.

On spectral Doppler, the portal vein and its major divisions will exhibit both red and blue color (Yin-Yang appearnce). This is due to the simultaneous capture of both blood flow going towards and away from the probe. However, the most essential characteristic is the monophasic wave pattern **(Figs. 3A to C)**. Portal vein velocity also helps to diagnose portal hypertension—normal portal flow velocity is 20–30 cm/s. In portal hypertension, it is <12 cm/s. Knowledge of the standard pulse wave pattern of the portal vein helps to diagnose abnormal wave patterns and identify the possible cause of the abnormality.

The pulse wave pattern of the hepatic artery is a biphasic wave **(Fig. 4)**. By assessing the pulse wave pattern, one can determine whether there is a flow in the artery or not. By measuring the velocity and resistance index, one can also determine whether an anastomotic stenosis or thrombosis has occurred following arterial reconstruction.

On IOUS, the hepatic vein appears as *anechoic* tubular structure with either a red or blue color signal on color Doppler. The characteristic pulse wave pattern is a periodic wave pattern **(Fig. 5A)**. Identification of the number of hepatic veins will help surgeons decide whether to preserve or resect them along with the tumors. It helps surgeons prevent inadvertent damage, particularly during minimally invasive surgery. Surgeons can mark

**TABLE 1:** Differences between portal vein, hepatic vein, hepatic artery, and bile ducts on ultrasound examination.

| *Features* | *Portal vein* | *Hepatic vein* | *Hepatic artery* | *Bile ducts* |
|---|---|---|---|---|
| Anechoic black tubular structure | Yes | Yes | Yes | |
| Has got thick echo-bright layer around it | Yes | Yes/No | No | No—except in cholangitis |
| Color | Yes | Yes | Yes | No |
| Doppler wave pattern | Monophasic | Periodic wave pattern | Biphasic wave pattern | No wave |

the exact location of the hepatic veins and their branches on the liver surface using IOUS-guided diathermy.

Intraoperative ultrasound will also help determine the extent of liver resection; for example, the surgeon can decide whether to proceed to the left or right side of the MHV in patients with left-sided liver tumors. Similarly, surgeons can also choose whether to preserve the right hepatic vein during planned posterior sectionectomy.

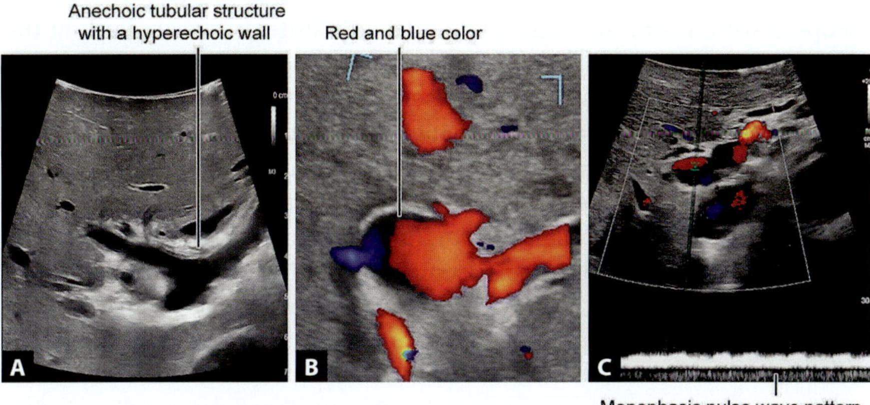


**Figs. 3A to C:** An IOUS feature of the portal vein. (A) Gray-scale image showing the portal vein as a black tubular structure with a hyperechoic wall; (B) Doppler examination demonstrating the characteristic "Yin-Yang" color pattern; (C) Spectral Doppler tracing illustrating the typical monophasic waveform.

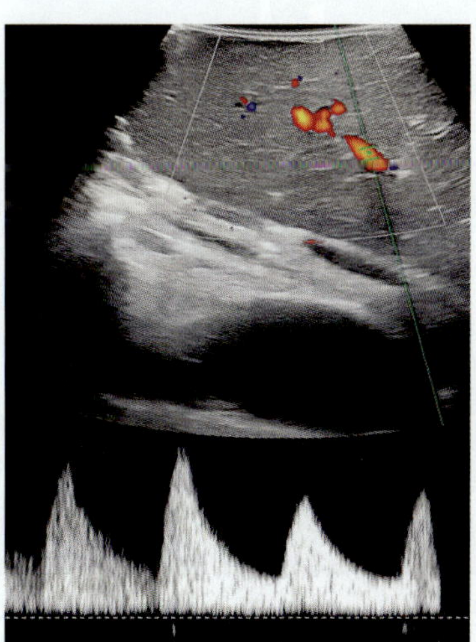

**Fig. 4:** An IOUS image of a liver demonstrating the typical biphasic pulse wave pattern of the normal hepatic artery.

## INTRAOPERATIVE ULTRASOUND IN ASSESSING THE RESECTABILITY AND PLANNING OF LIVER RESECTION

Despite the best available preoperative imaging, in some patients, it may not be sufficiently sensitive to inform surgeons whether tumors are resectable or not. Sometimes, tumors may compress rather than infiltrate the major hepatic veins, and this may not be obvious on preoperative CT and/or MRI. In such patients, IOUS helps assess their involvement and determine resectability. **Figure 5B** shows obvious compression/involvement of the MHV but sparing of the inferior vena cava (IVC) in a patient with a large primary liver tumor. Preoperative CT and MRI could not give a definite answer regarding the involvement of IVC and MHV in a patient with a large primary liver tumor.

Intraoperative ultrasound will help surgeons to determine the presence of a portal vein thrombus (PVT), narrowing of the portal or superior mesenteric anastomosis, and the involvement or compression of the portal vein by the tumor. **Figure 6** shows the thrombus in the left portal vein (LPV) on IOUS in a patient with resectable hilar cholangiocarcinoma, as identified based on preoperative imaging. IOUS is an essential tool for identifying the location of HCC tumors in a cirrhotic liver. It shows the IOUS appearance of cirrhotic liver and the tumor, which is not visible or palpable on inspection/examination of the liver.

Several studies have demonstrated that R0 resection improves disease-free and overall survival for patients with CRLM, HCC, and cholangiocarcinoma. IOUS will help surgeons identify the exact extent of the tumor and mark the

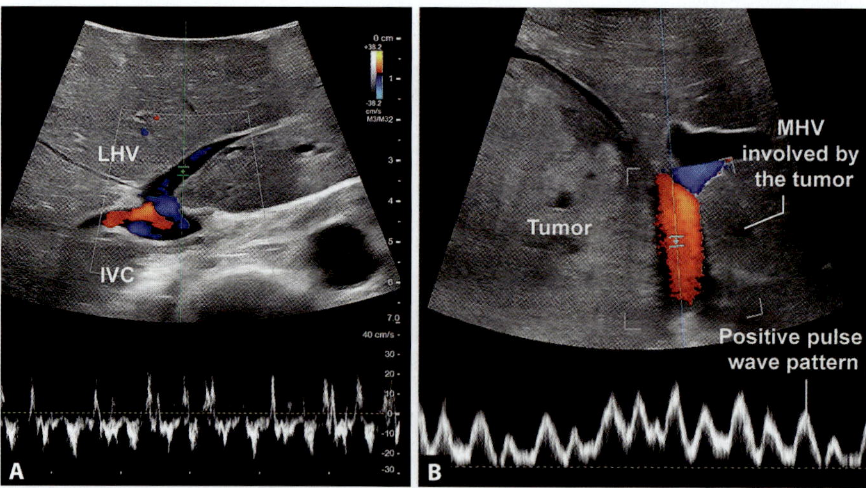


**Figs. 5A and B:** (A) An IOUS image of a liver demonstrating the typical periodic wave pattern of the normal hepatic venous pulse wave pattern; (B) An IOUS image shows a liver with a large HCC compressing/involving the MHV, resulting in loss of the periodic wave pattern. (LHV: Left hepatic vein)

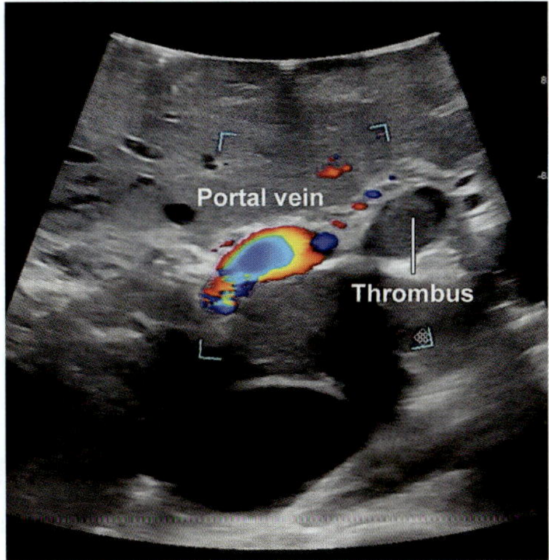


**Fig. 6:** An IOUS image of a liver demonstrating a filling defect from a thrombus in the left portal vein in a patient planned for right hepatectomy for hilar cholangiocarcinoma.

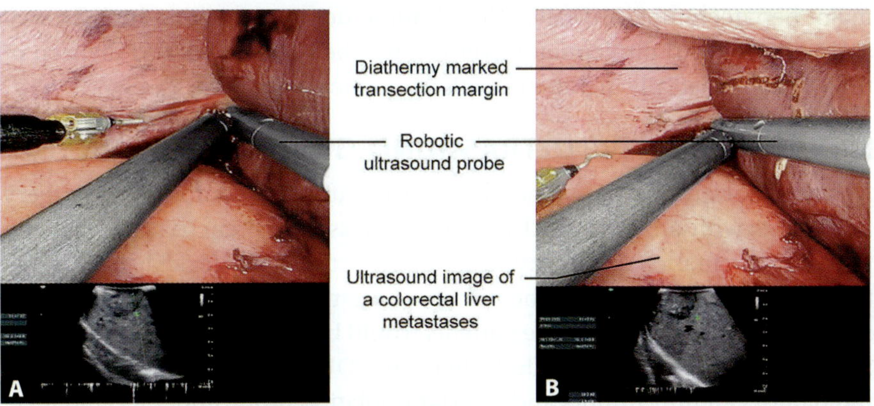


**Figs. 7A and B:** (A) Illustrating the visualization of a colorectal metastasis under a robotic ultrasound probe (bottom image). The tumor was not visible on visual inspection; (B) Robotic US probe (bottom image) confirming the presence of the tumor inside the marked transection margins.

resection margins. Marking of the resection level with diathermy is crucial in achieving a tumor-free margin (both circumferential and deep). **Figures 7A and B** illustrate the visualization of a CRLM under a robotic ultrasound probe (bottom image). The tumor was not visible on visual inspection.

Intraoperative ultrasound is crucial in identifying the tumor-free resection margin of the intrahepatic ducts in patients with mass-forming hilar cholangiocarcinoma. In minimally invasive surgery, surgeons must rely entirely on IOUS guidance to determine the ductal resection margin.

# THE ROLE OF INTRAOPERATIVE ULTRASOUND IN PARENCHYMAL-SPARING HEPATECTOMIES

Parenchymal-sparing hepatectomies (PSH) avoid the morbidity and mortality associated with major hepatectomies, while providing similar or comparable survival and recurrence rates. Therefore, it is preferable to perform PSH whenever it is possible and feasible. Studies have shown that PSH provides similar oncological outcomes to those of major liver resections.[4] IOUS facilitates PSH by allowing surgeons to accurately locate, mark, and remove each tumor. It is not possible to perform PSH without accurate and precise guidance provided by IOUS.

## IDENTIFICATION OF FLOW TO THE REMNANT LIVER

Intraoperative ultrasound helps to determine both arterial, portal venous and hepatic venous flow to the remnant liver. For example, when performing a right hepatectomy, portal flow to the left liver can be inadvertently compromised if the ligature or stapler applied to divide the RPV is moved to the left, narrowing the main and LPV and making it prone to PVT. To make major hepatectomies are safe, it is helpful to demonstrate that both arterial and portal flow to the remnant liver is intact before ligation and division of the vessels, especially in patients with anatomical variations.

## INTRAOPERATIVE ULTRASOUND-GUIDED ABLATION

Ablative therapy has shown equal survival outcomes compared to surgery in patients with one or two CRLM that are less than 3 cm in size.[5] In some patients, percutaneous ultrasound-guided ablation is not feasible or safe due to the superficial location of the tumors or their proximity to the diaphragm, stomach, or gallbladder. These patients would benefit from either minimally invasive or open IOUS-guided ablation. IOUS will help surgeons and radiologists identify tumors and insert the ablation probe under its guidance.

# THE ROLE OF INTRAOPERATIVE ULTRASOUND IN FLUORESCENCE IMAGE-GUIDED SURGERY

To accurately identify tumor-free margins and make liver surgery as anatomically precise as possible, surgeons are increasingly relying on fluorescence image-guided surgery (FIGS). ICG is a fluorescent dye that is exclusively taken up by the liver and excreted into bile. If injected either systemically or into the portal vein, it will be taken up by the liver, causing the liver to fluoresce and appear green under red light. This feature can be exploited, and ICG can be injected under IOUS guidance into segmental portal branches *(positive staining)* or systemically after ligating both the arterial and portal branches supplying the segment (s) *(negative staining),* which requires resection. FIGS is not possible without IOUS guidance.

## THE ROLE OF INTRAOPERATIVE ULTRASOUND IN DETECTING MISSED LIVER TUMORS

Intraoperative ultrasound is a sensitive investigation for detecting CRLM. It has changed surgical strategy in up to 40% of cases. IOUS has detected new metastases in 20–60% of cases. IOUS has also allowed for PSH compared to the non-IOUS group.[6,7] IOUS is more sensitive, with a diagnostic accuracy of 97% compared to 83% for MRI. The sensitivity of laparoscopic and open IOUS is similar, ranging from 94 to 99%.[6]

## THE ROLE OF INTRAOPERATIVE ULTRASOUND IN LIVER TRANSPLANTATION

Liver transplantation is a highly complex and technically challenging procedure, particularly living and re-do transplantation. Unfortunately, vascular complications are the most serious complications and one of the common reasons for graft failure within the immediate perioperative period. The reported incidence of vascular complications ranges from 8 to 20%.[8]

Intraoperative ultrasound will help surgeons assess not only patency but also flow velocity and resistance index. The use of IOUS has enabled surgeons to address vascular patency issues during surgery, thereby preventing graft loss simultaneously. IOUS also helps transplant surgeons in determining which hepatic veins to reimplant by accurately assessing the diameter of the veins.

## LIMITATIONS OF INTRAOPERATIVE ULTRASOUND IN LIVER SURGERY

Despite its various uses, there are limitations to the use of IOUS. The first and most significant limitation is the subjective nature and the time required to learn and master the technique and interpretation of the images. Most surgeons who use IOUS are self-taught surgeons, as there is no structured training pathway. Therefore, considerable subjectivity is involved in interpreting the IOUS.

The other limitations of the IOUS are that standard contact scanning of the liver can miss small, superficial tumors, particularly in cirrhotic livers and segments 7 and 8, as it can be difficult to perform IOUS in these scenarios. In these cases, it is better to perform the IOUS once the liver is mobilized, if not using the probe standoff technique, where the IOUS is performed through a saline or water-filled glove placed on the liver.

## THE LIVER INTRAOPERATIVE ULTRASOUND TECHNIQUE

To ensure surgeons can learn to perform liver IOUS using a specific and consistent landmark, the first author developed a technique called

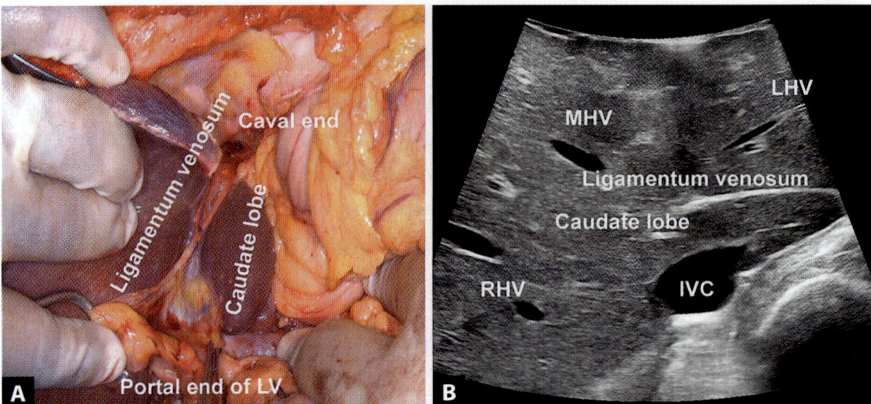


**Figs. 8A and B:** (A) An image of the ligamentum venosum between the left lateral liver and the caudate lobe; (B) An intraoperative ultrasound image of the liver illustrating the ligamentum venosum between the left lateral liver and the caudate lobe.

"Aroori Ligamentum Venosum (ALV)," which relies on the identification of the ligamentum venosum (LV) between the left lateral liver and the caudate lobe **(Figs. 8A and B)**. LV is the obliterated ductus venosum, which connects the LPV and IVC at the junction of the left and middle hepatic veins. It appears as an echo-bright band under IOUS. Surgeons can trace either the portal or the hepatic venous end of the LV and follow either the portal or hepatic veins to evaluate the entire liver. If they get lost, they can always go back to the LV and restart the procedure. The link to the ALV technique can be found at *https://pubmed.ncbi.nlm.nih.gov/40451418*.[9]

## ROLE OF INTRAOPERATIVE ULTRASOUND IN BILIARY SURGERY

### Detection of Bile Duct Stones

In 10–20% of patients with symptomatic gallstones, there are concurrent bile duct stones (BDS). The confirmation of suspected BDS and treatment is essential in preventing and treating BDS-associated complications. Compared to an intraoperative cholangiogram, IOUS is a non-invasive test with no risk of contrast, radiation, or damage to the bile duct. It provides information about the presence of BDS but also offers insights into the anatomy of the cystic duct **(Figs. 9A and B)**, the diameters of the cystic and bile ducts, the locations of the stones, their sizes, and the number of stones. This information can guide surgeons to decide regarding the best approach to BDS, i.e., transcystic versus transcholedochal approach.

Bile duct stone will cause posterior acoustic shadowing on IOUS **(Fig. 9C)**. Whereas biliary sludge or polyps will not give posterior acoustic shadowing, and surgeons can use this feature to diagnose BDS. We recommend selective

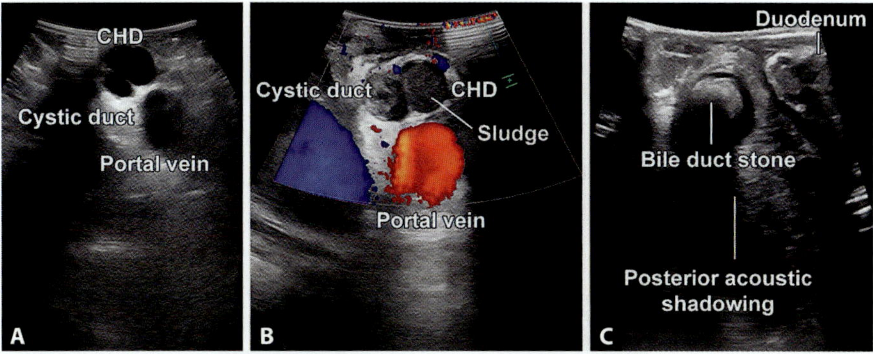


**Figs. 9A to C:** An intraoperative ultrasound image demonstrating variations in cystic duct insertion. (A) Shows the posterior location of the cystic duct; (B) Cystic and CHD next to each other in the retro-pancreatic area and filled with biliary sludge; (C) Bile duct stone with posterior acoustic shadowing. (CHD: common hepatic duct)

use in the following situations: in patients with gallstones and dilated bile duct on preoperative imaging, history of gallstone-induced acute pancreatitis, elevated transaminases, jaundice, and confirmed BDS on preoperative imaging. Limitations of IOUS include a subjective nature and reduced sensitivity in patients with a nondilated bile duct.

## Intraoperative Ultrasound in Assessing the Difficulty of Cholecystectomy and Identification of Remnant Gallbladder

In the hands of experienced surgeons, IOUS can help alleviate the challenges of cholecystectomy. By using IOUS, surgeons can pre-empt the difficulty of cholecystectomy, the need for conversion to an open operation or subtotal cholecystectomy (STC), and the anticipated duration of surgery.

A significant proportion of STC patients develop recurrent symptoms and require remnant cholecystectomy (RC). RC is a technically challenging and complex operation. IOUS can guide surgeons to the exact location of the gallbladder, as it is often shrunken, shriveled, and adherent to the omentum, duodenum, and bowel. By identifying the precise location and its proximity to the other structures, surgeons can direct the dissection into the appropriate area rather than unthinkingly dissecting out the area where it is supposed to be.[10] IOUS will also help surgeons to identify the bile duct and can prevent BDI.

## Diagnosis of Gallbladder Cancer

Gallbladder cancer can be challenging to differentiate from Xanthogranulomatous cholecystitis on preoperative imaging. However, IOUS can aid in identifying GBC and help determine the best course of action.

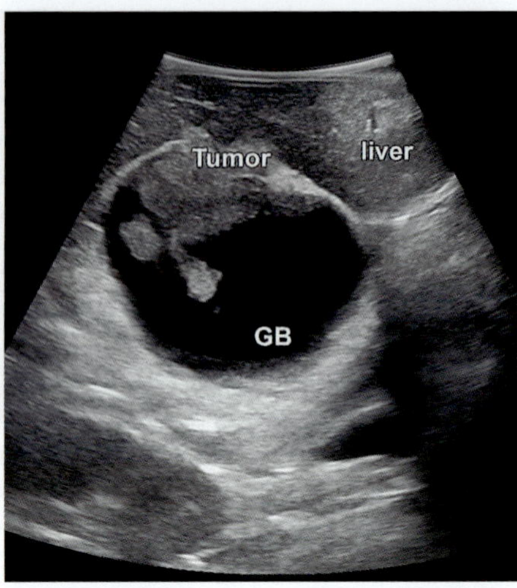


**Fig. 10:** An IOUS image of a gallbladder tumor with involvement of the cystic plate and tumor extension into the liver.

**Figure 10** shows the typical appearance of a gallbladder tumor on IOUS. GBC does not exhibit posterior acoustic shadowing, as it is a soft tissue mass that allows ultrasound waves to travel through with minimal reflection. IOUS also helps surgeons determine the involvement of the liver and the proximity of the tumor to the inflow.

## THE ROLE OF INTRAOPERATIVE ULTRASOUND IN PANCREATIC SURGERY

Intraoperative ultrasound can also guide surgeons in localizing small functional/nonfunctional neuroendocrine tumors (NET) **(Figs. 11A and B)**. It can also aid in targeting the dissection in that area and facilitate the enucleation of these tumors. IOUS allows surgeons to estimate the distance between the pancreatic duct and the tumor, enabling them to decide whether enucleation is feasible or not. Traditionally, tumors that are 3 mm or longer away from the PD are the ones chosen for enucleation. However, a study by Tang et al. has shown no increased pancreatic fistula rate, even in patients with tumors that are within a 3-mm distance from the PD.[11]

Intraoperative ultrasound helps with the identification and marking of the pancreatic transection margin in patients with various tumors. It also helps surgeons determine whether they can preserve the spleen on the splenic artery and vein in patients with benign or premalignant tumors. IOUS is highly sensitive and specific in assessing vascular involvement and, therefore, resectability status in both chemo-naive and post-neoadjuvant chemotherapy patients. The sensitivity and specificity in chemo-naive patients are 92% and 93%, respectively.[12,13]

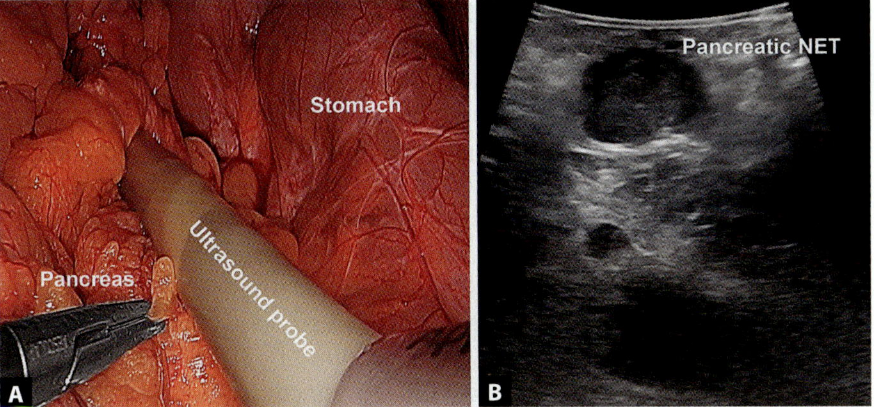


**Figs. 11A and B:** (A) Laparoscopic ultrasound examination of a patient with a functional neuroendocrine tumor; (B) IOUS shows a circumscribed hypoechoic tumor away from the pancreatic duct. Patient underwent enucleation.

Patients with symptomatic pseudocysts following acute pancreatitis requiring either endoscopic or surgical decompression would benefit from IOUS. In patients who require either cystogastrostomy or cystojejunostomy, IOUS can help surgeons identify and locate the pseudo-cyst, guiding the needle to aspirate the contents before opening the cyst and draining it. A small proportion of patients with chronic pancreatitis benefit from surgery. In these patients, IOUS facilitates the localization of the PD and cannulation of the same. This would allow surgeons to open the pancreatic parenchyma exactly at the level of identified PD on IOUS. IOUS also allows the localization of the tumor within the background of chronic pancreatitis, which can be otherwise difficult to find on inspection/palpation of the pancreas.

## THE ROLE OF CONTRAST-ENHANCED LIVER ULTRASOUND

Contrast-enhanced intraoperative ultrasound (CE-IOUS) is a relatively new imaging tool in liver surgery that enables the real-time assessment of liver parenchyma during surgery. Consequently, it enables surgeons to make more accurate adjustments intraoperatively. It is being increasingly used as an adjunct to CT, MRI, and conventional IOUS for patients undergoing liver surgery. Its role in this context can be important in two main settings: (1) discrimination of indeterminate lesions detected in cirrhotic livers by conventional IOUS, and (2) detection of CRLM that may be overlooked by other imaging modalities.[14]

From a technical perspective, the modality of CEUS and CE-IOUS utilizes ultrasound contrast agents, which are, in essence, gas-filled microbubbles.[15] Various types are used in different continents, and for liver assessment specifically, second-generation agents such as Sonovue and Sonazoid are the current standard.[16] These consist of—(1) a heavy-molecular-weight gas like sulfur hexafluoride (SF6) to reduce solubility and increase stability under high pressure, and (2) an encapsulating shell, typically a monolayer of phospholipids or protein coating, to stabilize the gas.[16] This composition makes the microbubble highly elastic.

As with other imaging modalities, following contrast injection in the context of CE-IOUS in liver surgery, an enhancement pattern emerges, which is crucial for diagnostic purposes. There are three phases of enhancement, namely the arterial phase (AP), the portal venous phase (PVP), and the late phase (LP), and their timings are of paramount importance to know. The AP commences 10–20 seconds post-contrast injection (PCI) and continues until 30–45 seconds PCI. The PVP follows, starting from 30–45 seconds PCI extending to 2 minutes PCI. The LP lasts from the end of the PVP until there is unequivocal clearance of microbubbles from the circulation, typically at around 4–6 minutes.[14]

## UTILITY OF LIVER CONTRAST-ENHANCED INTRAOPERATIVE ULTRASOUND

As liver CE-IOUS enables the sensitive detection of vascular morphology and perfusion in real-time with high temporal and spatial resolution, it allows for the detection and characterization of vascular lesions. This aids the determination of underlying malignancy as well as the establishment of specific diagnoses. The algorithms used for diagnosis are similar to those for noninvasive diagnosis of liver masses on CT and MRI scans and are based on enhancement characteristics in the AP and the PVP. According to the *CEUS Liver Imaging Reporting and Data System (CEUS LI-RADS),* there are major and ancillary features.[17]

*Early marked washout* is typical for metastases and intrahepatic cholangiocarcinoma, compared to *late marked washout, which* is suggestive of malignancy but not specific to any type. The same counts for early mild washout. *Late mild washout* is typical for HCC and HCC precursor nodules, and the *absence of washout* is indicative of benign lesions.

Liver CE-IOUS can be valuable in aiding the discrimination of indeterminate lesions detected in cirrhotic livers by conventional IOUS. It can be very helpful in detecting CRLM that other imaging modalities may overlook. It can aid in the differential diagnosis between benign and malignant lesions. It can be a valuable tool in the context of "disappearing" metastases (DLM). The rate of DLM in the literature ranges from 9 to 24%. Compared with palpation and intraoperative ultrasonography, CE-IOUS was reported to be more sensitive for detecting DLM, revealing an additional 10–15% of DLM.[18,19]

Finally, in the context of HCC, several studies have highlighted the benefits of liver CE-IOUS, demonstrating its utility in both benign pathologies, such as regenerative nodules, and malignant lesions. It offers the advantage of intraoperative characterization, based on vascularization patterns, of lesions that could not be diagnosed by preoperative imaging, resulting in modification of the surgical therapy decision and expansion of the resection or intraoperative ablation.[20,21]

## CONCLUSION

Intraoperative ultrasound is an essential adjunct to HPB surgeons. IOUS complements the currently available preoperative imaging. It is a noninvasive tool that not only confirms preoperative imaging findings but also provides additional information such as intrahepatic vascular anatomy and anatomical variations, accurately localizes all the tumors and facilitates parenchymal preservation hepatectomies, helps with identification and marking of transection margins, resectability, confirmation of flow to the remnant liver, and facilitates intraoperative ablation and fluorescence image-guided surgery. As it is a noninvasive test, it will allow surgeons to repeat the tests as many times as possible. It will also allow surgeons to orient anatomy following mobilization of the liver. In biliary surgery, it facilitates the detection of bile duct stones and the treatment approach. It also aids in differentiating chronic cholecystitis from gallbladder cancer, addressing the challenges of cholecystectomy, and identifying remnant gallbladders and cystic duct anatomical variations. In pancreatic surgery, IOUS aids in the assessment of resectability, location and marking of the resection margin, type of resection, and guides localization of the pancreatic duct. Although IOUS is a highly sensitive and specific complementary tool to the preoperative imaging, it comes with limitations such as a subjective nature, a learning curve, and the initial cost of the equipment.

## REFERENCES

1. Makuuchi M, Torzilli G, Machi J. History of intraoperative ultrasound. Ultrasound Med Biol. 1998;24(9):1229-42.
2. Makuuchi M, Hasegawa H, Yamazaki S. Intraoperative Ultrasonic Examination for Hepatectomy. Jpn J Clin Oncol. 1981;11(2):367-90.
3. Bismuth H, Castaing D, Garden OJ. The use of operative ultrasound in surgery of primary liver tumors. World J Surg. 1987;11(5):610-4.
4. Torzilli G, Montorsi M, Donadon M, Palmisano A, Del Fabbro D, Gambetti A, et al. 'Radical but conservative' is the main goal for ultrasonography-guided liver resection: Prospective validation of this approach. J Am Coll Surg. 2005;201(4):517-28.
5. van der Lei S, Puijk RS, Dijkstra M, Schulz HH, Vos DJW, De Vries JJJ, et al. Thermal ablation versus surgical resection of small-size colorectal liver metastases (COLLISION): an international, randomised, controlled, phase 3 non-inferiority trial. Lancet Oncol. 2025;26(2):187-99.

6. Viganò L, Ferrero A, Amisano M, Russolillo N, Capussotti L. Comparison of laparoscopic and open intraoperative ultrasonography for staging liver tumours. Br J Surg. 2013;100(4):535-42.
7. Kupke LS, Dropco I, Götz M, Kupke P, Jung F, Stroszczynski C, et al. Contrast-Enhanced Intraoperative Ultrasound Shows Excellent Performance in Improving Intraoperative Decision-Making. Life. 2024;14(9):1199.
8. Astarcıoglu I, Egeli T, Gulcu A, Ozbilgin M, Agalar C, Cesmeli EB, et al. Vascular Complications After Liver Transplantation. Exp Clin Transplant. 2023;21(6):504-11.
9. Amavasya VV, Aroori S. How I do it: the technique of intraoperative ultrasound of the liver using the ligamentum venosum as the landmark. J Gastrointest Surg. 2025;29(8):102104.
10. Ibrahim R, Abdalkoddus M, Mownah OA, Chanthu A, Yao L, Aroori S. Safety profile and outcomes of intraoperative ultrasound-guided remnant cholecystectomy. Ann R Coll Surg Engl. 2023;105(6):528-31.
11. Tang W, Gao Y, Zhao Z, Kang Y, Xu Y, An L. Intraoperative Ultrasound Guided Robotic Pancreatic Enucleation, Does a Distance of 3mm Still Matters? Surg Innov. 2023;30(2):166-75.
12. Shin LK, Brant-Zawadzki G, Kamaya A, Jeffrey RB. Intraoperative ultrasound of the pancreas. Ultrasound Q. 2009;25(1):39-48.
13. van Veldhuisen E, Walma MS, van Rijssen LB, Busch OR, Bruijnen RCG, van Delden OM, et al. Added value of intra-operative ultrasound to determine the resectability of locally advanced pancreatic cancer following FOLFIRINOX chemotherapy (IMAGE): a prospective multicenter study. HPB. 2019;21(10):1385-92.
14. Torzilli G, Del Fabbro D, Olivari N, Calliada F, Montorsi M, Makuuchi M. Contrast-enhanced ultrasonography during liver surgery. Br J Surg. 2004;91(9):1165-7.
15. Klibanov AL. Targeted delivery of gas-filled microspheres, contrast agents for ultrasound imaging. Adv Drug Deliv Rev. 1999;37(1–3):139-57.
16. Dijkmans PA, Juffermans LJM, Musters RJP, van Wamel A, ten Cate FJ, van Gilst W, et al. Microbubbles and ultrasound: from diagnosis to therapy. Eur J Echocardiogr. 2004;5(4):245-56.
17. American College of Radiology. ACR Liver Imaging Reporting & Data System (LI-RADS®). [online] Available from https://www.acr.org/Clinical-Resources/Clinical-Tools-and-Reference/Reporting-and-Data-Systems/LI-RADS. [Last accessed November, 2025]
18. Tsilimigras DI, Ntanasis-Stathopoulos I, Paredes AZ, Moris D, Gavriatopoulou M, Cloyd JM, et al. Disappearing liver metastases: A systematic review of the current evidence. Surg Oncol. 2019;29:7-13.
19. Tani K, Shindoh J, Akamatsu N, Arita J, Kaneko J, Sakamoto Y, et al. Management of disappearing lesions after chemotherapy for colorectal liver metastases: Relation between detectability and residual tumors. J Surg Oncol. 2018;117(2):191-7.
20. Lu Q, Luo Y, Yuan CX, Zeng Y, Wu H, Lei Z, et al. Value of contrast-enhanced intraoperative ultrasound for cirrhotic patients with hepatocellular carcinoma: a report of 20 cases. World J Gastroenterol. 2008;14(25):4005-10.
21. Torzilli G, Palmisano A, Del Fabbro D, Marconi M, Donadon M, Spinelli A, et al. Contrast-enhanced intraoperative ultrasonography during surgery for hepatocellular carcinoma in liver cirrhosis: is it useful or useless? A prospective cohort study of our experience. Ann Surg Oncol. 2007;14(4):1347-55.

CHAPTER 6

# Biobanking: Its Role from Biological Samples to Precision Medicine

*Rohit Kumar Singh, Ruby Gupta, Puneet*

## INTRODUCTION

Biobanking has emerged as a transformative force in modern biomedical research and clinical medicine. It involves the systematic collection, processing, storage, and use of biological specimens—such as blood, urine, tissues, and cerebrospinal fluid—along with related clinical and demographic data, to advance scientific discovery and medical innovation. Initially limited to small, investigator-driven repositories, biobanks have evolved into large, networked infrastructures integrating electronic health records (ERHs), genomic data, and standardized protocols. Global collaborations such as the International Society for Biological and Environmental Repositories (ISBER), Biobanking and Biomolecular Resources Research Infrastructure (BBMRI), and Pan-European Biobanking have enhanced quality assurance (QA), reproducibility, and ethical transparency in biospecimen management.[1]

Today, biobanks are pivotal in studying complex diseases such as cancer, diabetes, and cardiovascular disorders, supporting biomarker identification and personalized therapeutic strategies. Their role during the coronavirus disease 2019 (COVID-19) pandemic exemplified their critical importance in vaccine development and immunological research. Despite their immense value, challenges persist regarding informed consent, data privacy, ownership, and sustainable funding. Maintaining specimen integrity and harmonized data systems also remains demanding.

Nevertheless, biobanks have become central to precision medicine, bridging clinical care and molecular science. More than repositories, they represent dynamic infrastructures driving translational research, evidence-based healthcare, and innovation in the pursuit of individualized and population-level medical advancement.

## TYPES OF BIOBANKS

Biobanks can be classified according to their purpose, scale, source of biospecimens, and degree of integration with clinical or population data. This classification is crucial, as it determines their scientific, ethical, and operational value.[2]

## Population-based Biobanks

These collect biospecimens and epidemiological data from large cohorts of apparently healthy individuals. Their goal is to study how genetic, lifestyle, and environmental factors influence disease over time. Notable examples are the *UK biobank, Nordic biobanks,* and the *All of Us Research Program (USA).* Applications include genome-wide association studies (GWAS), identifying genetic predispositions, and developing predictive health models.

## Disease-oriented Biobanks

These repositories gather biological materials from patients with specific conditions and are usually hospital-based. Samples—collected before, during, or after treatment—are linked with detailed clinical, radiological, and pathological data. Examples include *the Cancer Genome Atlas (TCGA)* and *International Cancer Genome Consortium (ICGC).* They support biomarker discovery, patient stratification, and translational research in precision medicine.

## Tissue Biobanks

Tissue biobanks preserve samples from surgical resections, biopsies, or autopsies, using methods like formalin fixation or snap-freezing. Supported by corresponding slides and digital records, they advance histopathology and molecular research. Examples are the *NCI's Cooperative Human Tissue Network (CHTN)* and *HTA-regulated Biobanks (UK).*

## Virtual or Federated Biobanks

These digital infrastructures store specimen *data* rather than physical samples, allowing institutions to share and access information remotely. Platforms such as *the Biobanking and Biomolecular Resources Research Infrastructure-European Research Infrastructure Consortium (BBMRI-ERIC)* and *Cancer Human Biobank (caHUB)* integrate repositories under common ethical and technical standards. They facilitate large-scale data harmonization, remote collaboration, and meta-analyses.

## Commercial or Private Biobanks

Privately managed, these focus on client-based storage and genetic profiling, often for regenerative or personalized medicine. Examples include *cord blood banks* and *DNA storage companies.* Applications extend to stem cell therapy, pharmacogenomics, and genetic ancestry studies.

## Environmental and Animal Biobanks

These collect biological materials from animals and ecosystems to support comparative medicine, zoonotic surveillance, and biodiversity preservation.

They are vital for tracking diseases such as rabies and avian influenza and for studying host-pathogen interactions.

### Hybrid or Integrated Biobanks

Modern research favors hybrid models integrating population, disease, and digital biobanks. Linked with EHRs and genomic databases, they support multiomic, AI-driven analytics for predictive diagnostics and drug discovery.[3]

## ESTABLISHING A BIOBANK

Establishing a modern biobank involves far more than storage and refrigeration—it demands a multidisciplinary framework combining scientific rigor, ethical oversight, and advanced technology.[4] A biobank's integrity relies on skilled professionals and transparent governance. Scientific teams manage biospecimen procurement, processing, and preservation following standardized operating procedures (SOPs). A well-defined governance policy specifying accountability and ownership fosters trust, reproducibility, and ethical integrity.[5-7]

Biospecimens include blood, plasma, serum, urine, cerebrospinal fluid, saliva, DNA, RNA, and tissues—each requiring specific handling to maintain molecular fidelity. Blood should be centrifuged at 4°C and stored at –80°C for long-term use.[8] DNA can be stored at 4°C short-term or –80°C for longer durations.[9] RNA, being labile, demands immediate stabilization and cryopreservation in liquid nitrogen.[10] Every specimen must carry a unique identifier linked to coded clinical and demographic data. According to the Indian Council of Medical Research (ICMR) (2020) guidelines, all samples must be anonymized or pseudonymized before use. Secure linkage between identity and code is stored in restricted-access systems. Temperature control and stability are the foundation of biobanking. Biomolecules degrade variably with temperature, thus monitoring of preservation equipment is essential. Storage at –20°C is recommended for short-term, however, long-term storage is recommended at –80°C, e.g., DNA, RNA, plasma, and proteins. Cryopreservation at –196°C in liquid nitrogen is recommended for viable cells or gametes.

Regular QA and quality control (QC) checks confirm biospecimen integrity through barcode verification, pH and hemolysis testing, and nucleic acid analysis. A robust Biobank Information Management System (BIMS) integrates clinical, molecular, and demographic data for each specimen. It enables full traceability, EHR integration, secure access, and export for research. In essence, building a biobank is a scientifically meticulous and ethically demanding endeavor. From sample collection to data integration, every step must follow harmonized SOPs, ensure ethical compliance, and maintain technological precision.[11]

## STANDARDIZATION INITIATIVES

The US National Cancer Institute's *caHUB* introduced comprehensive SOPs for sample handling and annotation. Subsequently, Mendy et al. (2017)[12] integrated ethical, legal, and social dimensions into harmonized frameworks, promoting responsible collaboration and donor trust.[5,13] The ISO 20387:2018 standard, *Biobanking—General Requirements for Biobanking*, formalized international quality and harmonization norms. It ensures biobank competence, impartiality, and consistency while improving access to high-quality biospecimens.[14] In India, NABL (Quality Council of India) now accredits biobanks under this framework, aligning national repositories with international standards and enabling global collaboration.

## GUIDELINES AND ETHICS INVOLVED WITH BIOBANKING

The establishment and functioning of a biobank extend beyond technical aspects of biospecimen collection and storage. They encompass a complex matrix of ethical, legal, and regulatory responsibilities aimed at safeguarding the dignity, autonomy, and rights of human participants while advancing scientific knowledge **(Flowchart 1)**. Every step—from acquisition to storage, retrieval, and data sharing—must comply with internationally recognized ethical and operational frameworks.[9] Several global organizations have developed frameworks governing biobank operations. It includes NIH–NCI Best Practices (2018), ISBER Best Practices (2012, updated), BBMRI-ERIC (2013), Council for International Organizations of Medical Sciences (CIOMS), and World Health Organization (WHO).[10,12,14-20] The Declaration of Helsinki (WMA, 1964; Revised 2024) remains the foundation of ethical research.[20] The latest revision strengthens participant involvement across all research stages, requires explicit consent for storage and reuse of specimens, ensures protection during global health emergencies, and emphasizes minimizing material wastage.

In India, the ICMR National Ethical Guidelines (2018)[21] regulate all biobank-related research. Institutional Ethics Committee (IEC) approval is mandatory. Key principles include written informed consent in the local language, broad consent for future research, clear storage duration, the right to withdraw samples before anonymization, and strict confidentiality of data.

**Flowchart 1:** Algorithm representing the functioning of the biobank with support of mutidisciplinary team under regulatory bodies, ethical governance, and legal framework.

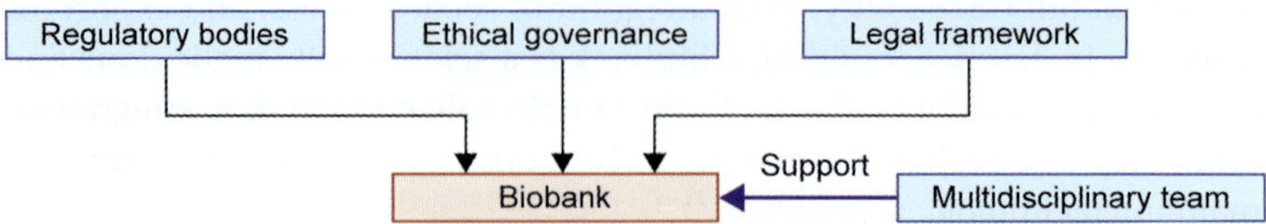

These align local ethics with global standards while respecting national legal frameworks.

## BIOBANK: FROM BIOLOGICAL SAMPLES TO PRECISION MEDICINE

The concept of biobanking has undergone a remarkable transformation over the past few decades, evolving from simple repositories of biological specimens to highly sophisticated, ethically governed, and technologically integrated systems that underpin the era of precision medicine. Biobanks are now indispensable infrastructures in medical research, linking biological samples with vast datasets encompassing clinical, genetic, lifestyle, and environmental information. This integration allows researchers to uncover novel biomarkers, understand disease mechanisms, and develop individualized therapeutic strategies—heralding a paradigm shift in modern healthcare.[18,21-23]

The term *biobank* is often used loosely to refer to any collection of biological materials. However, in its true scientific and regulatory sense, a biobank represents a systematically organized collection of biospecimens—including tissue, blood, urine, bone marrow, and other body fluids—accompanied by detailed and secure patient information. In essence, a biobank bridges the clinical and research domains. It is the foundation upon which translational research thrives—converting biological material into actionable knowledge that ultimately improves patient care. Among the various forms of biobanking, cancer-oriented biobanks hold particular prominence. These repositories collect and store biological materials from cancer patients at multiple stages—diagnosis, treatment, follow-up, and relapse. By correlating tissue changes with clinical outcomes, they provide invaluable resources for understanding tumor biology and therapeutic response.

Pathology laboratories play a pivotal role in this ecosystem. They serve as the gatekeepers of tissue integrity and quality. When required, advanced methods like macro- and microdissection are employed to enrich tumor content and reduce tissue heterogeneity.[18,22-24] This rigorous process guarantees that the samples stored in cancer biobanks can reliably support precision oncology—where therapies are tailored according to the genetic and molecular signature of each tumor. The emergence of next-generation biobanking reflects the dynamic landscape of biomedical science. The focus has shifted from static sample storage to living biobanks, encompassing vital cells, stem cell lines, and patient-derived models that remain biologically active.

Patient-derived xenografts (PDXs) and patient-derived organoids (PDOs) exemplify this evolution. PDX is the model developed following implantation of the tumor tissues from patients into immunocompromised or humanized mice. This model preserves the characteristics of cancer including its spatial structure and intratumor heterogeneity, PDX also retains the genomic features across different subtypes, stages, and backgrounds of diversified treatment. PDOs are the three-dimensional (3D) culture generated from various human cancers and it allows for deeper insights into tumor heterogeneity and spatial organization. These systems preserve the biological characteristics of the original tumor, allowing researchers to test therapeutic responses in preclinical settings. For example, the EurOPDX Consortium and the NCI's PDXNet have fostered international collaboration, enabling model sharing and standardization to accelerate cancer drug discovery. Similarly, the Princess Margaret Living Biobank (PMLB) in Canada has established a centralized repository of organoid and xenograft models from multiple organs, rigorously characterized for genomic fidelity and morphological accuracy. The successful creation of such living repositories depends heavily on rapid and controlled handling of tissues. Prolonged surgical time or delayed cooling can reduce cell viability and lower engraftment rates. Innovative technologies such as under-vacuum cold transport systems have emerged to minimize ischemic injury and preserve sample viability during transfer from the operating theater to the laboratory.

Additionally, biobanking now encompasses extracellular vesicles, metabolomic and lipidomic samples, and even longitudinal patient collections aimed at monitoring disease progression over time. These developments signify the dawn of functional biobanking, where preserved materials not only support molecular diagnostics but also fuel regenerative medicine, drug discovery, and individualized therapy design.

Ethical governance forms the moral backbone of biobanking. The process begins with obtaining informed consent, which must clearly describe the purpose of collection, the potential future use of biospecimens, privacy safeguards, and participants' rights to withdraw. Modern frameworks increasingly favor broad consent, allowing specimens to be used for unspecified future research within ethically approved boundaries. In addition to consent, confidentiality and data protection are paramount. Biobank databases must comply with national and international data protection laws such as the Health Insurance Portability and Accountability Act (HIPAA) and the General Data Protection Regulation (GDPR).[24]

In the modern context of personalized oncology, where treatment decisions hinge on molecular profiles, the pathologist's role transcends traditional microscopy. They become active collaborators in translational research, exploring the genomic profile. Personalized or precision medicine relies on the ability to stratify patients according to genetic, proteomic, or metabolic characteristics, and to design therapies that are both effective and minimally toxic. For example, epidermal growth factor receptor (EGFR) mutation testing in nonsmall cell lung cancer identifies patients eligible for tyrosine kinase inhibitors such as *gefitinib* or *erlotinib*. Similarly, detection of the BRAF V600E mutation in melanoma guides treatment with *vemurafenib*. These targeted therapies depend entirely on the availability of well-characterized biospecimens from biobanks. Large-scale initiatives like TCGA have demonstrated the power of biobanking in generating comprehensive molecular catalogues across cancer types. Such resources have laid the groundwork for molecular classification systems, drug development, and predictive biomarker validation.

The COVID-19 pandemic underscored both the challenges and the indispensability of biobanks. During the early outbreak of severe acute respiratory syndrome coronavirus 2 (SARS-CoV-2), biospecimen handling posed biosafety concerns due to unknown viral status. Organizations such as BBMRI-ERIC, WHO, and the Centers for Disease Control and Prevention (CDC) issued strict guidelines mandating that only accredited facilities with biosafety level 2 capacity handle COVID-related specimens. Many biobanks established dedicated repositories for pandemic-era samples, ensuring segregation and traceability.

Biobanks have become the lifeline of precision medicine, transforming raw biological samples into knowledge that informs prevention, diagnosis, and therapy. Their success depends on a delicate balance of scientific rigor, ethical governance, technological infrastructure, and multidisciplinary collaboration. The integration of biobanking with pathology, genomics, and clinical research has revolutionized the way we approach complex diseases, particularly cancer. Next-generation biobanks—housing organoids, xenografts, and high-throughput molecular datasets—now serve as dynamic laboratories that mirror human disease in real time **(Flowchart 2)**.[24-27]

## ARTIFICIAL INTELLIGENCE AND PREDICTIVE ANALYTICS

Artificial intelligence (AI)-driven analytics can process multimodal datasets—genomic, clinical, and imaging—to uncover hidden patterns and predict outcomes. Next-generation "Smart Biobanks" will integrate AI, robotics, and blockchain to enable real-time tracking, global data sharing, and automated operations. By uniting biobanking and big data analytics, healthcare is advancing toward a truly predictive, preventive, and personalized model—transforming patient care into a data-driven and precision-focused enterprise.[28]

## IMAGING BIOBANKS

Biobanks have become the backbone of translational and precision medicine by enabling the systematic collection and preservation of biological materials for clinical and research use. They support the discovery of disease markers, validation of therapeutic targets, and development of novel treatment

**Flowchart 2:** Algorithm: Biobanking from specimen to Individualized/precision therapy.

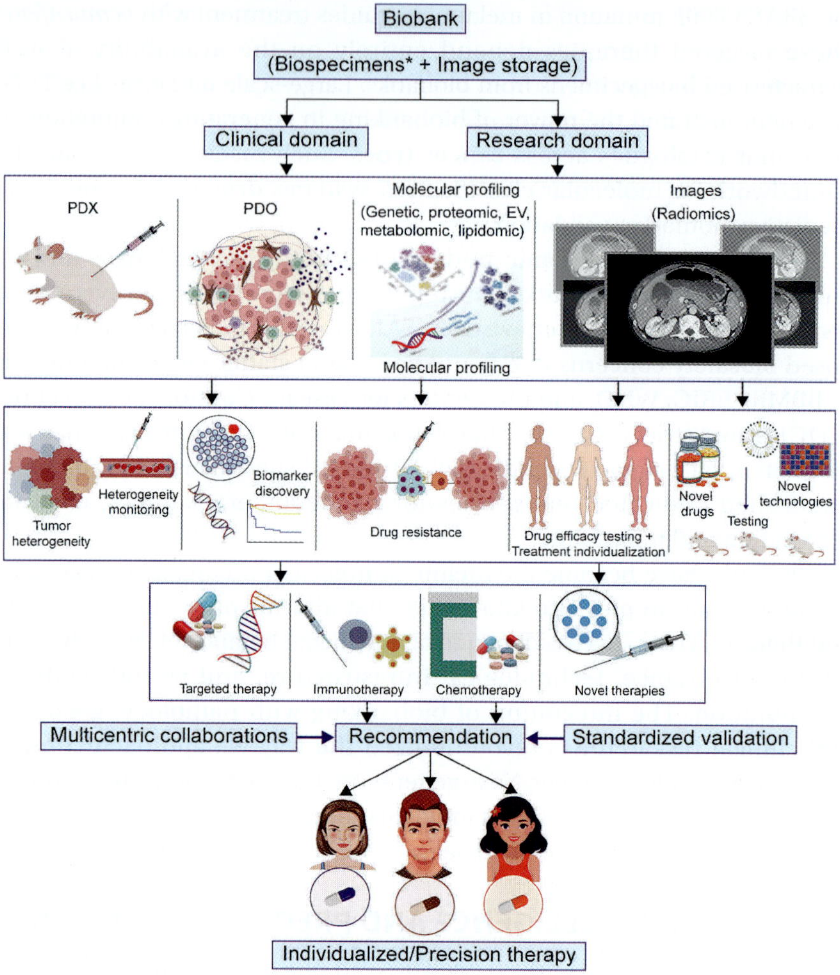

(*): It includes blood, plasma, serum, urine, CSF, saliva, DNA, RNA, and tissues. (EV: extracellular vesicles; PDO: patient-derived organoids; PDX: patient-derived xenograft)

strategies. An important and rapidly evolving extension of this concept is the imaging biobank, which seeks to curate and manage medical imaging data—computed tomography (CT), magnetic resonance imaging (MRI), positron emission tomography (PET), and other modalities—under the same structured, standardized, and ethical framework that governs biological specimen repositories.

The rationale for imaging biobanks arises from the recognition that images themselves are data-rich biospecimens. When processed through advanced computational tools, they reveal quantitative and qualitative information reflecting tissue microstructure, physiology, and metabolism.

These features—known as imaging biomarkers (IBs)—can serve as noninvasive surrogates of pathology, complementing or even replacing invasive tissue sampling. Thus, imaging biobanking represents a paradigm shift from storing physical biospecimens alone to preserving the digital phenotype of disease.

The foundation of imaging biobanking lies in the field of radiomics, which uses high-throughput computational analysis to extract numerous quantitative parameters from medical images obtained via CT, MRI, and PET. These radiomic features—texture, signal intensity, shape, perfusion indices, diffusion coefficients, and others—can be mathematically correlated with histopathological findings or treatment outcomes to identify reproducible IBs.[29]

Many such biomarkers are already used in clinical oncology, including tumor volume, vascular perfusion grade, diffusion patterns of water molecules, MR spectroscopy profiles, tissue stiffness on elastography, glucose metabolism on PET, and MR fingerprinting signatures. Because these features are derived from electromagnetic, photonic, or acoustic signals generated by the body, they represent a biophysical expression of disease phenotype. Importantly, they are noninvasive, repeatable, and suitable for longitudinal monitoring. According to latest researches, an imaging biobank should encompass raw image data, metadata, and derivative measurements, together with relevant clinical, pathological, and genomic annotations. The European Society of Radiology (2015) defines imaging biobanks as "organized databases of medical images and associated IBs shared among multiple researchers and linked to other biorepositories." This definition underscores their dual responsibility: maintaining the highest standards of data acquisition and analysis while promoting transparent data sharing and validation. Clinical translation depends upon this harmonization, as rigorous validation remains the critical bottleneck that distinguishes truly useful IBs from those lacking clinical relevance.

Most imaging biobanks have evolved within the oncology domain, where imaging plays a central role in disease detection, staging, and response assessment. A notable model is the Cancer Imaging Archive (TCIA) in the United States, a publicly accessible repository managed by the Frederick National Laboratory for Cancer Research. TCIA stores vast collections of de-identified DICOM-formatted images from patients with various malignancies. Each "collection" is organized by disease entity, imaging modality, or research focus, and many are accompanied by complementary data such as treatment details, outcomes, genomic mutations, and pathology results. Its open-access policy allows global researchers to download datasets for algorithm development, biomarker validation, and radiomics research.

While Europe lacks a centralized equivalent, several regional initiatives have recognized the urgent need to build interoperable imaging biobank networks. Such efforts must establish uniform acquisition protocols, metadata standards (e.g., MIABIS and FAIR principles), and legal frameworks for secure data exchange. Harmonization is essential to enable multicentric studies, reduce variability, and enhance reproducibility.[30-32]

A major frontier of modern biobanking is the integration of imaging and molecular data to explore relationships between phenotype and genotype. This emerging discipline, known as radiogenomics, merges radiomic descriptors with genomic, transcriptomic, and proteomic profiles to decode the biological basis of imaging patterns. High-throughput sequencing and bioinformatics have made it possible to integrate radiomic data with next-generation sequencing (NGS), DNA microarrays, and expression datasets. Through such analyses, radiogenomics can capture tumor heterogeneity and improve individualized therapy planning. Several studies have demonstrated these principles in glioblastoma multiforme, lung, prostate, and breast cancers, showing that imaging signatures can predict mutations and guide targeted therapy selection.

The convergence of certified biobanks containing biospecimens and imaging archives provides the necessary infrastructure for such integrative analyses. Hybrid biobanks, combining imaging with biological samples, offer an unprecedented opportunity to deliver fully personalized clinical management. A recurring limitation in the field is the gap between discovery and clinical validation. Many potential IBs demonstrate promise in retrospective analyses but fail when tested prospectively. To overcome this, multicentric collaborations and standardized validation frameworks must become routine practice. Looking ahead, the next decade will witness imaging biobanks evolving into multiomics and AI-driven ecosystems. AI and machine learning algorithms can mine massive image repositories to uncover subtle, predictive patterns invisible to human perception. These insights, when integrated with genomic and clinical data, can yield composite biomarkers with higher diagnostic and prognostic value. In the era of precision medicine, the strength of future research will rest not only on the quantity of biospecimens stored but also on the quality, interoperability, and accessibility of bioimages linked to them. Imaging biobanks thus represent the next frontier in translational research—an indispensable bridge from biological sample to clinical insight, from phenotype to genotype, and ultimately, from data to better patient care.[29-32]

## BIOBANKING AND SURGEON

Surgery, by its very nature, provides a unique and direct interface between clinical practice and biological material. Every operative procedure yields an opportunity to advance scientific knowledge—through tissues, fluids, or cellular samples that reflect the pathophysiological state of disease.

Biobanking, in this context, represents the organized extension of surgical science beyond the operating theater. It transforms routine surgical specimens into resources of enduring research value, linking clinical outcomes with molecular mechanisms and enabling precision-based interventions in the future.

The surgeon is central to the biobanking process. It is through the surgeon's judgment that appropriate samples are obtained—from tumor margins, resected organs, or diseased tissues—while ensuring patient safety, ethical compliance, and diagnostic adequacy. The modern biobank relies heavily on the surgical team for accurate documentation of intraoperative details, specimen origin, and patient consent. This multidisciplinary coordination between the surgeon, pathologist, and biobank custodian ensures that every specimen collected contributes meaningfully to translational research. From an academic standpoint, biobanking has transformed surgical research methodology. Traditional surgical studies were often limited by small sample sizes, heterogeneous data, and subjective interpretation. Biobanked specimens, coupled with clinical metadata, now allow for large-scale, longitudinal analyses of disease behavior, postoperative healing, and biomarker evolution. For instance, archived tumor tissues linked with patient follow-up data enable studies on recurrence patterns and therapeutic response, ultimately refining operative strategies and prognostic counseling. Similarly, biobanking of vascular, hepatic, or musculoskeletal samples has opened avenues for regenerative and reconstructive innovations.

In training environments, biobanks serve as invaluable teaching resources. They allow postgraduate trainees and surgical residents to correlate morphological observations with molecular and genetic data, fostering a deeper understanding of disease biology. Exposure to biobanking protocols also instils research discipline, documentation ethics, and respect for the scientific process—qualities essential for future academic surgeons. Thus, biobanking integrates seamlessly with the educational mission of medical colleges, bridging the gap between surgical skill and scientific inquiry.[33]

The impact of biobanking on surgical innovation is equally profound. Advances in organ preservation, cryobiology, and graft viability are rooted in biobanked research. Likewise, the development of patient-specific implants, stents, and biologically derived scaffolds often begins with data derived from well-curated biorepositories. Surgeons who engage with biobanking initiatives thus contribute not only to research but also to the evolution of surgical technology itself. Moreover, as the global emphasis shifts toward precision medicine, the surgeon's ability to align operative data with genomic or proteomic findings will determine the future of individualized surgical care.

Ethical stewardship remains paramount. Every specimen entrusted to a biobank originates from a patient's body and thus carries with it a moral obligation of confidentiality, respect, and responsible use. Surgeons, as custodians of these samples, must ensure that informed consent, traceability, and compliance with national regulations are rigorously maintained.

In essence, biobanking redefines the surgeon's role—from a technical expert to a contributor in the continuum of discovery. It symbolizes the fusion of clinical excellence with scientific curiosity, ensuring that what is excised in the operation theater becomes a building block for future breakthroughs. For the modern surgeon, participation in biobanking is not a luxury but a professional responsibility—an enduring commitment to advance surgical science and serve humanity through evidence, ethics, and innovation.

## CONCLUSION

In the surgical sciences, progress has always depended on observation, innovation, and evidence derived from meticulous study of human tissues. Biobanking represents the natural extension of that tradition—an organized, ethical, and scientifically rigorous method of preserving the biological narrative of our patients. For surgeons, biobanks are not merely repositories of specimens; they are living archives that connect operative experience with molecular understanding and clinical outcomes.

Modern surgery no longer ends when the wound is closed. Every excised specimen, every tissue biopsy, and postoperative fluid sample carries the potential to unravel mechanisms of disease, refine operative techniques, and personalize postoperative care. The emergence of standardized biobanking has therefore transformed surgical practice from being purely procedural to profoundly translational—enabling integration of genomic, proteomic, and histopathological data with operative findings.

Future surgical success will depend not only on technical mastery in the operating theater but also on our commitment to preserve, understanding and learning from the biological material entrusted to us. In essence, biobanking empowers the surgeon to transcend the operating table—from treating individual patients to contributing to the collective advancement of surgical science. The tissues we preserve today will illuminate the surgical solutions of tomorrow.

## REFERENCES

1. Vaz M, Vaz M, Srinivasan K. Ethical challenges in bio-banking: moving the agenda forward in India. Indian J Med Ethics. 2014;11(2):79-88.
2. National Cancer Institute. (2016). NCI Best Practices for Biospecimen Resources. [online] Available from https://dctd.cancer.gov/data-tools-biospecimens/biospecimens-biobanks/resources/best-practices/best-practices-2016.pdf [Last accessed November, 2025].
3. Campbell LD, Astrin JJ, DeSouza Y, Giri J, Patel AA, Rawley-Payne M, et al. The 2018 revision of the ISBER best practices: summary of changes and the editorial team's development process, Biopreserv Biobank. 2018;16:3-6.

4. 2012 best practices for repositories collection, storage, retrieval, and distribution of biological materials for research international society for biological and environmental repositories. Biopreserv Biobank. 2012;10(2):79-161.
5. Kirwan JA, Brennan L, Broadhurst D, Fiehn O, Cascante M, Dunn WB, et al. Preanalytical Processing and Biobanking Procedures of Biological Samples for Metabolomics Research: A White Paper, Community Perspective (for "Precision Medicine and Pharmacometabolomics Task Group"-The Metabolomics Society Initiative). Clin Chem. 2018;64(8):1158-82.
6. Slamon DJ, Clark GM, Wong SG, Levin WJ, Ullrich A, McGuire WL. Human breast cancer: correlation of relapse and survival with amplification of the HER-2/neu oncogene. Science. 1987;235(4785):177-82.
7. Tomczak K, Czerwińska P, Wiznerowicz M. The Cancer Genome Atlas (TCGA): an immeasurable source of knowledge. Contemp Oncol (Pozn). 2015;19(1A): A68-77.
8. Hsieh SY, Chen RK, Pan YH, Lee HL. Systematical evaluation of the effects of sample collection procedures on low-molecular-weight serum/plasma proteome profiling. Proteomics. 2006;6(10):3189-98.
9. Nederhand RJ, Droog S, Kluft C, Simoons ML, de Maat MP; Investigators of the EUROPA trial. Logistics and quality control for DNA sampling in large multicenter studies. J Thromb Haemost. 2003;1(5):987-91.
10. von Ahlfen S, Missel A, Bendrat K, Schlumpberger M. Determinants of RNA quality from FFPE samples. PLoS One. 2007;2:1261.
11. Hallmans G, Vaught JB. Best practices for establishing a biobank. Methods Mol Biol. 2011;675:241-60.
12. Mendy M, Caboux E, Lawlor RT, Wright J, Wild CP. Common Minimum Technical Standards and Protocols for Biobanks Dedicated to Cancer Research. Lyon (FR): International Agency for Research on Cancer; 2017.
13. Kirwan JA, Kaddurah-Daouk R, Mitchell T, Pischon T, Schmidt MA, Velagapudi V. Biobanking for Metabolomics and Lipidomics in Precision Medicine. Clin Chem. 2019;65(7):827-32.
14. Dagher G. Quality matters: International standards for biobanking. Cell Prolif. 2022;55(8):e13282.
15. Fortier I, Burton PR, Robson PJ, Ferretti V, Little J, L'Heureux F, et al. Quality, quantity and harmony: the DataSHaPER approach to integrating data across bioclinical studies. Int J Epidemiol. 2010;39(5):1383-93.
16. Peakman T, Elliott P. Current standards for the storage of human samples in biobanks. Genome Med. 2010;2(10):72.
17. International Organizations for Standardization (ISO). (2018). ISO 20387:2018 Biotechnology–biobankingy–general requirements for biobanking. [online] Available from https://www.iso.org/standard/67888.html [Last accessed November, 2025].
18. CLSI. (2025). CLSI PRE02: Collection of Diagnostic Venous Blood Specimens. [online] Available from https://clsi.org/shop/standards/pre02/ [Last accessed November, 2025].
19. International Ethical Guidelines for Health-related Research Involving Humans: Prepared by the Council for International Organizations of Medical Sciences (CIOMS) in collaboration with the World Health Organization (WHO) [Internet]. 4th edition. Geneva: Council for International Organizations of Medical Sciences; 2016.

20. World Medical Association. World Medical Association Declaration of Helsinki: Ethical Principles for Medical Research Involving Human Participants. JAMA. 2025;333(1):71-4.
21. Indian Council of Medical Research. (2018). Handbook on National Ethical Guidelines for Biomedical and Health Research Involving Human Participants. [online] Available from https://www.icmr.gov.in/icmrobject/uploads/Guidelines/1724914217_handbook_on_icmr_ethical_guidelines_2018.pdf [Last accessed November, 2025].
22. Yassin R, Lockhart N, González del Riego M, Pitt K, Thomas JW, Weiss L, et al. Custodianship as an ethical framework for biospecimen-based research. Cancer Epidemiol Biomarkers Prev. 2010;19(4):1012-5.
23. Gabelloni M, Faggioni L, Borgheresi R, Restante G, Shortrede J, Tumminello L, et al. Bridging gaps between images and data: a systematic update on imaging biobanks. Eur Radiol. 2022;32(5):3173-86.
24. CLSI. (2023). CLSI PRE04: Handling, Transport, Processing, and Storage of Blood Specimens for Routine Laboratory Examinations. [online] Available from https://clsi.org/shop/standards/pre04/ [Last accessed November, 2025].
25. Caulfield T, McGuire AL, Cho M, Buchanan JA, Burgess MM, Danilczyk U, et al. Research ethics recommendations for whole-genome research: consensus statement. PLoS Biol. 2008;6(3):e73.
26. National Heart, Lung, and Blood Institute working group; Fabsitz RR, McGuire A, Sharp RR, Puggal M, Beskow LM, et al. Ethical and practical guidelines for reporting genetic research results to study participants: updated guidelines from a National Heart, Lung, and Blood Institute working group. Circ Cardiovasc Genet. 2010;3(6):574-80.
27. Kocarnik JM, Fullerton SM. Returning pleiotropic results from genetic testing to patients and research participants. JAMA. 2014;311(8):795-6.
28. U.S. Department of Health and Human Services. Presidential Commission for the Study of Bioethical Issues, Anticipate and Communicate: ethical management of incidental and secondary findings in the clinical, research, and direct-to-consumer contexts. Washington, DC: U.S. Department of Health and Human Services; 2013.
29. Black L, Avard D, Zawati MH, Knoppers BM, Hebert J, Sauvageau G. Funding considerations for the disclosure of genetic incidental findings in biobank research. Clin Genet. 2013;84:397-406.
30. Wolf SM, Crock BN, Van Ness B, Lawrenz F, Kahn JP, Beskow LM, et al. Managing incidental findings and research results in genomic research involving biobanks and archived data sets. Genet Med. 2012;14:361-84.
31. McDonald SA, Watson MA, Rossi J, Becker CM, Jaques DP, Pfeifer JD. A new paradigm for biospecimen banking in the personalized medicine era. Am J Clin Pathol. 2011;136:679-84.
32. Rosenberg RN. Translating biomedical research to the bedside: a national crisis and a call to action. JAMA. 2003;289:1305-6.
33. Thasler WE, Thasler RM, Schelcher C, Jauch KW. Biobanking for research in surgery: are surgeons in charge for advancing translational research or mere assistants in biomaterial and data preservation? Langenbecks Arch Surg. 2013;398(4):487-99.

CHAPTER 7

# Liquid Biopsy: The Future of Cancer Detection

*Pranab Dey*

## INTRODUCTION

Since decades, the surgeons are habituated to do excision and incisional biopsy for histopathological evaluation of the tissue. The biopsy is considered the gold standard for the diagnosis and classification of the tumor. The biopsy is often difficult to collect as it is an invasive technique. The repeated surgical biopsy is also not convenient for continuous monitoring of the patient. Moreover, many times the early tumor is difficult to detect as they may not be visible by radiology or other techniques. Recently, a newer technology known as "Liquid biopsy"[1,2] is becoming popular.[1,2] It is defined as "A type of laboratory test which is done on the blood, urine, or other body fluids to study the circulating cancer cells or circulating DNA, RNA or other molecules that are released by the tumor cells."[3] Unlike conventional biopsy, the liquid biopsy can supply vast amount of essential information regarding early tumor diagnosis, detection of minimal residual disease (MRD), identification of drug resistance, personalized therapy, monitoring of therapy, and early recurrence. It is now the cornerstone of the oncology service, particularly in precision medicine. The current study is focused on the detection and isolation of the various components of liquid biopsy along with its precise clinical applications.

## CONVENTIONAL BIOPSY VERSUS LIQUID BIOPSY: WHY TO DO LIQUID BIOPSY?

In case of conventional biopsy, the surgeon takes incisional or excisional biopsy from the tumor tissue **(Table 1)**. The surgical technique is invasive and needs specialization for the procurement of deeper tissue from the internal organ. Unlike the conventional biopsy, the liquid biopsy is totally noninvasive and can be repeated at different intervals. So, it may detect the emergence of treatment resistant clone. The liquid biopsy can be done without the presence of visibly detected mass. The conventional biopsy represents the part of the tumor tissue that has been taken for examination. The tumor is usually heterogeneous that means the distinct genetic and other molecular techniques in the different areas of the tumor and biopsy may not represent the true nature of the tumor. In contrast, the liquid biopsy avoids heterogeneity of the tumor. In the deeply situated tumor, the liquid biopsy is very effective as there is no need to access the tumor mass because simple collection of blood and/or body fluid contain the circulating tumor cells (CTCs) or circulating DNA, RNA, or other molecules is enough. So, the liquid biopsy has emerged as a game-changer in cancer diagnosis and management.

The difference between the conventional and liquid biopsy is mentioned in **Table 1** and **Figure 1**.

**TABLE 1:** Conventional biopsy versus liquid biopsy.

| *Features* | *Liquid biopsy* | *Conventional biopsy* |
|---|---|---|
| Technique | Noninvasive | Invasive |
| Collection of sample | Indirect. Collection of blood, urine, or body fluid | Direct. The tissue is directly collected from the tumor |
| Presence of tumor | No need of visible tumor | Visible tumor is needed |
| Multiple sampling | Multiple sampling at different time intervals is possible | Multiple sampling is not always possible |
| Tumor burden | Tumor burden is directly proportional to size of the primary tumor. | Quantity of CTC/ctDNA is directly proportional to tumor burden |
| Tumor heterogeneity | Not affected by tumor heterogeneity | Affected by tumor heterogeneity |
| Mode of processing | Difficult to process and needs special skill | Easy to process |
| Cost | Very costly | Low cost |

(CTC: circulating tumor cell; ctDNA: circulating tumor DNA)

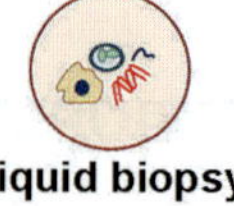

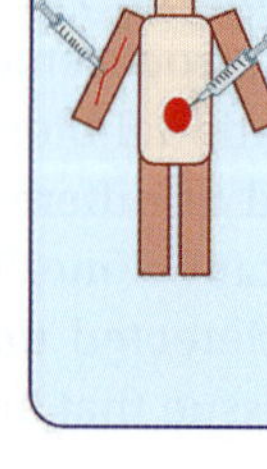

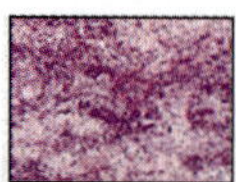



**Fig. 1:** Comparison of liquid biopsy and conventional biopsy.

## LIQUID BIOPSY: CONSTITUENTS

*Sample:* The liquid biopsy samples are taken from (1) Blood, (2) Broncho-alveolar lavage, gastric lavage, urine, effusion fluid, sputum, or any other body fluids.

The components of liquid biopsy are as follows **(Fig. 2)**:

- Circulating tumor cells
- Circulating tumor DNA (ctDNA)
- Cell-free DNA (cfDNA)
- Cell-free RNA (cfRNA)
- Extracellular vesicles (EVs)

*Circulating tumor cells:* In recent years, it has been noted that the initial level and rising number of CTC is related with the evolvement of cancer and metastasis. CTCs are heterogeneous in nature and carry the specific genetic characteristic of the tumor cell. CTC comes to blood circulation mainly from primary tumor tissue. Occasionally it is derived from the metastatic site. CTCs have a very short life span of 1–2 hours and they are quickly cleared by the liver and spleen. CTCs are remarkably less in blood circulation ranging from 1 to 10 CTCs per mL of blood.[4] It is a challenge for the pathologists to isolate CTCs from the circulation. The isolation of CTC is done by many complex technologies. The presence of the cell surface antigen is an important way to recognize the tumor cells and isolation. The cell membrane of CTCs contains epithelial cell adhesion molecule (EpCAM). The antibody against EpCAM binds to the cell membrane of CTCs and so helps to isolate CTCs.

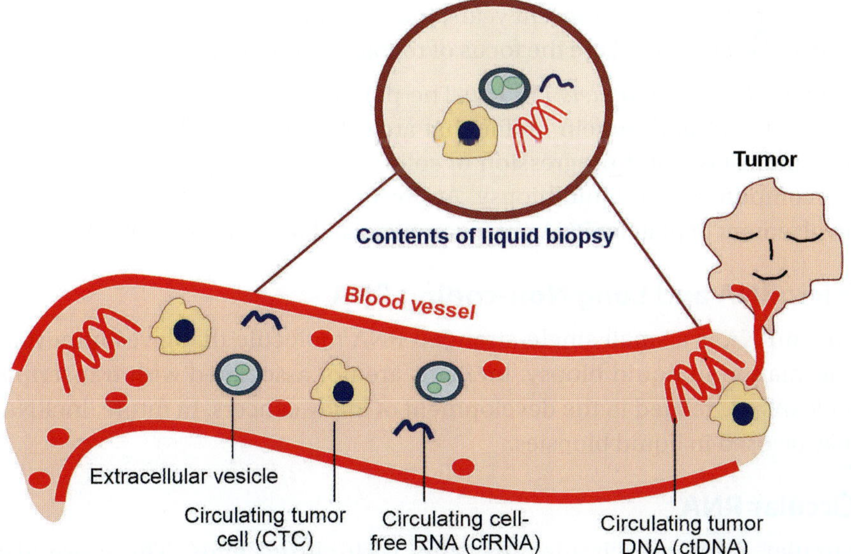


**Fig. 2:** Schematic diagram showing major constituents of the liquid biopsy.

*Circulating tumor DNA:* ctDNA comes to the circulation by cell death (both apoptosis and necrosis) and active secretion by normal and cancer cells. ctDNA is a type of circulating extracellular nucleic acids derived from tumor. The concentration of ctDNA is only <0.01% of total cfDNA and constituted of small DNA fragments (180–200 bp). It has a short half-life of few minutes to couple of hours because it is rapidly cleared from circulation through nucleosomes in the liver (liver macrophages), or by circulating nucleases and in kidney. Circulating tumor DNA (ctDNA) is one of the important components of liquid biopsy. ctDNA may be either double-stranded or single-stranded and carries all the genetic information as that of CTCs. The rising level of ctDNA is an important marker of metastasis. ctDNA shedding in circulation depends on various factors such as tumor site, disease burden, and tissue cell turnover.

*Cell-free DNA:* cfDNA is primarily derived from normal leukocytes and stromal cells, released in the blood circulation. Unlike ctDNA, the cfDNA are derived both from normal and tumor tissue. They also may be nuclear or mitochondrial origin.

*Circulating cfRNA:* cfRNA consists of messenger RNA (mRNA), microRNA (miRNA), long non-coding RNA (lncRNA), small nuclear and nucleolar RNAs (snRNA, snoRNA) and circular RNA (circRNA). This cfRNA is actively released from the tumor tissue and also from apoptotic and necrotic cells.

*Extracellular vesicles:* Extracellular vesicles are membrane covered particles of size around 30–120 nm in diameter. The vesicles have lipid bilayer membrane and carry proteins, DNA, RNA, small non-coding RNAs [microRNA (miRNA)], and lipids. There are three types of EV: (1) exosomes, (2) microvesicles, and (3) apoptotic bodies. In recent years, the exosomes and its products (nucleic acid and metabolites) are the focus of research attraction.

*Tumor-educated platelets (TEPs):* The platelets in cancer patients have a different RNA and protein profile that are called TEPs. TEPs may be related with metastasis and progression of solid tumors. It may be used as one of the components of liquid biopsy. At present, the exact mechanisms of the involvement of platelet RNA are incomplete and further research is needed.

## microRNA and Long Non-coding RNA

The miRNA is a small single-stranded RNA molecule that gives important information in liquid biopsy. lncRNAs are not associated with transcripts. lncRNAs are related in the development of many cancers. In future, lncRNAs may be used in liquid biopsies.

## Circular RNA

Circular RNAs are circular in shape with closed ends. These are also nonprotein-coding transcripts and resist degradation by nuclease enzyme.

CircRNAs work as proto-oncogenes, and are involved in the growth, proliferation, invasion, and metastasis of cancer.

## Circulating Tumor Cell Enrichment: Searching "a Needle in Haystack"

In the advanced cancer, the concentration of CTC in the blood is about 1 CTC per $10^7$ of WBC. So, it is a challenge to find out and collect CTC from this extremely low concentration.[5] CTC enrichment can be done by: (1) on the basis of immunological method, (2) physical properties, and (3) microfluidic immunocapture. **Table 2** highlights the different types of cell enrichment technique.

- *Immunological method:*
  - *Positive selection:* CTCs are usually epithelial cells that are coated with EpCAM. So, antibody against EpCAM is used to identify and subsequently separation of CTC. The magnetic nanoparticles coated with anti-EpCAM antibodies are used **(Fig. 3)**. Subsequently, the

**TABLE 2:** Different types of cell enrichment technique.

| *Category* | *Commercially available techniques* | *Mode of enrichment* | *Capture efficiency (%)* | *Comments* |
|---|---|---|---|---|
| *Immunological* | Cell search, Adna test, magnetic-activated cell sorting (MACS test) | Target antibody against epithelial cell adhesion molecule (EpCAM) is used to separate the cells | 40–90 | • Only EpCAM-positive circulating tumor cells (CTCs) are detected<br>• Cell search system is Food and Drug Administration (FDA) approved |
| *Physical property based Density based* | • OncoQuick<br>• AccuCyte | • Density separation<br>• Buffy coat preparation to separate CTCs | • 25–80<br>• 90 | • Low recovery rate<br>• Multiple samples can be processed |
| *Microfluidic immuno-capture* | • CTC-Chip<br>• HB-Chip geometrically enhanced differential immunocapture (GEDI chip) | The sample flows in an antibody coated channel to capture the CTC | 60–90 | Only EpCAM-positive cells are recovered |

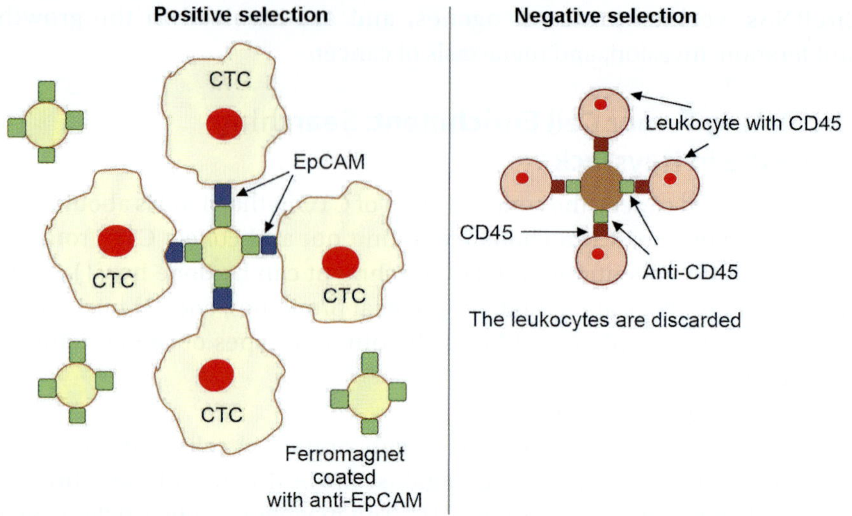


**Fig. 3:** Immunological method of cell enrichment. In positive selection, magnetic nanoparticles coated with anti-epithelial cell adhesion molecule (anti-EpCAM) antibodies are used to capture the tumor cells. In negative selection, the CD45 positive cells are removed from the sample.

magnetic field is applied to isolate those CTC. Cell-search system is based on this principle.

- *Negative selection:* The leukocytes have CD45 antibodies on the surface and so by using anti-CD45 antibody, they can be isolated **(Fig. 3)**.

- *Physical properties:* The CTCs can also be separated on the basis of various physical properties such as large size, deformation of CTCs, density, and surface electrical charges **(Fig. 4)**.
- *Microfluidic-based enrichment:* The sample flows in an antibody-coated (anti-EpCAM) channel to capture the CTC **(Fig. 4)**.

## ANALYSIS OF LIQUID BIOPSY: MOLECULAR TECHNIQUES

The different types of molecular techniques are shown in **Flowchart 1**.

### Genetic Study

*Mutational detection:* The demonstration of the mutation in ctDNA provides valuable information. The following techniques are used to detect the mutations.

### Polymerase Chain Reaction-based Technologies

- *Droplet digital polymerase chain reaction (ddPCR):* It is an extremely sensitive technique which can quantify the target nucleic acid with high precision.[6]

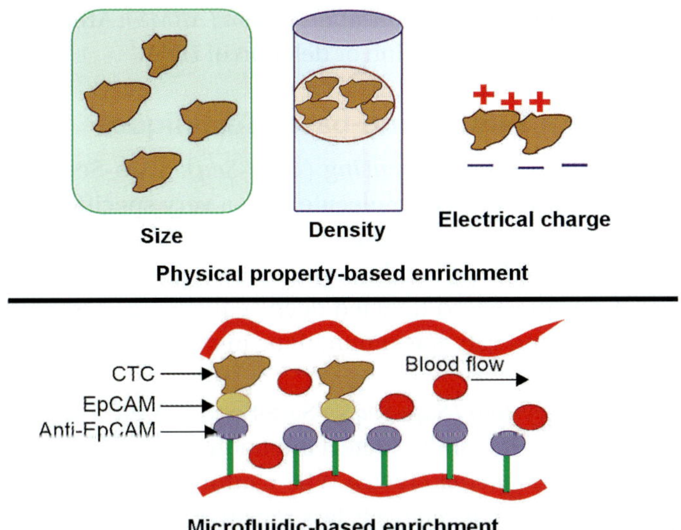


**Fig. 4:** Physical and microfluidic-based technique of cell separation. (CTC: circulating tumor cell; EpCAM: epithelial cell adhesion molecule)

**Flowchart 1:** Different technologies to detect genetic and epigenetic abnormalities in liquid biopsy specimen.

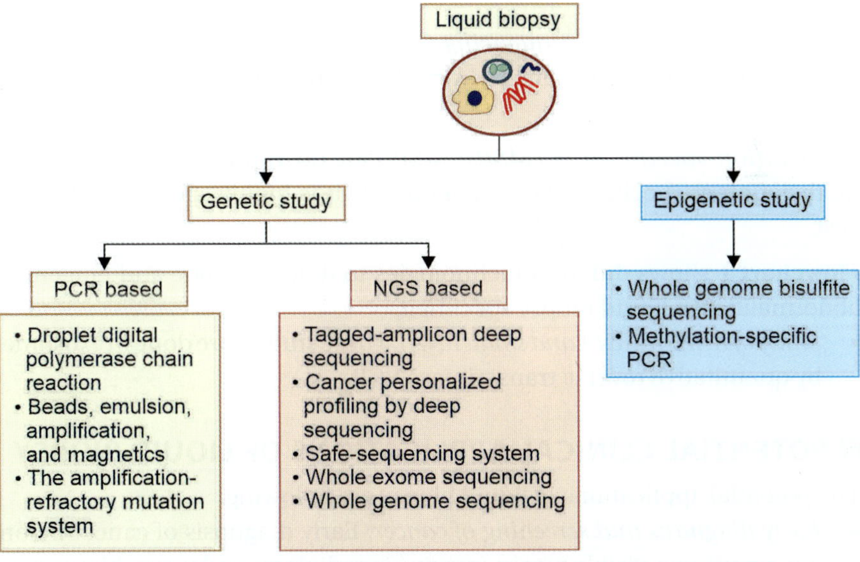


(NSG: next-generation sequencing; PCR: polymerase chain reaction)

- *Beads, emulsion, amplification, and magnetics (BEAMing):* In this technology, the PCR is combined with flow cytometry. BEAMing is also very sensitive and can identify 0.01% mutation.[6]

- *The amplification-refractory mutation system (ARMS)*: ARMS can identify the single base change mutation or deletion of DNA.[7]

## Next-generation Sequencing-based Techniques

- *Tagged-amplicon deep sequencing (TAm-Seq):* TAm-Seq uses unique tag (barcode) to label DNA molecule. It is a very specific and sensitive technique and can low allele frequencies (0.1–2%).[8]
- *Cancer personalized profiling by deep sequencing (CAPP-Seq):* CAPP-Seq is a hybrid-capture-based targeted deep sequencing. It is very powerful NGS technique and can detect mutations in ctDNA with high sensitivity and specificity.[9]
- *Safe-sequencing system (Safe-SeqS):* Safe-SeqS has ultra-high sensitivity and specificity and it is able to detect mutations at <0.1% allele frequency.
- *Whole exome sequencing (WES):* WES captures all the exons (coding) regions of the DNA. It is relatively less sensitive. However, it provides the comprehensive mutation profiling.[10]
- *Whole genome sequencing (WGS):* WGS sequences both coding and noncoding regions of ctDNA. It has low sensitivity in detecting point mutations.

## Epigenetic Study

*Whole-genome bisulfite sequencing (WGBS-Seq):* It is considered as gold standard method for assessing DNA methylation. It gives epigenetic profiling of ctDNA.[11]

*Methylation-specific PCR (MSP):* MSP can do rapid detection of DNA methylation at specific CpG sites of ctDNA. It is highly specific and of low cost.

**Flowchart 1** shows different technologies to detect genetic and epigenetic abnormalities in liquid biopsy specimen.

- *Study of RNA (miRNA and small RNA):* These studies are done in exosomes by quantitative reverse transcriptase PCR.

# POTENTIAL CLINICAL APPLICATIONS OF LIQUID BIOPSY

The potential applications of liquid biopsy are following:

- *Early diagnosis and screening of cancer:* Early diagnosis of cancer before any symptoms, visible tumor, imaging in radiology, and tumor biomarkers is of intense clinical interest. Is it possible that the liquid biopsy can fulfil this expectation? The main challenges in early detection by liquid biopsy are as follows:
    - Low shedding of tumor cells in the circulation and extremely low amount of ctDNA in the early cancer

- Limited cancer-specific mutations
- Demonstration of driver gene mutations in aged individual has added complication.[12]

Early detection of cancer and cancer screening can be done by the following ways:

- *Quantitation of cfDNA:* There was attempt to assess the presence of cancer by quantitating cfDNA/ctDNA in the blood. Numerous studies have shown the raised cfDNA/ctDNA level in the cancer patients compared to normal healthy persons.[13-15] In a meta-analytic study on prostate carcinoma, it was noted that the sensitivity and specificity of quantitative cfDNA is higher than serum prostate-specific antigen (PSA). So, cfDNA can be for prostate cancer screening.[16]

  The sensitivity of cfDNA to detect various cancer varies widely from 50 to 90%. The wide range of variation of sensitivity may be due to the mode of detection techniques and variable cut off value for the diagnosis in different studies. Moreover, cfDNA concentration may also depend on the tumor type, tumor volume, and metastasis.[17] So to determine threshold of the cancer detection needs more studies. The large case–control studies are needed before the clinical application of cancer detection by cfDNA quantitation.
- *Tumor-specific mutation:* The cancer specific DNA mutation has been highlighted by various studies. The detection of those specific mutational changes may be helpful in early diagnosis of cancer or cancer screening **(Table 3)**.[18-23] In addition, epigenetic changes such distinct DNA methylation patterns, DNA hydroxymethylation, DNA fragment length are also related in identification of cancer.[24]
- *Tumor-specific miRNA and s-RNA:* Tumor-specific miRNA and s-RNA are helpful in the detection of carcinomas.[23] Mensah et al.[25] studied miRNA in plasma by microfluidic cards and quantitative real-time PCR for screening of lung carcinoma cases. They suggested miRNA-based liquid biopsy in lung cancer screening. Association of several small RNAs is found with colorectal adenomas and can be used as useful biomarker to detect colorectal adenoma.[24]

Recently, the Food and Drug Administration (FDA) has approved some liquid biopsy tests for the cancer screening, such as the Epi proColon® for colorectal cancer (CRC). Epi proColon® detects methylated *SEPT9* DNA in CRC. The Epi proColon® is a qualitative test and uses real-time PCR. It is recommended in the patients with high risk of CRC and those patients who have not undergone in CRC screening.[26]

The CancerSEEK helps in screening of eight cancers (breast, colon, esophagus, lung, liver, ovary, pancreas, and stomach). It detects the mutation of 16 genes and combines both genetic and protein biomarkers analysis.[27]

**TABLE 3:** Cancer-specific mutation.

| *Tumor* | *Common mutations* | *Early diagnosis and screening* | *Early diagnosis and management* | *References* |
|---|---|---|---|---|
| Lung | EGFR, KRAS, ALK, BRAF, and TP53 | *SHOX2* gene hypermethylation is related to screening of squamous cell carcinoma | • *EGFR T790M mutation in NSCLC:* Resistance to EGFR inhibitor therapy<br>• *Greater expression of Ep-CAM, PIK3CA, AKT2, TWIST* and *ALDH1*: Metastasis and aggressiveness | 19 |
| Breast cancer | PIK3CA, TP53, ESR1, and HER2 (ERBB2) | *PIK3CA* gene mutation: Associated with early diagnosis of breast cancer | *PIK3CA* gene mutation: Resistance to HER2-targeting therapy | 20 |
| Colorectal cancer | APC, KRAS, BRAF, TP53, and PIK3CA | Methylated SEPT9 related with early cancer screening[22] | Mutated *KRAS* genes may escape anti-EGFR therapy[23] | 21 |
| Prostate cancer | AR, TP53, PTEN, and BRCA1/2 | *GSTP1 promoter methylation:* For prostate cancer screening | Androgen receptor L702H and AR-T878A mutations related with acquired drug resistance | 22 |

- *Targeted therapy by assessing specific molecular alterations:* In case of solid tumor, the demonstration of certain mutations indicates targeted chemotherapy. CTC and ctDNA/cfDNA contain all the molecular footprints of the tumor. So instead of going for traditional conventional biopsy, these mutations can be demonstrated by liquid biopsy. FDA has given approval for several tests on ctDNA to detect the actionable mutations. In cases of carcinoma of unknown primary (CUP), the actionable genetic mutation in ctDNA of liquid biopsy has been demonstrated in more than two-thirds of the patients, and so, they can be treated by specific therapy.

  The Food and Drug Administration (FDA) has approved several diagnostic tests on ctDNA such as Cobas EGFR mutation test V2 in non-small cell lung cancer, the therascreen PIK3CA RGQ PCR kit to detect PIK3CA mutation in carcinoma of the breast, and Guardant 360 for the detection of molecular profiling. It is a challenge to decide on chemotherapy protocols in the CUP and many times empirical chemotherapy regimens are given.

  Kato et al.[28] studied ctDNA alteration of the CUP by NGS. They noted that 66% of patients had pathogenic alterations and almost all the patients had actionable alterations.[28] The demonstrations of actionable genetic mutations have also been highlighted in liquid biopsies of esophageal carcinoma, gastric adenocarcinomas gynecological cancers, and non-small cell lung carcinomas. Therefore, liquid biopsy plays a significant role in individualized or precision medicine therapy.[29-32]
- *Monitoring the therapy:* Liquid biopsy plays an important role in monitoring the chemotherapeutic response and also the assessment of drug resistance. The fall of CTC count is directly related with the adequate response of chemotherapy.[33] Variant allele frequency (VAF) indicates ratio of DNA fragments with the specific mutation to the total number of DNA fragments at that locus. The higher pretreatment VAF is related with reduced survival and lower on-treatment VAF means the good chemotherapy response and better survival.[34] Genome instability number (GIN) refers to the degree of genomic instability in a tumor. Continuously reduced level of GIN measured in ctDNA indicates the good response to chemotherapy.[35]
- *Detection of drug resistance:* In colorectal cancer, the clonal evolution of the mutated *RAS* gene is responsible for resistance of anti-EGFR antibody therapy.[36] In breast carcinomas, PIK3CA gene mutation is associated with resistance to HER2-targeting therapy.[20] The loss of function PTEN mutations and ESPR1-activating mutations cause resistance to PI3K-α inhibitor therapy.[37] In non-small cell lung carcinoma cases, EGFR T790M mutation causes resistance to anti-EGFR therapy.[19] The expression of AR-V7 splice variant on the CTCs of metastatic prostate cancer patients strongly predicts the resistance to abiraterone and enzalutamide.

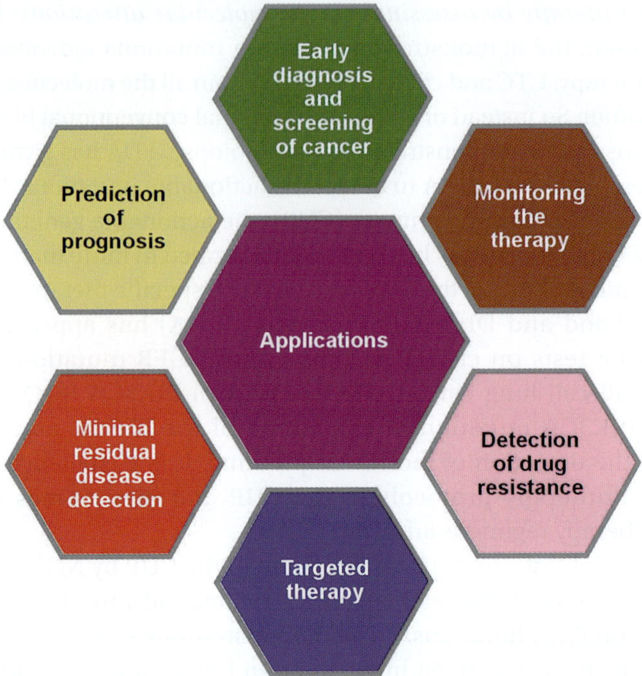


**Fig. 5:** Major applications of liquid biopsy.

- *Identifying MRD:* Liquid biopsy is useful in the detection of MRDs in various carcinomas.[38,39] Real-time monitoring of CTC and cfDNA may be helpful to detect MRD. Interestingly, the molecular relapse is demonstrated many months before the detection by standard radiological imaging or other biomarkers.[40]
- *Prediction of prognosis:* The preoperative and postoperative level of CTC and ctDNA/cfDNA may help in prognostic assessment. The increased number of CTC in the postoperative period indicates poor disease-free survival.[41] In a study with a variety of cancer, the patients with more than 5% *ctDNA* gene alteration had poor prognosis.[42] Certain mutations such as KRAS hotspot mutations or hypermethylation of CDKN2A in colorectal carcinomas have bad prognosis.[43] **Figure 5** highlights the major applications of liquid biopsy.

Circulating tumor DNA detection predicts the response of drugs such as palbociclib and fulvestrant in metastatic breast cancer.[44] ctDNA detection can also predict the response of neoadjuvant chemotherapy and prognosis in patients with early breast cancer. In patients with advanced pancreatic cancer on therapy, decreases of KRAS mutant ctDNA are considered as early tumor response.

## CHALLENGES IN THE IMPLEMENTATION OF LIQUID BIOPSY: ARE WE READY?

Liquid biopsy is a noninvasive technique that has intense impact of cancer diagnosis, treatment, monitoring, and prognostic prediction. In spite of its vast potential, liquid biopsy faces several technological, biological, and clinical challenges **(Table 4)**.

- *Extremely low concentration:* As mentioned repeatedly, the concentration of ctDNA and CTC is extremely low. The concentration of ctDNA may be <0.01% of cfDNA. Therefore, there may be problem in distinguishing real mutation versus background noise.
- *Lack of standardization:* There are considerable variations in the collection of sample, processing, and interpretation. This may be responsible for significant variation of the result, and so it is difficult to compare results across the laboratories.
- *Fallacy in CTC detection:* CTC is usually detected and isolated on the basis of surface EpCAM of the tumor cells. However, many tumor cells may not show surface EpCAM expression.
- *Sensitivity and specificity:* The sensitivity of detecting ctDNA or CTCs on liquid biopsy is low particularly in low tumor burden and early-stage cancers. Thus, the chances of false-negative reporting are high. The presence of ctDNA from benign tumors and other nonmalignant conditions are responsible for false-positive reporting.
- *Tumor heterogeneity:* The liquid biopsy may not fully capture the tumors genetic heterogeneity and thus, it may lead to incomplete profiling and inappropriate treatment planning.

**TABLE 4:** Challenges and solutions of liquid biopsy.

| *Challenges* | *Impact* | *Solution* |
|---|---|---|
| Extremely low concentration of ctDNA and CTC | Reduction of sensitivity | Deep sequencing |
| Lack of standardization | Reproducibility is low | Written strict guidelines |
| Fallacy in CTC detection | Low sensitivity | Multiple epithelial markers |
| Clonal hematopoiesis of indeterminate potential (CHIP) | Misinterpretation as tumor mutations | Parallel sequencing of WBC to filter out CHIP mutations |
| Clinical validation | Slow acceptance | More large prospective real-world study |
| Cost | Reduced accessibility | Cheaper and cost-effective techniques |

(CTC: circulating tumor cell; ctDNA: circulating tumor DNA)

- *Clonal hematopoiesis of indeterminate potential (CHIP):* The presence of driver gene mutations in elderly individuals may be misinterpreted as tumor mutations.[13]
- *Cost and accessibility:* Liquid biopsy is very costly and is inaccessible to many laboratories.
- *Clinical validation:* Many techniques need large-scale prospective validation before its clinical applications.
- *Ethical and psychological concerns:* The application of liquid biopsy in cancer screening is a debatable issue. As no visible tumor is detected, so, the management may be difficult to decide. Informed consent explaining the implications of the liquid biopsy and its limitations should be explained to the patient and also crucial for ethical practice.

## CONCLUSION

In conclusion, the liquid biopsy is a cutting-edge technology that has vast potential. This is a noninvasive technique, and the samples are easy to collect independent of the visible tumor. The potential clinical applications of liquid biopsy are the cancer screening, monitoring therapy, precision medicine for individual patients, the detection of MRDs, prognosis prediction. The liquid biopsy provides the sequential information of tumor life and provides new insight of the disease. Currently, there is a great need of strict guidelines in the liquid biopsy. The guidelines are helpful mainly for the maintenance of the standard and interpretation of its results, such as European Society for Medical Oncology (ESMO) recommendations[45] and National Comprehensive Cancer Network (NCCN) guidelines.[46] In spite of huge potential, it is not implemented in the laboratories because of technical complexity, lack of standardization, prospective validation, and high cost. We expect that the rapid progression of technology will make the liquid biopsy cheap and accessible to the laboratories.

## REFERENCES

1. Ghosh RK, Pandey T, Dey P. Liquid biopsy: A new avenue in pathology. Cytopathology. 2019;30(2):138-43.
2. Dey P. Liquid biopsy: Research Laboratory to Clinical applications. In: Dey P (Ed). Recent advances in Pathology-1. New Delhi; Jaypee Brothers medical Publishers Pvt Ltd. 2024.
3. https://www.cancer.gov/publications/dictionaries/cancer-terms/def/liquid-biopsy
4. Yang YP, Giret TM, Cote RJ. Circulating Tumor Cells from Enumeration to Analysis: Current Challenges and Future Opportunities. Cancers (Basel). 2021;13(11):2723.
5. Alix-Panabières C, Pantel K. Challenges in circulating tumour cell research. Nat Rev Cancer. 2014;14(9):623-31.

6. Zhang BO, Xu CW, Shao Y, Wang HT, Wu YF, Song YY, et al. Comparison of droplet digital PCR and conventional quantitative PCR for measuring *EGFR* gene mutation. Exp Ther Med. 2015;9(4):1383-8.
7. Little S. Amplification-refractory mutation system (ARMS) analysis of point mutations. Curr Protoc Hum Genet. 2001;Chapter 9:Unit 9.8.
8. Feng YJ, Liu QF, Chen MY, Liang D, Zhang P. Parallel tagged amplicon sequencing of relatively long PCR products using the Illumina HiSeq platform and transcriptome assembly. Mol Ecol Resour. 2016;16(1):91-102.
9. Newman AM, Lovejoy AF, Klass DM, Kurtz DM, Chabon JJ, Scherer F, et al. Integrated digital error suppression for improved detection of circulating tumor DNA. Nat Biotechnol. 2016;34(5):547-55.
10. Imperial R, Nazer M, Ahmed Z, Kam AE, Pluard TJ, Bahaj W, et al. Matched Whole-Genome Sequencing (WGS) and Whole-Exome Sequencing (WES) of Tumor Tissue with Circulating Tumor DNA (ctDNA) Analysis: Complementary Modalities in Clinical Practice. Cancers (Basel). 2019;11(9):1399.
11. Lee EJ, Luo J, Wilson JM, Shi H. Analyzing the cancer methylome through targeted bisulfite sequencing. Cancer Lett. 2013;340(2):171-8.
12. Chan HT, Nagayama S, Chin YM, Otaki M, Hayashi R, Kiyotani K, et al. Clinical significance of clonal hematopoiesis in the interpretation of blood liquid biopsy. Mol Oncol. 2020;14:1719-30.
13. Tang Z, Li L, Shen L, Shen X, Ju S, Cong H. Diagnostic Value of Serum Concentration and Integrity of Circulating Cell-Free DNA in Breast Cancer: A Comparative Study with CEA and CA15-3. Lab Med. 2018;49(4):323-8.
14. Agah S, Akbari A, Talebi A, Masoudi M, Sarveazad A, Mirzaei A, et al. Quantification of Plasma Cell-Free Circulating DNA at Different Stages of Colorectal Cancer. Cancer Invest. 2017;35(10):625-32.
15. Chen H, Sun LY, Zheng HQ, Zhang QF, Jin XM. Total serum DNA and DNA integrity: diagnostic value in patients with hepatitis B virus-related hepatocellular carcinoma. Pathology. 2012;44(4):318-24.
16. Yin C, Luo C, Hu W, Ding X, Yuan C, Wang F. Quantitative and Qualitative Analysis of Circulating Cell-Free DNA Can Be Used as an Adjuvant Tool for Prostate Cancer Screening: A Meta-Analysis. Dis Markers. 2016;2016:3825819.
17. Bronkhorst AJ, Ungerer V, Holdenrieder S. The emerging role of cell-free DNA as a molecular marker for cancer management. Biomol Detect Quantif. 2019;17:100087.
18. Pessoa LS, Heringer M, Ferrer VP. ctDNA as a cancer biomarker: A broad overview. Crit Rev Oncol Hematol. 2020;155:103109.
19. Revelo AE, Martin A, Velasquez R, Kulandaisamy PC, Bustamante J, Keshishyan S, et al. Liquid biopsy for lung cancers: an update on recent developments. Ann Transl Med. 2019;7(15):349.
20. Alimirzaie S, Bagherzadeh M, Akbari MR. Liquid biopsy in breast cancer: A comprehensive review. Clin Genet. 2019;95(6):643-60.
21. Ding Y, Li W, Wang K, Xu C, Hao M, Ding L. Perspectives of the Application of Liquid Biopsy in Colorectal Cancer. Biomed Res Int. 2020;2020:6843180.
22. Riaz IB, Wang L, Kohli M. Liquid biopsy approach in the management of prostate cancer. Transl Res. 2018;201:60-70.
23. Hoadley KA, Yau C, Hinoue T, Wolf DM, Lazar AJ, Drill E, et al. Cancer Genome Atlas Network; Stuart JM, Benz CC, Laird PW. Cell-of-Origin Patterns Dominate

the Molecular Classification of 10,000 Tumors from 33 Types of Cancer. Cell. 2018 Apr 5;173(2):291-304.e6.

24. Roberts BS, Hardigan AA, Moore DE, Ramaker RC, Jones AL, Fitz-Gerald MB, et al. Discovery and Validation of Circulating Biomarkers of Colorectal Adenoma by High-Depth Small RNA Sequencing. Clin Cancer Res. 2018;24(9):2092-9.
25. Mensah M, Borzi C, Verri C, Suatoni P, Conte D, Pastorino U, et al. MicroRNA Based Liquid Biopsy: The Experience of the Plasma miRNA Signature Classifier (MSC) for Lung Cancer Screening. J Vis Exp. 2017;(128):56326.
26. Shirley M. Epi proColon® for Colorectal Cancer Screening: A Profile of Its Use in the USA. Mol Diagn Ther. 2020;24(4):497-503.
27. Killock D. Diagnosis: CancerSEEK and destroy - a blood test for early cancer detection. Nat Rev Clin Oncol. 2018;15(3):133.
28. Kato S, Weipert C, Gumas S, Okamura R, Lee S, Sicklick JK, et al. Therapeutic actionability of circulating cell-free DNA alterations in carcinoma of unknown primary. JCO Precis Oncol. 2021;5:PO.21.00011.
29. Kato S, Okamura R, Baumgartner JM, Patel H, Leichman L, Kelly K, et al. Analysis of Circulating Tumor DNA and Clinical Correlates in Patients with Esophageal, Gastroesophageal Junction, and Gastric Adenocarcinoma. Clin Cancer Res. 2018;24(24):6248-56.
30. Charo LM, Eskander RN, Okamura R, Patel SP, Nikanjam M, Lanman RB, et al. Clinical implications of plasma circulating tumor DNA in gynecologic cancer patients. Mol Oncol. 2021;15(1):67-79.
31. Shatsky R, Parker BA, Bui NQ, Helsten T, Schwab RB, Boles SG, et al. Next-Generation Sequencing of Tissue and Circulating Tumor DNA: The UC San Diego Moores Center for Personalized Cancer Therapy Experience with Breast Malignancies. Mol Cancer Ther. 2019;18(5):1001-11.
32. Schwaederlé MC, Patel SP, Husain H, Ikeda M, Lanman RB, Banks KC, et al. Utility of Genomic Assessment of Blood-Derived Circulating Tumor DNA (ctDNA) in Patients with Advanced Lung Adenocarcinoma. Clin Cancer Res. 2017;23(17):5101-11.
33. Li Y, Wu S, Bai F. Molecular characterization of circulating tumor cells-from bench to bedside. Semin Cell Dev Biol. 2018;75:88-97.
34. Zhang Q, Luo J, Wu S, Si H, Gao C, Xu W, et al. Prognostic and Predictive Impact of Circulating Tumor DNA in Patients with Advanced Cancers Treated with Immune Checkpoint Blockade. Cancer Discov. 2020;10(12):1842-53.
35. Jensen TJ, Goodman AM, Kato S, Ellison CK, Daniels GA, Kim L, et al. Genome-Wide Sequencing of Cell-Free DNA Identifies Copy-Number Alterations That Can Be Used for Monitoring Response to Immunotherapy in Cancer Patients. Mol Cancer Ther. 2019;18(2):448-58.
36. Siravegna G, Mussolin B, Buscarino M, Corti G, Cassingena A, Crisafulli G, et al. Clonal evolution and resistance to EGFR blockade in the blood of colorectal cancer patients. Nat Med. 2015;21(7):795-801. Erratum in: Nat Med. 2015;21(7). Erratum in: Nat Med. 2015;21(7):827.
37. Razavi P, Dickler MN, Shah PD, Toy W, Brown DN, Won HH, et al. Alterations in PTEN and ESR1 promote clinical resistance to alpelisib plus aromatase inhibitors. Nat Cancer. 2020;1(4):382-93.
38. Ignatiadis M, Reinholz M. Minimal residual disease and circulating tumor cells in breast cancer.Breast Cancer Res. 2011;13(5):222.

39. Kasimir-Bauer S. Circulating tumor cells as markers for cancer risk assessment and treatment monitoring. Mol Diagn Ther. 2009;13(4):209-15.
40. Chaudhuri AA, Chabon JJ, Lovejoy AF, Newman AM, Stehr H, Azad TD, et al. Early detection of molecular residual disease in localized lung cancer by circulating tumor DNA profiling. Cancer Discov 2017;7:1394-403.
41. Cristofanilli M, Budd GT, Ellis MJ, Stopeck A, Matera J, Miller MC, et al. Circulating tumor cells, disease progression, and survival in metastatic breast cancer. N Engl J Med. 2004;351(8):781-91.
42. Schwaederle M, Husain H, Fanta PT, Piccioni DE, Kesari S, Schwab RB, et al. Use of Liquid Biopsies in Clinical Oncology: Pilot Experience in 168 Patients. Clin Cancer Res. 2016;22(22):5497-505.
43. Lecomte T, Berger A, Zinzindohoue F, Micard S, Landi B, Blons H, et al. Detection of free-circulating tumor associated DNA in plasma of colorectal cancer patients and its association with prognosis. Int J Cancer. 2002;100:542-8.
44. Darrigues L, Pierga JY, Bernard-Tessier A, Bièche I, Silveira AB, Michel M, et al. Circulating tumor DNA as a dynamic biomarker of response to palbociclib and fulvestrant in metastatic breast cancer patients. Breast Cancer Res. 2021;23(1):31.
45. Pascual J, Attard G, Bidard FC, Curigliano G, De Mattos-Arruda L, Diehn M, et al. ESMO recommendations on the use of circulating tumour DNA assays for patients with cancer: a report from the ESMO Precision Medicine Working Group. Ann Oncol. 2022;33(8):750-68.
46. https://www.nccn.org/professionals/physician_gls/pdf/nscl.pdf

CHAPTER 8

# Radiomics and Radiogenomics for Precision Medicine

*Ishan Kumar, Ashish Verma, Pramod K Singh, Ritu Ojha*

## INTRODUCTION

Precision medicine identifies and accepts the fact that each individual has a unique biological makeup. Hence, the apparently similar appearing natural history of same disease in two different individuals may be intricately different. The more logical way should therefore be aiming at treating individuals than just treating diseases. The former approach has been presumably implicated as the cause of most treatment failures and disease relapses. These mandates understanding the complex interaction between the genetic, molecular, and environmental aspects of an individual's disease.[1] Objective validation of these nuances may best be achieved by a comparison of prospective and retrospective investigations and laboratory parameters, medical imaging being in the forefront and most convincing hence one should understand the verbatim related to this science **(Table 1)**.

**TABLE 1:** Important terminology related to precision medicine.

| | |
|---|---|
| Precision medicine (PM) | • Utilizing a patient's genetic profile to guide prevention, diagnosis, and treatment<br>• Focuses on classifying patients into subpopulations<br>• Also called as precision medicine |
| Pharmacogenomics | Tells about how a person's genes affect their response to drugs |
| Genomic medicine | The use of genetic information to improve health outcomes and guide care decisions |
| Stratified medicine | Identifies subgroups of patients: (1) Those who respond to a specific drug, (2) those at risk of side effects from a certain treatment |
| Theranostics | • Combines therapeutic and diagnostic tools into a single approach<br>• To tailor treatment to an individual based on diagnostic information |
| Radiogenomics | Studies the relationship between imaging features and genetic/molecular traits |

*Contd...*

*Contd...*

| | |
|---|---|
| Companion diagnostics | An in vitro diagnostic or imaging tool essential for the safe/effective use of a specific therapeutic product |
| Radiomics | • High-throughput extraction of a large number of quantitative features from medical images (CT/MRI/ ultrasound/radiographs)<br>• Uses machine learning and artificial intelligence to analyze large datasets |

(CT: computed tomography; MRI: magnetic resonance imaging)

Radiomics refers to the process of extracting large amounts of quantitative features from medical images using data-characterization algorithms, hence, understanding disease biology in a noninvasive way than just reading the altered anatomy. It uses advanced algorithms and artificial intelligence (AI) to analyze image features such as shape, texture, and intensity which may extrapolate to structural, functional, metabolic, and even molecular aspects of disease.[2,3] These features hidden in the numbers that constitute the computer algorithm used for generation of medical images can reveal important insights into tumor behavior beyond what radiologists can see. This in turn may assist in early diagnosis, classification, staging, prognosis, evaluate response to therapy, and monitor for recurrence with remarkable precision. In simpler terms, it turns images into data that computers can analyze to detect patterns linked to a disease's behavior or its underlying biology.[1-3] This imaging data when correlated with gene expression profiles or molecular markers, is known as radiogenomics.

**How does radiomics work?**

Radiomics studies typically follow a few key steps **(Fig. 1)**:

- *Image acquisition:* High-quality scans are collected using standard imaging protocols. Clinical, genetic, and laboratory data may also be included.
- *Image segmentation:* Radiologists or software outline the area of interest—for example, the tumor—so that only the relevant part of the image is analyzed.
- *Feature extraction and selection:* Dozens or even hundreds of features are pulled from the images. Special statistical tools are used to pick the most important ones.
- *Model building and validation:* Machine learning models—like random forests or neural networks—are trained to look for patterns. These models used should be validated before it is used for scientific and clinical purposes.

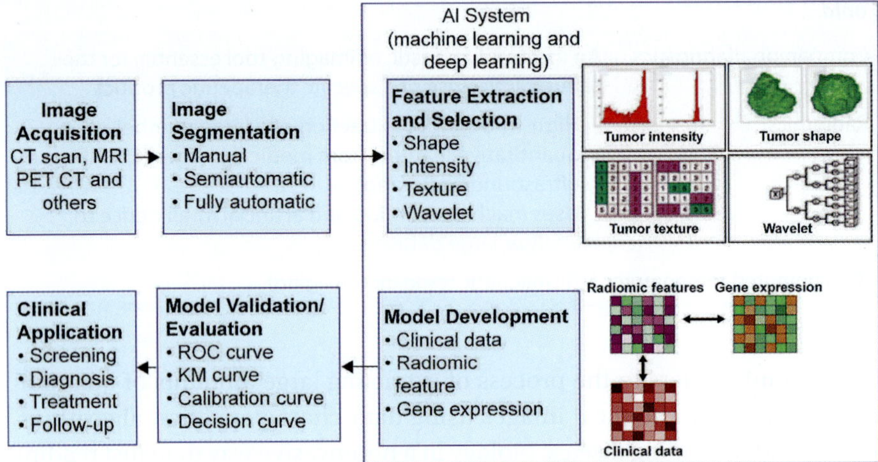


**Fig. 1:** Overview of radiomics workflow. (AI: artificial intelligence; KM: Kaplan-Meier; ROC: receiver-operating characteristic)

## INTRODUCTION TO RADIOMIC FEATURE CATEGORIES

Radiomics papers often include technical terms that can feel overwhelming. These terms simply describe different ways of measuring what a tumor looks like on imaging. Broadly, radiomic features are grouped into categories **(Table 2)**:

- *Shape based* → How the tumor looks (round, irregular, big, and small)?
- *First order* → How bright or dark the pixels are (basic intensity statistics)?
- *Second order (texture)* → How pixels are arranged in relation to each other (smooth vs. patchy vs. heterogeneous)?
- *Higher order* → patterns revealed after applying filters or mathematical methods.
- *Advanced/integrated* → combinations with clinical or genetic data to predict outcomes.

## APPLICATION OF RADIOMICS IN CANCER

In radiomics, understanding tumor biology is also feasible as it allows the extraction of quantitative information of the tumor based on spatial and temporal heterogeneity of the acquired images. This information obtained should be further correlated with the tumor's phenotype which may either reflect genomic and molecular traits/signature or outcomes. Similarly, texture features may also be used in predicting various oncogenic processes as tumor proliferation, angiogenesis, hypoxia, and tumor invasion. Radiomics also provides diagnostics and prognostic imaging biomarkers in various solid tumors. These imaging biomarkers are used to differentiate healthy, benign, and malignant tissue. The other important application of radiomics is the

**TABLE 2:** Categories of radiomic features.

| *Category* | *Key terms* | *Explanation* |
|---|---|---|
| Morphological (shape-based) | • Volume—size of the lesion<br>• Surface area—outer boundary<br>• Compactness—how tightly packed the shape is<br>• Sphericity—how close to a sphere | Shape features describe the geometry of a tumor. For example, an irregular, spiculated mass is often more aggressive than a smooth, round one |
| First order (intensity/ histogram) | • Mean, max, min—average and extreme voxel intensities<br>• Percentiles, e.g., 10th or 90th brightness level<br>• Skewness—whether intensity distribution is lopsided.<br>• Kurtosis—"peakedness" of the distribution<br>• Entropy—randomness/complexity of signal<br>• Uniformity—similarity of intensities | • These features summarize the brightness distribution inside the tumor (like reading a histogram)<br>• High entropy = more heterogeneity, often seen in malignant tumors. High kurtosis = sharp peaks, linked with certain textures |
| Second order (texture) | • Gray-level co-occurrence matrix (GLCM)—how often pairs of pixels with specific intensities occur together<br>• Run-length matrix (RLM)—how many consecutive voxels share the same intensity<br>• Gray-level size zone matrix (GLSZM)—size of uniform-intensity regions | Texture features capture the spatial arrangement of voxels. They tell us if tissue is coarse, smooth, patchy, or heterogeneous. Example: a tumor with high GLCM entropy is more disorganized inside |
| Higher order (filtered/ transformed) | • Wavelet transform—breaks the image into low- and high-frequency components (like separating outlines from fine detail)<br>• Laplacian of Gaussian (LoG)—highlights edges and spots<br>• Fractal analysis—measures repeating complex patterns<br>• Minkowski functionals—describe structure/shape in 3D | These features enhance hidden patterns not visible to the naked eye. Think of them as mathematical "filters" that reveal subtle textures or heterogeneity |

disease monitoring and prediction of treatment response. Thus, it is used as precision medicine based on specific biomarkers for particular cancer and selecting the best treatment option. The radiomics biomarkers may also predict the high risk of recurrence of tumor, suggesting intense post-treatment surveillance **(Fig. 2)**. The fusion of genomic molecular data with imaging data reflecting quantitative disease phenotypes and analysis to establish the links

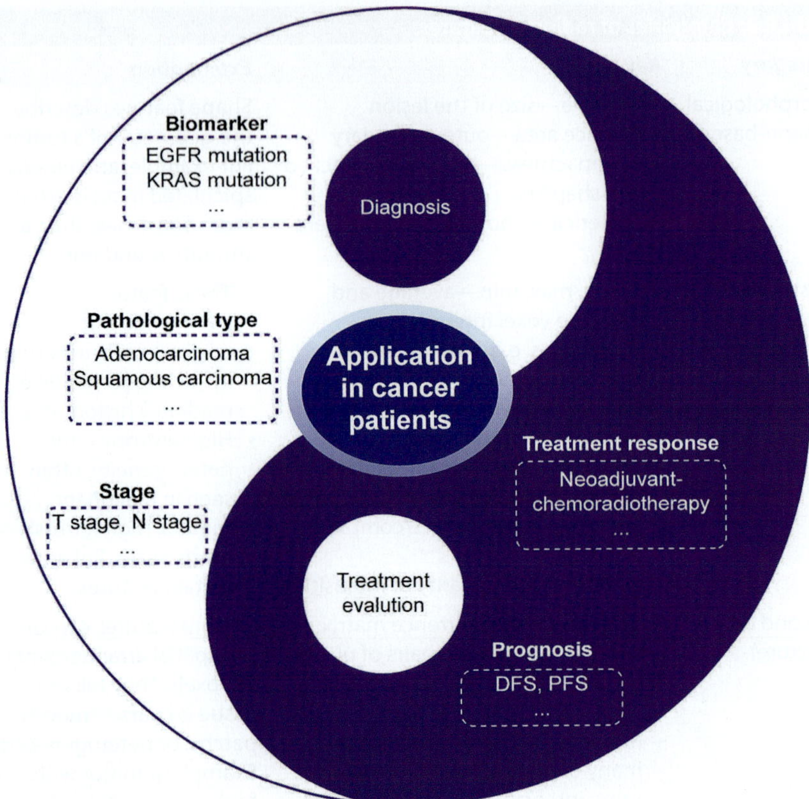


**Fig. 2:** Application of radiomics and radiogenomics in cancer patients. (DFS: disease-free survival; EGFR: epidermal growth factor receptor; KRAS: Kirsten rat sarcoma viral oncogene; PFS: progression-free survival)

between imaging features and genomics which give insight to the genetic background of the disease **(Fig. 3)**. Recent studies have shown the potential of radiomics in evaluating the genomic feature and tumor subtype, thus, it may improve or surpass the present diagnostic methods. Radiomics has also demonstrated its ability in predicting the prognosis of various cancers.

## APPLICATIONS IN BREAST CANCER

Breast cancer has been recognized to be a collection of genetically distinct subtypes, each with its own biological behavior and response to therapy. Subtypes designated by histopathology and immunohistochemistry, viz., luminal A, luminal B, are human epidermal growth factor receptor 2 (HER2)-enriched, and basal or triple-negative, are typically determined by the presence or absence of estrogen receptor (ER), progesterone receptor (PR), and HER2 status. Tissue biopsy samples do not give a global overview of the tumor, especially in metastatic or multifocal disease. The use of dynamic

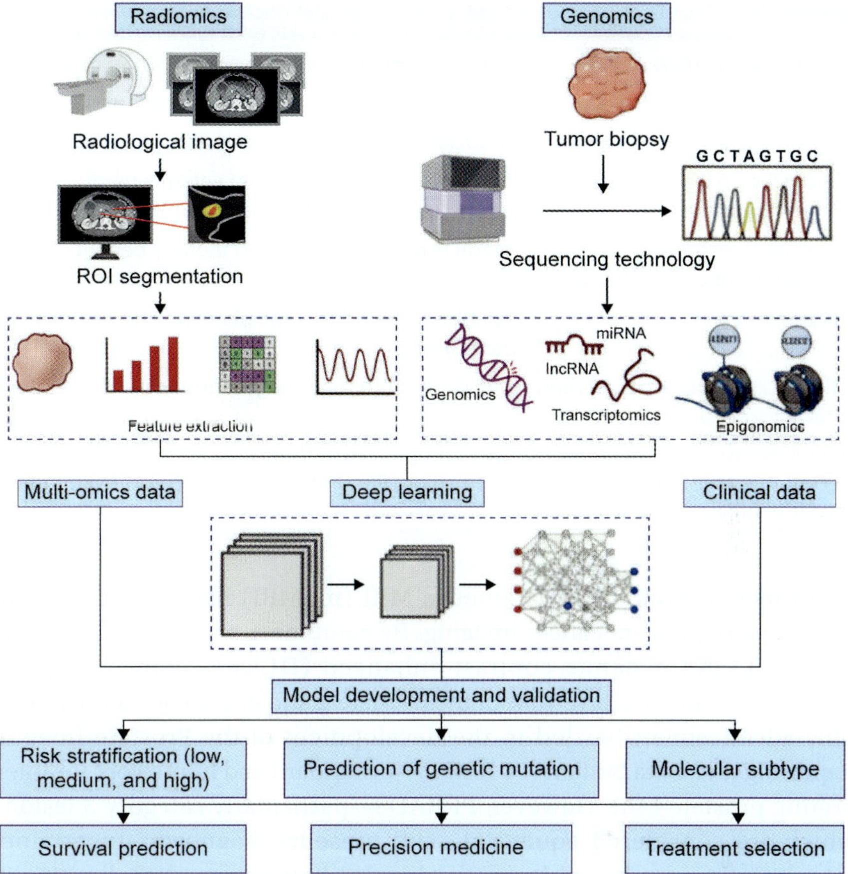


**Fig. 3:** Radiogenomics: Schematic representation showing integration of genetic molecular data with imaging features.

contrast-enhanced magnetic resonance imaging (DCE-MRI), can give a global picture of tumor microstructural heterogeneity, hence acknowledging the possibility of consequential anomalous treatment response is a good example of the application of radiogenomics.[4-6] HER2-overexpressed cancers respond to drugs such as trastuzumab and pertuzumab; a feature which may be detected by DCE-MRI and hence guide the treatment.[5,6] Many such examples exist in relation to breast cancers **(Table 3)**.

## APPLICATIONS IN PROSTATE CANCER

Prostate cancer is one of the most commonly diagnosed malignancies in men, and its global burden continues to rise with aging populations and improved screening. Clinically, it presents a significant challenge due to its wide spectrum of behavior, ranging from indolent tumors that may never cause harm to highly aggressive forms requiring immediate intervention.

**TABLE 3:** Clinical applications of the radiomics and radiogenomics in breast cancer.

| *Clinical application* | *Role of radiomics* |
|---|---|
| Molecular subtype prediction | Differentiates ER, PR, HER2 status and tumor grade |
| Triple-negative breast cancer | Associated with aggressive phenotype (TNBC) |
| Luminal vs. basal subtype differentiation | *Luminal B:* High background enhancement<br>*Basal:* Necrosis and vascular variability |
| Treatment response (neoadjuvant chemotherapy) | Predicts recurrence risk and therapy benefit |
| Radiogenomics | Enables targeted therapy planning and response assessment |
| High-risk population screening (BRCA carriers) | MRI superior to mammography in early detection |

(BRCA: breast cancer gene; ER: estrogen receptor; HER2: human epidermal growth factor receptor 2; MRI: magnetic resonance imaging; PR: progesterone receptor; TNBC: triple-negative breast cancer)

In recent years, multiparametric MRI (mpMRI) has transformed the landscape of prostate cancer imaging. By combining anatomical, diffusion-weighted, and dynamic contrast-enhanced (DCE) sequences, mpMRI provides a comprehensive view of the prostate gland and the lesions within it. This advancement has led to the development of the Prostate Imaging Reporting and Data System (PI-RADS)—a standardized framework for interpreting prostate MRI. However, PI-RADS—particularly category 3 lesions, which are considered equivocal—still presents diagnostic uncertainty. Interpretation can be subjective and varies between readers, limiting its consistency and precision. This is where radiomics has emerged as a powerful complement to conventional MRI interpretation. Radiomics enables the extraction of large volumes of quantitative data from mpMRI images—features related to tumor texture, intensity, shape, and heterogeneity—that may be invisible to the human eye but rich in diagnostic value.[7,8]

A recent study compared two radiomic models for prostate cancer detection: a standard model based on T2-weighted and apparent diffusion coefficient (ADC) maps, and an advanced model that incorporated diffusion kurtosis imaging (DKI) and quantitative DCE parameters.

- Interestingly, although all models performed well the simpler model using just T2 and ADC features actually outperformed the more complex one.
- 3D lesion segmentation yielded greater diagnostic accuracy than 2D analysis, emphasizing the importance of capturing the full spatial complexity of tumors. This underscores a key principle: effective radiomic models do not necessarily require complex inputs, but rather thoughtful feature selection and robust analytical design.

Another practical application lies in resolving the ambiguity of PI-RADS 3 lesions, which often leave both radiologists and urologists uncertain about the need for biopsy. Radiomic models applied to mpMRI data have demonstrated the ability to predict which of these lesions are more likely to harbor clinically significant cancer (Gleason score ≥6). In a study analyzing PI-RADS 3 and upgraded PI-RADS 4 lesions, radiomic features—particularly those derived from T2-weighted and ADC images—were able to classify malignancy with high accuracy. The models achieved area under the curves (AUCs) ranging from 80 to 89%, outperforming the diagnostic performance of PI-RADS alone.

Radiomics in prostate cancer also has potential beyond diagnosis. Advanced MRI techniques like DKI offer insights into tissue microstructural complexity, while quantitative DCE parameters can reflect vascular properties such as perfusion and permeability, both of which are indicators of tumor aggressiveness. Although still in early stages, radiogenomic studies are exploring correlations between imaging features and underlying genetic alterations in prostate cancer. This could open the door to imaging-driven predictions of molecular behavior, potentially guiding not just whether to treat, but how.

## APPLICATIONS IN BRAIN TUMOR

The field of neuro-oncology has seen significant advances in recent years, particularly with the integration of molecular biology and imaging. Next-generation sequencing has revolutionized our understanding of the genetic and molecular underpinnings of primary brain tumors.[9-11] Building on this, researchers are now aiming to translate these molecular insights into imaging-based tools, allowing for noninvasive classification of tumors. Glioblastoma multiforme (GBM), one of the most aggressive brain tumors, is divided into two main categories: (1) isocitrate dehydrogenase (IDH)-wild-type and (2) IDH-mutant. This distinction has significant prognostic value—patients with IDH1-mutant GBMs tend to have better outcomes than those with wild-type tumors. This molecular difference can be captured noninvasively through magnetic resonance spectroscopy (MRS), which can detect a specific metabolite, D-2-hydroxyglutarate (D-2HG), which is uniquely produced by IDH1/2-mutant gliomas **(Table 4)**.

Medulloblastomas, the most common malignant brain tumors in children, are now classified into four molecular subtypes: (1) sonic hedgehog (SHH), (2) Wingless pathway (WNT), (3) group 3, and (4) group 4. These subgroups differ in terms of prognosis and therapeutic targets. MRS again plays a role here—SHH medulloblastomas typically show high choline and lipid levels with low taurine, while group 3 and 4 tumors are associated with elevated taurine and reduced lipid/creatine. This distinction can influence

**TABLE 4:** Clinical applications of radiomics in brain tumors.

| *Application* | *Radiomic features* | *Key findings* |
|---|---|---|
| IDH1/2 mutation detection | D-2HG metabolite on MRS | Distinguishes IDH-mutant from wild-type GBM; prognostic and predictive marker |
| IDH1 mutation prediction on MRI | Tumor size, cysts, enhancement, and satellite lesions | Routine MRI findings predict IDH1 mutation with 97.5% accuracy |
| Aggressiveness assessment | Proliferation-to-invasion ratio (ρ/D) from diffusion MRI | Lower ρ/D in IDH-mutant gliomas; more diffuse but less aggressive |
| Molecular-genetic associations | Necrosis/enhancement ratio | Linked with: *KLK3* and *RUNX3* genes |
| | Subventricular-zone involvement | *RAP2A* and *TYMS* genes |
| | Vasogenic edema | FOXP1 and PIK3IP1 expression |
| Prognosis stratification | Volume class, hemorrhage, and T1/FLAIR-envelope ratio | • MRI-based signatures stratify<br>• GBM into prognostic subgroups |
| Invasion gene signature prediction | FLAIR signal intensity | Classifies GBM based on gene signatures related to cell migration and invasion |
| Tumor metabolism imaging | PET tracer 11C-DASA-23 uptake | Targets pyruvate kinase M2; selectively accumulates in GBM, mapping metabolic activity |

(11C-DASA-23: carbon-11 labeled DASA-23 (pyruvate kinase M2 ligand); D-2HG: D-2-hydroxyglutarate; FLAIR: fluid-attenuated inversion recovery; FOXP1: Forkhead box protein P1; GBM: glioblastoma multiforme; IDH: isocitrate dehydrogenase; KLK3: kallikrein-related peptidase 3; MRI: magnetic resonance imaging; MRS: magnetic resonance spectroscopy; PET: positron emission tomography; PIK3IP1: phosphoinositide-3-kinase interacting protein 1; RUNX3: runt-related transcription factor 3;TYMS: thymidylate synthase)

therapy selection. For instance, the drug vismodegib, which inhibits the SHH pathway, has been shown to be effective only in SHH-subtype tumors, making early and accurate molecular classification critically important.

## LUNG CANCER AND OTHER PULMONARY DISEASES

Lung cancer remains the leading cause of cancer-related deaths in the United States and the second most commonly diagnosed malignancy in both men and women. Prognosis is closely linked to tumor stage. Unfortunately, over 75% of lung cancers are diagnosed at an advanced stage, underscoring the critical need for early detection, which significantly improves the potential for curative treatment.

**TABLE 5:** Current applications of radiomics in lung cancer and other pulmonary diseases.

| *Clinical application* | *Results* |
|---|---|
| Pulmonary nodule characterization | Sensitivity up to 88% in distinguishing adenocarcinoma from granuloma; noncontrast CT often superior to contrast (due to reduced confounding from vascular structures) |
| Prognosis in NSCLC | Strong correlation with survival; texture features predict poor response to chemoradiotherapy |
| Quantification of diffuse lung disease | Correlates with lung function and fibrosis severity; aids preoperative evaluation |
| Prediction of nodal metastasis | Radiomics of the primary tumor helps predict lymph node involvement when nodes are inconspicuous. |
| Radiogenomics (e.g., EGFR, KRAS, and ALK) | Associations between imaging patterns and gene expression/metagenes; potential for noninvasive genotyping |

(ALK: anaplastic lymphoma kinase; CT: computed tomography; EGFR: epidermal growth factor receptor; KRAS: Kirsten rat sarcoma viral oncogene; NSCLC: nonsmall cell lung cancer)

Radiomics is increasingly being integrated into thoracic oncology, offering noninvasive, quantitative imaging biomarkers that aid in the evaluation of pulmonary nodules, tumor characterization, treatment stratification, and even the exploration of molecular signatures. Given the lung's complex anatomical and functional environment, radiomics provides a way to decode imaging beyond morphology, capturing intratumoral heterogeneity, microarchitecture, and pathophysiologic changes that are otherwise imperceptible on routine computed tomography (CT) or positron emission tomography (PET) imaging.[12-14] Radiomics has demonstrated clinical utility across various domains **(Table 5)**.

## GENITOURINARY MALIGNANCIES

The role of imaging in renal cell carcinoma (RCC) has evolved beyond just serving as a roadmap for surgery. Preliminary radiogenomic studies of clear cell RCC indicate that imaging features may correlate with the presence of certain characteristic genetic alterations.[15,16] Also, radiomics has shown promising results in gynecological tumors such as cervical cancers and ovarian masses **(Table 6)**.[17-19]

## LIVER MASSES

In terms of clinical applications, several studies have shown the potential of radiomics in liver tumor characterization and treatment planning **(Table 7)**.[19-24]

**TABLE 6:** Application of radiogenomics in renal and other gynecological tumors.

| *Clinical application* | *Key findings* |
|---|---|
| VHL mutation in clear cell RCC | Well-defined margins and nodular enhancement are associated with VHL mutations |
| BAP1/KDM5C mutation in RCC | BAP1/KDM5C mutation associated with renal vein invasion |
| BAP1 mutation in RCC | Ill-defined tumor margins, calcification related to BAP1 mutation which has poor prognosis |
| MUC4 mutation in RCC | Exophytic tumor growth suggests phenotypic link with tumor expansion pattern |
| Cervical cancer treatment response prediction | Lower apparent diffusion coefficient (ADC) on MRI associated with better chemotherapy response |
| Ovarian cancer prognosis and subtype prediction | Mesenteric infiltration on CT is correlated with CLOVAR mesenchymal subtype and shorter progression-free survival |

(BAP1: BRCA1 associated protein-1; CLOVAR: classification of ovarian cancer; CT: computed tomography; KDM5C: lysine (k)-specific demethylase 5C; MRI: magnetic resonance imaging; MUC4: mucin 4; RCC: renal cell carcinoma; VHL: Von Hippel-Lindau gene)

**TABLE 7:** Application of radiomics in liver tumors.

| *Clinical application* | *Key findings* |
|---|---|
| Classify liver tumors using MRI | Topological features improved tumor classification beyond standard texture analysis |
| Differentiate hemangioma, HCC, and metastasis | Radiomics distinguished hemangiomas from metastases and HCC |
| Distinguish benign vs. malignant liver lesions | Combined radiomics and clinical factors improved accuracy for adenomas, cysts, hemangiomas, HCC, and metastases |
| Predict nonbeneficial resection in ICC | Radiomic model outperformed clinical models in identifying futile surgeries |
| Predict early recurrence after liver surgery | Integrated model (18,000+ features) predicted early recurrence with high accuracy |
| Predict treatment response to TARE in ICC | Higher iodine uptake in arterial phase linked to better response, PFS, and OS |

(HCC: hepatocellular carcinoma; ICC: intrahepatic cholangiocarcinoma; MRI: magnetic resonance imaging; OS: overall survival; PFS: progression-free survival; TARE: transarterial radioembolization)

## RADIOMICS IN GALLBLADDER CARCINOMA

Gallbladder carcinoma (GBC) remains a challenging malignancy to diagnose and manage, largely due to its subtle early presentation and anatomical

**TABLE 8:** Application of radiomics in gallbladder carcinoma.

| *Clinical application* | *Radiomic features* | *Key findings* |
|---|---|---|
| Predict overall survival | Kurtosis (medium texture scale) using TexRAD software | Higher kurtosis associated with worse survival |
| Differentiate tumor grade | Mean intensity, kurtosis | Mean intensity can distinguish moderately from poorly differentiated adenocarcinoma |
| Identify malignant gallbladder polyps | Skewness, contrast (GLCM) from high-resolution ultrasound | Combined with US features: Specificity improved to 93.8%, identifies polyps that warrant surgery |
| Predict histological grade (preoperative) | CT texture (especially kurtosis) | Kurtosis showed consistent correlation with grade and outcome |
| Predict lymph node metastases | Arterial phase CT texture | Preoperative prediction possible; useful for surgical planning |
| Predict early recurrence | Radiomic score + stage + grade | High-risk patients identified for surveillance or adjuvant therapy |
| Differentiate GBC from XGC | Deep learning + triphasic CT | Higher radiomics scores, poor differentiation, and advanced pathological staging (pT3/4, pN2): More likely to have early recurrence |

(CT: computed tomography; GBC: gallbladder carcinoma; GLCM: gray-level co-occurrence matrix; TexRAD: Texture Analysis Software; XGC: xanthogranulomatous cholecystitis)

proximity to critical hepatobiliary structures. Conventional imaging helps to identify suspicious features, but often lacks the granularity to assess tumor biology. Radiomics offers a new layer of information by quantifying texture and structural features from imaging, potentially aiding in diagnosis, risk stratification, and treatment planning **(Table 8)**.[25-31]

On imaging, gallbladder lesions can appear in various forms—ranging from a mass replacing the gallbladder fossa, to a polypoidal intraluminal lesion, or simply as diffuse wall thickening. Along with morphology, radiologists assess tumor size, local invasion into the liver or biliary tree, presence of gallstones or ascites, and evidence of metastatic spread to the liver, lymph nodes, or omentum. These anatomical features not only guide clinical decision-making but also form the basis for region of interest (ROI) selection in radiomics analysis.

## RADIOMICS IN PANCREATIC TUMORS

Radiomics is proving to be a valuable tool in the evaluation of pancreatic tumors, offering quantitative, noninvasive insights that complement

**TABLE 9:** Application of radiomics in pancreatic masses.

| *Clinical application* | *Utility of radiomics* |
|---|---|
| Differentiate cancer vs. autoimmune pancreatitis | Sensitivity up to 90.6% and specificity up to 100% |
| Detect pancreatic adenocarcinoma vs. normal tissue | Sensitivity 100% and specificity 98.5% |
| Classify cystic lesions (SCN, MCN, IPMN, and SPN) | 84% accuracy using radiomics; improved further with clinical/demographic data |
| Stratify IPMN by malignancy risk | Accuracy up to 96% in distinguishing low- vs. high-grade dysplasia |
| | 92% accuracy for malignancy risk stratification |
| Differentiate PNETs from accessory spleen | Improved diagnostic confidence; better differentiation |
| Predict PNET grade (G1 vs. G2/G3) | High-grade tumors associated with lower sphericity, higher skewness |
| Distinguish atypical PNETs from adenocarcinomas | Helps in difficult differential diagnosis |
| Assess early response to chemoradiotherapy in adenocarcinoma | Early changes observed within 2 weeks; predicted nonresponders |
| Evaluate post-treatment response in adenocarcinoma | Detected subtle response changes not visible on routine imaging |
| Link with genetic mutations (radiogenomics) of adenocarcinoma | Associated with KRAS, TP53, SMAD4 mutations, and overall survival |

(IPMN: intraductal papillary mucinous neoplasm; KRAS: Kirsten rat sarcoma viral oncogene; MCN: mucinous cystic neoplasm; PNET: pancreatic neuroendocrine tumors; SCN: serous cystadenoma; SMAD4: mothers against decapentaplegic homolog 4; SPN: solid pseudopapillary neoplasm; TP53: tumor protein 53)

conventional imaging and clinical assessment. With the pancreas being a complex organ affected by a wide spectrum of benign, inflammatory, and malignant processes, radiomics may help to overcome the diagnostic challenges posed by overlapping imaging features **(Table 9)**.[32-39]

## RADIOMICS IN PANCREATITIS

Radiomics has emerged as a valuable imaging biomarker in the evaluation of pancreatitis, showing promising potential in diagnostic differentiation, risk stratification, and early prediction of complications. By extracting high-dimensional features from CT and MRI images, radiomics models can noninvasively quantify pancreatic tissue characteristics, offering insights beyond the scope of conventional imaging interpretation.[40-45] Radiogenomics has shown promise in evaluation of pancreatitis.

*Predicting recurrence in acute pancreatitis (AP):* Recurrent acute pancreatitis (RAP), defined as two or more distinct episodes of AP at least 3 months apart, is clinically challenging due to its multifactorial etiology and variable prognosis. Texture features extracted from the entire pancreatic parenchyma on arterial and venous phase CT scans have been used to develop models that can predict recurrence risk in patients after a first episode. These models may help to guide closer surveillance and early interventions in high-risk patients.

*Clinical severity of acute pancreatitis:* MRI-based radiomics, particularly from the portal venous phase, have outperformed traditional scoring systems such as APACHE II, BISAP, and MRSI in predicting clinical severity, enabling more accurate early risk stratification.

*Prediction of extrapancreatic necrosis (EXPN):* Radiomics models using T2-weighted MRI images of peripancreatic collections and contrast-enhanced arterial phase images of the pancreatic parenchyma have shown improved accuracy in early prediction of EXPN compared to standard imaging scores.

*To distinguish between mass-forming chronic pancreatitis and pancreatic ductal adenocarcinoma (PDAC):* These two entities may appear similar on imaging, especially when chronic pancreatitis (CP) presents as a focal mass or when PDAC is associated with chronic changes. Texture features and shape-based parameters extracted from CT images can help to delineate the underlying pathology with greater precision, potentially reducing diagnostic uncertainty and avoiding both overtreatment and undertreatment.

*Focal autoimmune pancreatitis (AIP):* In particular, the localized form of type I or II poses another diagnostic challenge. Radiomics models based on multiphase contrast-enhanced CT have shown good discriminatory power in separating focal AIP from PDAC, providing a valuable adjunct to serology, clinical criteria, and endoscopic evaluation.

## COLORECTAL CANCERS

In colorectal cancer, the molecular landscape is highly heterogeneous and significantly impacts prognosis and treatment response. Alterations in genes such as Kirsten rat sarcoma viral oncogene (KRAS), NRAS, BRAF, and ABCC2 influence not only tumor behavior but also resistance to targeted therapies. Notably, the expression of ABCC2, which encodes a transporter protein associated with multidrug resistance, has been found to correlate with both nodal involvement and advanced metastatic stages. Furthermore, genes such as *CDH6, CDKNV1,* and *INHBB* show significant associations with radiomic features such as tumor flatness, texture entropy, and gray-level nonuniformity.[46]

Certain imaging-derived features, such as flatness, sum entropy, and entropy from the gray level co-occurrence matrix (GLCM), have been linked with progression-free survival (PFS). These correlate with molecular markers, nodal status, and histological stage. In contrast, features such as 3D surface-to-volume ratio, inverse difference moment, and high expression of ALDH1A1 are more predictive of overall survival. These findings suggest that radiogenomic profiling can capture complex biological signals that go beyond conventional imaging and staging methods.

When examining modality-specific insights, fluorodeoxyglucose-positron emission tomography (FDG-PET)/CT has been particularly useful in evaluating KRAS mutation status. Tumors with KRAS mutations tend to show significantly higher SUVmax and SUVpeak, indicative of more aggressive behavior and poorer prognosis. MRI has also demonstrated utility in identifying KRAS mutations, with mutant tumors showing longer axial dimensions, lower ADC values (both mean and maximum), reduced true diffusion, and higher pseudodiffusion coefficients, reflecting more restricted water movement, and greater cellular density. Interestingly, CT texture analysis has been shown to outperform PET-derived SUVmax in predicting KRAS mutation status.

Magnetic resonance imaging-based radiomics has been the most extensively studied in colorectal cancer. Various studies have demonstrated strong predictive performance when radiomics is combined with clinical parameters or traditional radiology. Below is a summary of key findings on the application of radiomics **(Table 10)**.

Beyond prediction, radiomics has also shown promise in identifying genetic mutations that traditionally require tissue biopsies. Noninvasive detection of RAS (KRAS/NRAS) and BRAF mutations has been demonstrated

**TABLE 10:** Application of radiomics in colorectal carcinoma.

| *Clinical goal* | *Performance/outcome* |
|---|---|
| Predict response to chemotherapy | Radiomics improved prediction; agreement $\kappa = 0.82$ vs. 0.25 with standard imaging |
| Predict pathological complete response | Texture features such as skewness and entropy showed AUCs of 0.73–0.75 |
| Assess nodal metastases | Clinical radiomics models achieved AUCs up to 0.83 |
| Predict tumor differentiation | Radiomic features identified low- vs. high-grade tumors with AUC $\approx$ 0.80 |
| Evaluate T and N staging | SVM-based radiomic models achieved AUC $\approx$ 0.86 |
| Detect synchronous liver metastases | Combined models reached AUCs up to 0.92, with >80% accuracy |
| Predict overall survival and recurrence | Second-order features predicted recurrence risk with up to 90% accuracy |

(AUC: area under the curve; SVM: support vector machine)

**TABLE 11:** Application of radiomics in gastric tumors.

| *Clinical application* | *Key radiomic findings* |
|---|---|
| Differential diagnosis (e.g., adenocarcinoma vs. lymphoma, autoimmune vs. malignant lesions) | Improved accuracy in distinguishing malignant from benign/inflammatory masses (AUC up to 0.86–0.92) |
| Histological grading | Moderate correlation with tumor differentiation; ability to separate low- vs. high-grade tumors |
| T and N staging | Predicted nodal positivity with AUC ≈ 0.79–0.80; staging accuracy comparable to radiologists |
| Vascular invasion | Higher entropy associated with vascular invasion (AUC ~0.82) |
| Occult peritoneal or liver metastasis | High predictive performance (AUC > 0.9), aiding surgical planning |
| Response to chemotherapy/ radiotherapy | Distinguishes responders vs. nonresponders; associated with survival outcomes |
| Prognosis (OS, DFS, and recurrence) | Combined models improve prediction of recurrence and survival; HR ~3.0–3.7, C-index ~0.82 |

(AUC: area under the curve; DFS: disease-free survival; HR: hazard ratio; OS: overall survival)

using CT and MRI-based radiomic models. These mutations are typically associated with resistance to epidermal growth factor receptor (EGFR)-targeted therapies and poorer survival outcomes.

## GASTRIC CANCER

Gastric cancer is the second leading cause of cancer deaths and shows high recurrence despite standard treatment. Traditional AJCC tumor, node, metastasis (TNM) staging does not fully explain outcome differences. Radiomics and radiogenomics provide noninvasive and repeatable biomarkers that link imaging traits with tumor biology, improving prediction of staging, metastasis, treatment response, and survival **(Table 11)**. Integrating radiomic features with molecular markers and clinical data offers more accurate personalized prognostic models than TNM staging alone.[47]

## CHALLENGES IN CURRENT USE OF RADIOMICS AND RADIOGENOMICS IN CLINICAL PRACTICE

As we know in each radiological image, various quantitative radiomics features are present from which deep learning algorithms in AI automatically select and extract the data. Thus, the development of robust deep learning algorithms is important. The number of inputs should be reduced to develop sensitive machine learning algorithms and should be properly assessed.

The main limitations involve variability in feature extraction and lack of reproducibility. Thus, emphasis is on standardizing the present imaging methodology in relation to dose administered, use of acquisition parameters, and reconstruct kernels. The genomics studies are complex and expensive, hence cannot be used on a large scale. The correlation of feature extraction and image analysis requires software and imaging equipment. Most of the studies are single center with small sample size. The testing datasets and validation are inadequate, which may have detrimental impact on the model adaption, optimization, and assessment processes.

## CONCLUSION

Imaging has become an indispensable tool in the precision medicine era for genitourinary and gynecological malignancies. Advanced modalities such as mpMRI, PET CT, and diffusion-weighted imaging not only improve tumor detection and characterization but also enable noninvasive insights into tumor genetics and biology through radiogenomics. These imaging techniques facilitate better risk stratification, guide targeted biopsies, monitor treatment response, and predict patient outcomes. As imaging continues to integrate with molecular profiling, it holds the promise to further personalize treatment, optimize therapeutic strategies, and ultimately improve survival and quality of life for patients with these cancers. Continued research and validation of imaging biomarkers are essential to fully realize their potential in routine clinical practice.

## REFERENCES

1. European Society of Radiology (ESR). Medical imaging in personalized medicine: a white paper. Insights Imaging. 2015;6:141-55.
2. EFPIA. Precision Medicine: Giving the Right Medicine, to the Right Patient, at the Right Time. [online] Available from https://www.efpia.eu/about-medicines/development-of-medicines/precision-medicine [Last accessed October, 2025].
3. Lambin P, Leijenaar RTH, Deist TM, Peerlings J, de Jong EEC, van Timmeren J, et al. Radiomics: the bridge between medical imaging and personalized medicine. Nat Rev Clin Oncol. 2017;14(12):749-62.
4. Incoronato M, Aiello M, Infante T, Cavaliere C, Grimaldi AM, Mirabelli P, et al. Radiogenomic Analysis of Oncological Data: A Technical Survey. Int J Mol Sci. 2017;18(4):805.
5. Monti S, Aiello M, Incoronato M, Grimaldi AM, Moscarino M, Mirabelli P, et al. DCE-MRI Pharmacokinetic-Based Phenotyping of Invasive Ductal Carcinoma: A Radiomic Study for Prediction of Histological Outcomes. Contrast Media Mol Imaging. 2018;2018:5076269.
6. Sharma P, Kumar I, Ojha R, Khanna S, Verma A. Prediction of genetic profile of breast carcinoma on MRI using a combination of DCE-MRI, DWI, and MR spectroscopy: A prospective observational study. Malig Spect. 2024;1:290-9.
7. Monti S, Brancato V, Di Costanzo G, Basso L, Puglia M, Ragozzino A, et al. Multiparametric MRI for Prostate Cancer Detection: New Insights into the

Combined Use of a Radiomic Approach with Advanced Acquisition Protocol. Cancers (Basel). 2020;12(2):390.
8. Brancato V, Aiello M, Basso L, Monti S, Palumbo L, Di Costanzo G, et al. Evaluation of a multiparametric MRI radiomic-based approach for stratification of equivocal PI-RADS 3 and upgraded PI-RADS 4 prostatic lesions. Sci Rep. 2021;11(1):643.
9. Jena B, Saxena S, Nayak GK, Balestrieri A, Gupta N, Khanna NN, et al. Brain Tumor Characterization Using Radiogenomics in Artificial Intelligence Framework. Cancers (Basel). 2022;14(16):4052.
10. Singh G, Manjila S, Sakla N, True A, Wardeh AH, Beig N, et al. Radiomics and radiogenomics in gliomas: a contemporary update. Br J Cancer. 2021; 125(5):641-57.
11. Beig N, Correa R, Thawani R, Prasanna P, Badve C, Gold D, et al. MEDU-48. MRI TEXTURAL FEATURES CAN DIFFERENTIATE PEDIATRIC POSTERIOR FOSSA TUMORS. Neuro Oncol. 2017;19(Suppl 4):iv47.
12. Lee G, Park H, Bak SH, Lee HY. Radiomics in Lung Cancer from Basic to Advanced: Current Status and Future Directions. Korean J Radiol. 2020;21(2):159-71.
13. Beig N, Khorrami M, Alilou M, Prasanna P, Braman N, Orooji M, et al. Perinodular and Intranodular Radiomic Features on Lung CT Images Distinguish Adenocarcinomas from Granulomas. Radiology. 2019;290(3):783-92.
14. Zhong Y, Yuan M, Zhang T, Zhang YD, Li H, Yu TF. Radiomics Approach to Prediction of Occult Mediastinal Lymph Node Metastasis of Lung Adenocarcinoma. AJR Am J Roentgenol. 2018;211(1):109-13.
15. Liu L, Yi X, Lu C, Qi L, Zhang Y, Li M, et al. Applications of radiomics in genitourinary tumors. Am J Cancer Res. 2020;10(8):2293-308.
16. Goyal A, Razik A, Kandasamy D, Seth A, Das P, Ganeshan B, et al. Role of MR texture analysis in histological subtyping and grading of renal cell carcinoma: a preliminary study. Abdom Radiol (NY). 2019;44(10):3336-49.
17. Wang H, Hu D, Yao H, Chen M, Li S, Chen H, et al. Radiomics analysis of multiparametric MRI for the preoperative evaluation of pathological grade in bladder cancer tumors. Eur Radiol. 2019;29(11):6182-90.
18. Tong Y, Udupa JK, Wang C, Chen J, Venigalla S, Guzzo TJ, et al. Radiomics-guided therapy for bladder cancer: Using an optimal biomarker approach to determine extent of bladder cancer invasion from t2-weighted magnetic resonance images. Adv Radiat Oncol. 2018;3(3):331-8.
19. Yang R, Wu J, Sun L, Lai S, Xu Y, Liu X, et al. Radiomics of small renal masses on multiphasic CT: accuracy of machine learning-based classification models for the differentiation of renal cell carcinoma and angiomyolipoma without visible fat. Eur Radiol. 2020;30(2):1254-63.
20. Granata V, Fusco R, Setola SV, Simonetti I, Cozzi D, Grazzini G, et al. An update on radiomics techniques in primary liver cancers. Infect Agent Cancer. 2022;17(1):6.
21. Chu H, Liu Z, Liang W, Zhou Q, Zhang Y, Lei K, et al. CT radiomics for prediction of futile resection in intrahepatic cholangiocarcinoma. Eur Radiol. 2021;31:2368-76.
22. Qin H, Hu X, Zhang J, Dai H, He Y, Zhao Z, et al. Machine-learning radiomics for recurrence in perihilar cholangiocarcinoma. Liver Int. 2021;41:837-50.
23. Li Z, Mao Y, Huang W, Li H, Zhu J, Li W, et al. Texture-based classification of liver lesions on T2 MRI. BMC Med Imaging. 2017;17:42.

24. Jansen MJA, Kuijf HJ, Veldhuis WB, Wessels FJ, Viergever MA, Pluim JPW. Automatic classification of focal liver lesions with MRI. PLoS One. 2019; 14:e0217053.
25. Gupta P, Rana P, Ganeshan B, Kalage D, Irrinki S, Gupta V, et al. CT texture-based radiomics in gallbladder cancer. Clin Exp Hepatol. 2021;7:406-14.
26. Choi TW, Kim JH, Park SJ, Ahn SJ, Joo I, Han JK. Risk stratification of gallbladder polyps with US texture analysis. Eur Radiol. 2018;28:196-205.
27. Chen M, Cao J, Bai Y, Tong C, Lin J, Jindal V, et al. Nomogram for early detection of malignant gallbladder lesions. Clin Transl Gastroenterol. 2019;10: e0098.
28. Xiang F, Liang X, Yang L, Liu X, Yan S. Contrast-enhanced CT radiomics for prediction of recurrence-free survival in gallbladder carcinoma after surgical resection. Eur Radiol. 2022;32(10):7087-97.
29. Zhang W, Wang Q, Liang K, Lin H, Wu D, Han Y, et al. Deep learning nomogram for preoperative distinction between Xanthogranulomatous cholecystitis and gallbladder carcinoma: A novel approach for surgical decision. Comput Biol Med. 2024;168:107786.
30. Baishya NK, Baishya K. Radiomic nomograms in CT diagnosis of gallbladder carcinoma: a review. Discov Oncol. 2024;15:844.
31. Gupta P, Dutta N, Tomar A, Singh S, Choudhary S, Mehta N, et al. Deep learning-based segmentation of gallbladder cancer on abdominal computed tomography scans: a multicenter study. Abdom Radiol (NY). 2025;50(10):4615-24.
32. de la Pinta C. Radiomics in pancreatic cancer for oncologist: Present and future. Hepatobiliary Pancreat Dis Int. 2022;21(4):356-61.
33. Cheng MF, Guo YL, Yen RF, Chen YC, Ko CL, Tien YW, et al. Clinical Utility of FDG PET/CT in Patients with Autoimmune Pancreatitis: a Case-Control Study. Sci Rep. 2018;8(1):3651.
34. Chu LC, Park S, Kawamoto S, Fouladi DF, Shayesteh S, Zinreich ES, et al. Utility of CT Radiomics Features in Differentiation of Pancreatic Ductal Adenocarcinoma From Normal Pancreatic Tissue. AJR Am J Roentgenol. 2019;213(2):349-57.
35. Dmitriev K, Kaufman AE, Javed AA, Hruban RH, Fishman EK, Lennon AM, et al. Classification of Pancreatic Cysts in Computed Tomography Images Using a Random Forest and Convolutional Neural Network Ensemble. Med Image Comput Comput Assist Interv. 2017;10435:150-8.
36. Hanania AN, Bantis LE, Feng Z, Wang H, Tamm EP, Katz MH, et al. Quantitative imaging to evaluate malignant potential of IPMNs. Oncotarget. 2016;7(52):85776-84.
37. Lin X, Xu L, Wu A, Guo C, Chen X, Wang Z. Differentiation of intrapancreatic accessory spleen from small hypervascular neuroendocrine tumor of the pancreas: textural analysis on contrast-enhanced computed tomography. Acta Radiol. 2019;60(5):553-60.
38. Choi TW, Kim JH, Yu MH, Park SJ, Han JK. Pancreatic neuroendocrine tumor: prediction of the tumor grade using CT findings and computerized texture analysis. Acta Radiol. 2018;59(4):383-92.
39. Li J, Lu J, Liang P, Li A, Hu Y, Shen Y, et al. Differentiation of atypical pancreatic neuroendocrine tumors from pancreatic ductal adenocarcinomas: Using whole-tumor CT texture analysis as quantitative biomarkers. Cancer Med. 2018;7(10):4924-31.

40. Guo CG, Ren S, Chen X, Wang QD, Xiao WB, Zhang JF, et al. Pancreatic neuroendocrine tumor: prediction of the tumor grade using magnetic resonance imaging findings and texture analysis with 3-T magnetic resonance. Cancer Manag Res. 2019;11:1933-44.
41. Yan G, Yan G, Li H, Liang H, Peng C, Bhetuwal A, et al. Radiomics and Its Applications and Progress in Pancreatitis: A Current State of the Art Review. Front Med (Lausanne). 2022;9:922299.
42. Zhang Y, Cheng C, Liu Z, Pan G, Sun G, Yang X, et al. [Differentiation of autoimmune pancreatitis and pancreatic ductal adenocarcinoma based on multi-modality texture features in 18F-FDG PET/CT]. Sheng Wu Yi Xue Gong Cheng Xue Za Zhi. 2019;36(5):755-62.
43. Frøkjær JB, Lisitskaya MV, Jørgensen AS, Østergaard LR, Hansen TM, Drewes AM, et al. Pancreatic magnetic resonance imaging texture analysis in chronic pancreatitis: a feasibility and validation study. Abdom Radiol (NY). 2020;45(5):1497-506.
44. Yu B, Li J, Li N, Zhu Y, Chen Y, He W, et al. Progression to recurrent acute pancreatitis after a first attack of acute pancreatitis in adults. Pancreatology. 2020;20(7):1340-6.
45. Gupta P, Siddiqui R, Singh S, Pradhan N, Shah J, Samanta J, et al. Application of deep learning models for accurate classification of fluid collections in acute necrotizing pancreatitis on computed tomography: a multicenter study. Abdom Radiol (NY). 2025;50(5):2258-67. Erratum in: Abdom Radiol (NY). 2025;50(5):2268-9.
46. Inchingolo R, Maino C, Cannella R, Vernuccio F, Cortese F, Dezio M, et al. Radiomics in colorectal cancer patients. World J Gastroenterol. 2023;29(19): 2888-904.
47. Wang Y, Jin ZY. Radiomics in gastric cancer: a frontier in decision making. Chin Med J (Engl). 2019;132:1983-9.

CHAPTER 9

# Thoracic Trauma

*Dinesh Bagaria, Shristi Rathore, Subodh Kumar*

## INTRODUCTION

Trauma is a manmade pandemic of modern world amounting to 5.8 million deaths and loss of >130 million of disability adjusted life years (DALYs) in all ages and economic groups annually. Thoracic trauma is one of the most common injuries found in around 60% of patients with polytrauma. These injuries present in 10% or more of all trauma admissions and significantly contributing in up to 35% of all trauma-related deaths. Prompt evaluation and timely intervention are the key to prevent majority of these deaths. Majority of chest injuries can be managed with simple lifesaving interventions in emergency department (ED) only. Operative interventions are needed in 7–8% of blunt injuries and 15–25% of penetrating injuries.

All trauma patients require a protocolized approach in the initial assessment and management irrespective of mechanism of injuries and their patterns. On arrival, all patients with trauma are assessed and managed according to recent Advanced Trauma Life Support (ATLS®) guidelines which prioritize emergent management of eXsanguinating eXternal hemorrhage followed by early identification of other life-threatening conditions by clinical examination using a "look, listen, feel" (inspection, auscultation, and palpation) approach, and adhering to the following sequence:[1]

- eXsanguinating eXternal hemorrhage
- Airway assessment with cervical spine motion restriction
- Breathing and ventilation
- Circulation with hemorrhage control
- Disability—brief neurologic assessment
- Exposure/environmental control

Specific imaging used as adjuncts to primary survey are chest and pelvic X-rays and extended-focused assessment with sonography in trauma (e-FAST). Depending upon the response to resuscitation, trauma patients are categorized as rapid responders, transient responders, and nonresponders. Nonresponders are immediately subjected to damage control surgery (DCS) for hemorrhage control and contamination prevention. Hemodynamically stable patients are further evaluated by detailed secondary survey and use of more advanced imaging like contrast-enhanced computed tomography (CECT) scan to diagnose other injuries.

Following life-threatening thoracic injuries need to be diagnosed and managed promptly in trauma patients:

## AIRWAY OBSTRUCTION AND TRACHEOBRONCHIAL TREE INJURIES

Airway obstruction in trauma patients may occur either due to the tongue fall in unconscious patients, or due to loosen teeth, secretions, and blood. Besides, expanding neck hematomas may also cause airway obstruction due to compression of the trachea.

Tracheobronchial tree injuries, though life-threatening, are rare, and occur due to penetrating injuries in majority of cases. These injuries are usually associated with major intrathoracic vascular, esophageal, and/or pulmonary injuries. Blunt injuries, due to rapid deceleration or compressive forces, primarily occur within 2 cm of carina.

Majority of these patients present with features suggestive of tension pneumothorax or severe subcutaneous emphysema. Persistent air leak after intercostal drainage tube (ICD) insertion may be another presentation of such injuries. The air leak from the ICD is graded as per the Cerfolio classification **(Table 1)**. Patients with major air leak who do not respond to nonoperative management strategies such as negative suction and/or insertion of second ICD require emergency thoracotomy.

Chest X-ray features suggestive of tracheobronchial injuries are subcutaneous or mediastinal emphysema, pneumothorax, parabronchial air, and dropped lung (lung apex rests at the level of hilum) **(Fig. 1)**. In stable patients with adequate oxygenation, further evaluation with CECT scan of chest/torso helps in assessing the extent of tracheobronchial injuries.

Airway stabilization is of utmost importance in the management of these injuries. Fiberoptic bronchoscopy may be useful for diagnosing an injury and in guiding the endotracheal tube to bridge the tracheal defect if any, and selective intubation of the mainstem bronchus of the uninjured lung in select group.[2] In patients with penetrating neck injuries or cut throat injuries, where distal end of trachea could be visualized, under vision intubation of distal trachea through the neck wound is a lifesaving strategy to buy time to arrange for definitive management **(Fig. 2)**.

**TABLE 1:** Cerfolio classification of air leak through intercostal drainage tube (ICD).

| | |
|---|---|
| Grade 1 | On coughing |
| Grade 2 | During expiration only |
| Grade 3 | During inspiration only |
| Grade 4 | Continuous bubbling during whole breath cycle |

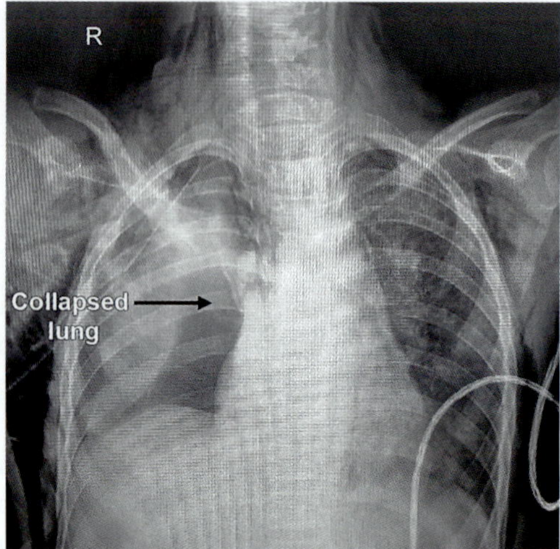


**Fig. 1:** Chest X-ray showing persistent pneumothorax with fallen lung sign.

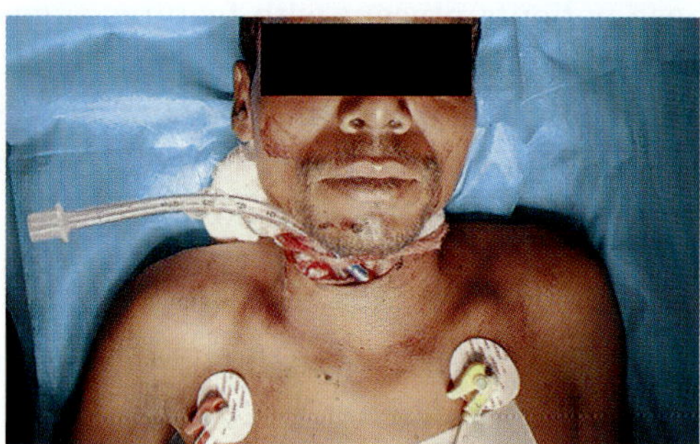

**Fig. 2:** Endotracheal intubation through visible tracheal defect.

Majority of tracheobronchial injuries in hemodynamically stable patients will be managed nonoperatively. The important surgical principles are minimum debridement, minimize lateral dissection, buttressing with vascularized flaps of strap or intercostal muscles, pericardium, or pleura. Covered self-expanding metal tracheal stents are useful alternative for poor surgical candidates. Recently, few case reports showed successful utilization of bronchoscopic application of cyanoacrylate glue in management of small tracheal lacerations.

## TENSION PNEUMOTHORAX

Pneumothorax is the accumulation of air in the pleural space originating mostly from lung parenchyma, but sometimes from tracheobronchial tree. One uncommon but life-threatening situation is tension pneumothorax occurring in 5–6% of chest trauma patients. It occurs when a one-way "flutter valve" mechanism forms, resulting in leakage of air into the pleural

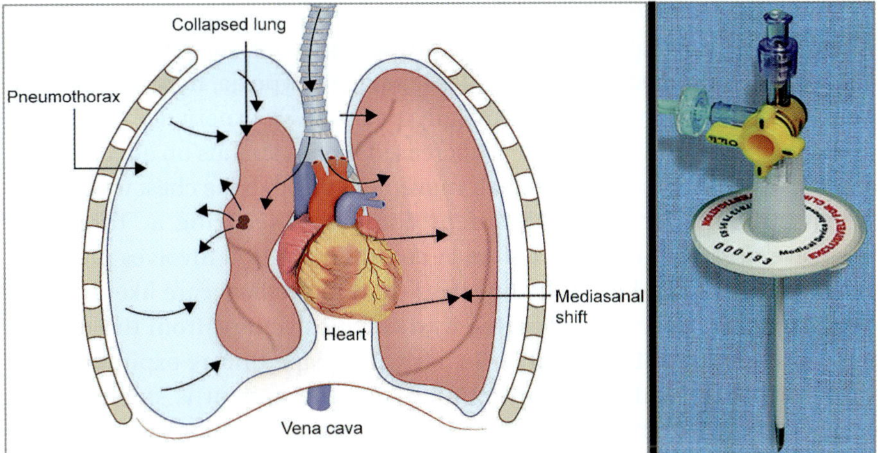


**Fig. 3:** Diagrammatic representation of consequences due to tension pneumothorax along with commercially available needle for thoracic decompression.

space with each breath cycle leading to continuously increase in pleural air volume and pressure. This increased pressure results into ventilatory or hemodynamic compromise due to compression of the great vessels, lung, heart, and trachea and shifting of mediastinum **(Fig. 3)**. More frequently, it occurs in patients with simple pneumothorax who are put on positive pressure ventilation without putting ICD. Spontaneously breathing patients complain of chest pain, inability of breath normally, and respiratory distress. Features suggestive of shock due to decreased cardiac output along with a silent and hyperresonant chest on the side of injury are diagnostic of tension pneumothorax. The classical signs such as distended neck veins and tracheal deviation are found infrequently.

Tension pneumothorax is an exclusive clinical diagnosis, and no imaging is required to diagnose and treat it. Hemodynamically stable patients with significant air in pleural cavities on chest X-ray should not be diagnosed as a case of tension pneumothorax. Once clinically detected, immediate next step is needle thoracocentesis. The latest evidence recommends needle thoracocentesis in the second intercostal space (ICS) over midclavicular line or fifth ICS over midaxillary line, depending upon clinical setting. After needle decompression ICD should be inserted in the fifth ICS in these patients.

## OPEN PNEUMOTHORAX

In open pneumothorax, a full-thickness chest wall defect, equal or larger than the two-thirds of diameter of patient's trachea allows communication of the pleural cavity with the external environment. This communication will be the path of least resistance for the air to travel compared to natural airway during a breathing cycle. With each breath, air is "sucked in" through this wound, so commonly referred as sucking chest wounds. This communication will cause loss of physiological negative intrapleural pressure thus impairing effective lung expansion on both sides leading to hypoxia, hypercapnia, and rapid respiratory compromise. Clinically, patients will experience chest pain, difficulty in breathing, tachypnea, decreased breath sounds on affected side, and noisy "hissing" sound due to air movement through the chest wall defect.

The initial specific management comprises securing a "three-way occlusive dressing" over the defect. A common method involves placing a clean sheet prepared from various bags used in medical care like drainage bags, etc. over defect and securing it with adhesive tape from three sides, making it act like a flutter valve. So, air will escape during expiration, but valve will occlude during inspiration. Once the patient is stable and in controlled environment, a chest tube is placed at a remote site from the defect. Subsequently to it, definitive wound closure needs to be done.

## MASSIVE HEMOTHORAX

Hemothorax is the presence of blood in the pleural cavity. When the amount of this blood is significant enough to cause hemodynamic instability, it is considered massive hemothorax. Massive hemothorax occurs primarily due to penetrating trauma leading to hilar and systemic vascular injuries mainly due to aortic, subclavian, and internal mammary arteries or sometimes due to penetrating cardiac injuries. Massive hemothorax can be defined as "immediate drainage of blood volume >1,500 mL or 30% of total blood volume from the chest tube, or drainage of >200 mL per hour for 2–4 consecutive hours". These criteria were based on observational studies in penetrating military injuries and were also considered as indications for urgent thoracotomy. There was no consideration of time elapsed since injuries and hemodynamic effect of intrathoracic bleeding.

Presently, though, the criteria to define massive hemothorax are still the same, the decision of further management is determined by the hemodynamic status of patient and response to the resuscitative measures. Literature suggests that considering the ICD output alone will lead to 20–25% nontherapeutic thoracotomies.

Increased opacity/whiteout lung in chest X-ray is suggestive of significant hemothorax **(Fig. 4)**. Patients who respond to the resuscitative measures need to be evaluated further by CECT scan to assess source of hemorrhage as well as to rule out other injuries. Any obvious contrast extravasation from identifiable vessels can be managed by angioembolization. The aortic injuries have been discussed later in this chapter.

Nonresponders should immediately be shifted to operation room for emergency thoracotomy.[3] Clamshell thoracotomy is preferred approach in majority of such patients for easy bilateral access. Recently, several reports

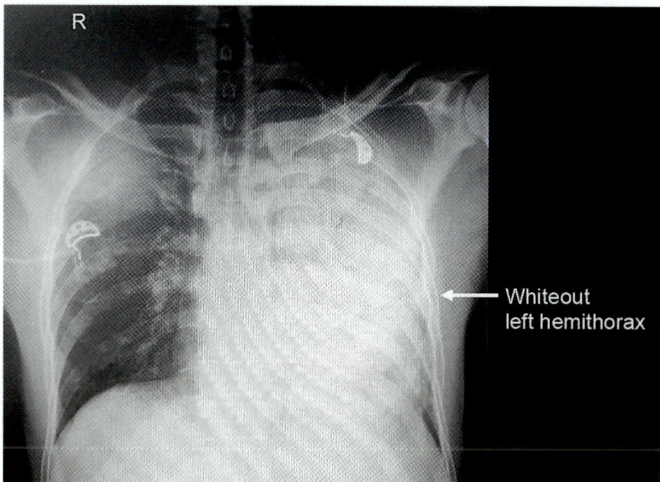


**Fig. 4:** Chest X-ray anteroposterior (AP) supine film showing significant left hemothorax.

suggested that, it is safe to process the blood drained out of circulation in massive hemothorax through cell saver systems and can be autotransfused.

## CARDIAC TAMPONADE

Cardiac tamponade is acute collection of blood in the pericardial cavity not able to egress. The fibrous pericardium does not have much tensile strength. So, the accumulated blood compresses the heart chambers leading to a decrease in cardiac filling, end-diastolic dysfunction, decrease preload; and stroke volume causing decreased cardiac output and eventually global hypoperfusion.

The most common (80–90%) mechanism is penetrating injuries. There should be high index of suspicion in patients who present with penetrating injuries to "cardiac box", a rectangular region on the anterior chest, marked by the sternal notch superiorly, the xiphoid process inferiorly, and the nipples bilaterally. The most common (43%) chamber which gets injured the right ventricle due to its maximal anterior exposure. Other cardiac chambers which get injured are left ventricle (33%), right atrium (15%), and left atrium (6%).

If the pericardial laceration is sealed off by surrounding fatty tissues and blood clots, blood continues to collect in the pericardium, leading to pressure build up inside and results in tamponade. Clinical presentation of cardiac tamponade is shock characterized by profound tachycardia and hypotension. The classical description of clinical triad known as Beck's triad, which includes increased central venous pressures leading to distended neck veins, widening pulse pressure, and muffled heart tones is rarely found in trauma patients. Few patients with cardiac injury may present with massive

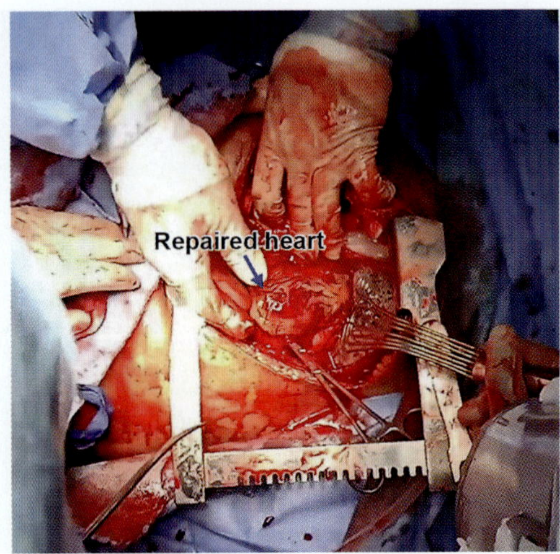


**Fig. 5:** Clamshell thoracotomy followed by pericardiotomy to release cardiac tamponade.

hemothorax if pericardial rent is big enough allowing the blood to leak into pleural cavity.

Classically, diagnosis of cardiac tamponade is made in a patient who presents with penetrating injury near the heart, with features of profound shock and presence of pericardial fluid in extended-focused assessment with sonography for trauma (e-FAST) examination. Management principles consist of initiation of aggressive circulatory support by rapid intravenous fluid infusion to increase venous pressure and improve cardiac output along with emergent pericardial decompression. This may be done by a subxiphoid needle cardiocentesis, a temporalizing measure to buy time in low resource setting, followed by emergency thoracotomy by left anterolateral or clamshell approach for definitive repair **(Fig. 5)**. Recent reports propose use of a diagnostic subxiphoid window into pericardium, in hemodynamically stable cases, with a diagnostic dilemma of hemopericardium.

## TRAUMATIC CARDIAC ARREST

This is an extreme situation where cardiac arrest occurs in a trauma patient, secondary to physiological insult rather than cardiac pathology. The major etiologies are blocked airway, tension pneumothorax, hemorrhagic shock, and cardiac tamponade. Due to intravascular hypovolemia, cardiopulmonary resuscitation (CPR) alone is futile in traumatic cardiac arrest (TCA) **(Flowchart 1)**. Treatment protocols in ED include secured airway, supplemental oxygen support, control of external hemorrhage, decompression of both chest cavities by finger thoracostomy, and restoration of intravascular volume which is of paramount importance and

**Flowchart 1:** Algorithm for management of TCA.

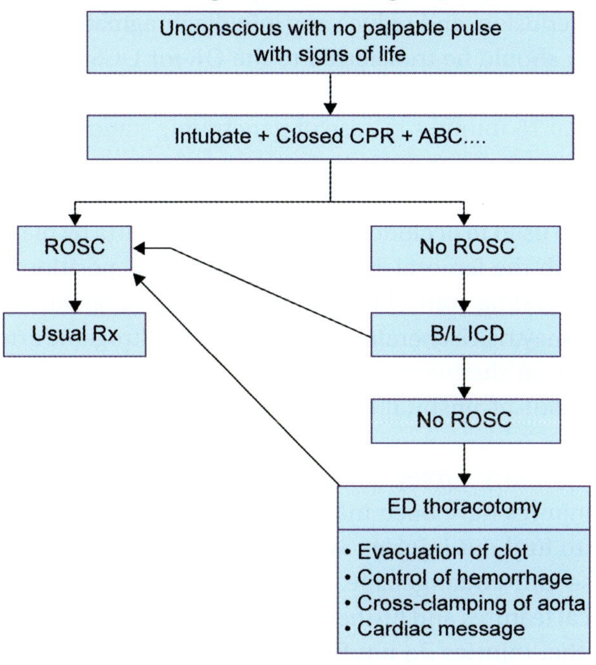


(ABC: airway, breathing, and circulation; CPR: cardiopulmonary resuscitation; ED: emergency department; ICD: intercostal drainage tube; ROSC: return of spontaneous circulation; TCA: traumatic cardiac arrest)

**BOX 1:** Recent indications for ED thoracotomy.

*Current indications for ED thoracotomy*

- *Penetrating trauma:*
  - Thoracic <15 minutes of prehospital CPR
  - Nonthoracic <5 minutes of prehospital CPR

*Blunt trauma <10 minutes of prehospital CPR*

- *Persistent severe postinjury hypotension (SBP <60):*
  - Cardiac tamponade
  - *Hemorrhage:* Intrathoracic, intra-abdominal, extremity, and cervical
  - Air embolism

(CPR: cardiopulmonary resuscitation; ED: emergency department; SBP: systolic blood pressure)

takes priority over chest compressions and advanced cardiac life support (ACLS) measures. A resuscitative thoracotomy may be indicated if there is no return of spontaneous circulation (ROSC), but there are signs of life in form of pupillary response, spontaneous respiratory efforts, spontaneous extremity movement, and pulseless electrical cardiac activity (PEA) **(Box 1)**. Resuscitative thoracotomy allows open cardiac massage, any thoracic hemorrhage control, and cross clamping of thoracic aorta.

Aortic cross-clamping will lead to improve afterload, increase coronary and cerebral perfusion, and reduce any infradiaphragmatic bleeding. If ROSC achieved, they should be transferred to the OR for DCS or definitive repair. Resuscitation is considered futile beyond 10 minutes following blunt trauma, and longer than 15 minutes in case of penetrating trauma if no ROSC could be achieved.

Recently, resuscitative endovascular balloon occlusion of the aorta (REBOA) is also used to occlude the lower thoracic aorta by placing a balloon catheter through the femoral artery. Inflation in this position will buy time for definitive bleeding control by slowing infradiaphragmatic bleeding. The use of REBOA may risk ischemia of distal tissue or iatrogenic arterial damage and thrombosis at the insertion site. Survival from TCA is comparable to nontraumatic out-of-hospital cardiac arrest, but with better neurological outcome.

Once the primary survey has been completed and all immediate life-threatening injuries have been managed, further detailed clinical examination is done to find out injuries, which if not treated on time may worsen in due course and endanger life. Sometimes, these injuries do not show specific clinical features and further imaging in form of CECT scan is needed. As we know that injuries do not follow anatomical boundaries, so a CECT scan of torso scan is advisable in patients with blunt trauma and in majority of penetrating injuries, where involvement of both chest and abdomen is a possibility. These potential life-threatening thoracic injuries are as follows:

## Simple Pneumothorax

In majority, injury to pulmonary parenchyma leads to pneumothorax. Most often, intrapleural air leak is self-limiting. The management of pneumothorax which is diagnosed on chest X-ray is insertion of ICD tube. Recent studies suggest that asymptomatic pneumothoraxes <35 mm from the chest wall, as measured on the CT scan, can be managed without tube thoracostomy at a facility where such patients can be closely monitored for any deterioration.[4] Another specific situation is occult pneumothorax, in which chest X-ray also does not reveal pneumothorax and the same is diagnosed on CECT scan. However, if patients with occult pneumothorax need to be transferred to another center, especially by air, or require positive pressure ventilation, it is advisable to insert ICD in them. The change in transpleural pressure with altitude can potentially result in enlargement of the pneumothorax and conversion from asymptomatic to symptomatic during flight.

## Hemothorax

Intrapleural hemorrhage leading to a hemothorax can originate from the chest wall, intercostal vessels, internal mammary arteries, great vessels, mediastinum, lung parenchyma, diaphragm, or abdomen. Majority patients with hemothorax remain asymptomatic and hemodynamically stable. Supine chest X-ray in a trauma patient reveals homogenous ground glass opacity on the affected side. Latest literature suggests, e-FAST examination being more accurate in diagnosing hemothorax, as ultrasound has consistently been shown to be more sensitive than chest X-ray for the detection of hemothorax. Once the primary survey has been completed, CECT scan will reveal presence of hemothorax especially in asymptomatic patients. Ultrasound and CT scan can also be used to quantify the hemothorax and plan further treatment. Recently, hemothorax <300 mL (1.5 cm pleural stripe) has been defined as occult hemothorax which is diagnosed on CT scan and not on chest X-ray following blunt trauma. These patients may be observed without ICD insertion.[5]

Management of hemothorax requires ICD insertion which allows lung expansion and compression of the bleeding vessel to stop the ongoing bleed, if any. If the patient is hemodynamically stable, and the hemothorax is diagnosed on CECT scan, nonoperative management with close observation, active respiratory care, and adequate pain control can be attempted. These patients need to be monitored clinically and with chest X-ray for any deterioration and timely intervene undrained large intrapleural blood might lead to retained hemothorax. Recent reports suggested that use of bedside saline irrigation early through ICD in these patients helped in reducing the incidence of retained hemothorax.

Retained hemothorax has been defined as blood clots of volume 500 mL or more occupying the pleural space that cannot be drained by ICD after 72 hours. The incidence is estimated between 5 and 30%. The consequences of retained hemothorax include fibrothorax, empyema, and pneumonia.

Management options for retained hemothorax are, intrapleural fibrinolytic therapy (IPFT) or surgical evacuation by video-assisted thoracoscopic surgery (VATS) **(Fig. 6)** or open thoracotomy.[6]

## Principles of Intercostal Drainage Tube Management

Intercostal drainage tube insertion is one of the most critical and most frequent intervention done in patients with chest trauma. Recently, a term nonoperative intervention (NOI) is used to refer management of patients with chest trauma with ICD alone. Following are the evidence-based tenets guiding various aspects of ICD care:

- The ICD insertion being an invasive procedure must be performed under all aseptic precautions, whenever possible, and clinical condition of the patient may provide enough time for aseptic precaution.
- The usual size is 24 French (Fr) to 28 Fr. Recent literature suggests that a 14 Fr tube is as effective as larger size in select cases of pneumothorax and hemothorax.[7]

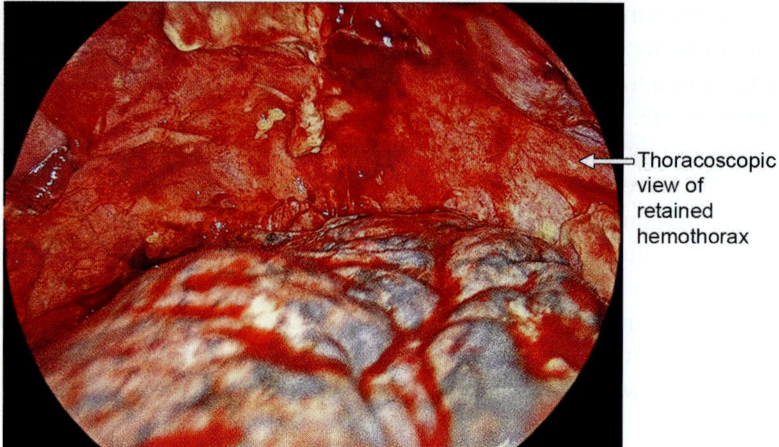


**Fig. 6:** Video-assisted thoracoscopic surgery (VATS) for retained hemothorax.

- The usual site is fifth ICS. It approximately corresponds to inframammary folds. ICD is inserted just anterior to midaxillary line.
- There is no preference for direction of the ICD tip in the pleural cavity in cases of pneumothorax or hemothorax.
- The ICD must be connected to an underwater seal system or to a system with one-way valve mechanism to prevent sucking in of environmental air into the pleural cavity.
- A routine postprocedure chest X-ray is recommended to assess proper placement of ICD.
- Length of the drainage tube should be sufficient to allow movement of the patient in the bed to prevent accidental pull out of the tube. At the same time, it should not be too long tube otherwise work of breathing will increase which will hamper the drainage.
- The practice of routine pleural lavage through the ICD might help in early clearance of hemothorax in selected cases.
- Routing use of negative suction with underwater seal system has not been found beneficial.[8]
- Role of routine daily follow-up X-ray is not clear, and studies are underway to define it better.
- Routine use of prophylactic antibiotics after ICD insertion in patients with isolated chest trauma is not recommended. Only one dose of prophylactic antibiotic at the time of ICD insertion is sufficient, except in penetrating injuries, gross breach in asepsis, and if antibiotics therapy is warranted for other associated conditions.[9]
- It is the nature of ICD content, not the amount only, which should be taken into consideration before removing ICD. There is no consensus for a threshold amount, but current best practices are to plan ICD removal

when output is <100 mL/day and serous in nature. Removal at end of expiration or maximal inspiration appears to make no difference.

- There is no consensus regarding role of routine chest X-ray after ICD removal. Such practices vary from institution to institution. However, if required then it should be done 4–6 hours after ICD removal.

## Rib Fractures

Chest wall injuries in the form of rib fractures are one of the most encountered injuries. The chest wall helps in ventilation by volumetric expansion of pleural cavity and protection of underlying visceral structures. Presence of rib fractures is a marker of derangement of both these two functions depending upon number and severity of rib fractures leading to hypoxemia and hypercarbia. Rib fractures at multiple places in the adjacent ribs may result in a radiographic flail segment or clinical flail chest. A radiographic flail segment is defined as three or more contiguous ribs broken at two or more places as visualized on imaging. Clinical flail chest is defined as paradoxical movement of the segment of chest wall independently during respiration. Paradoxical movement occurs because the flail segments are no longer attached to the chest wall, causing the injured portion of the chest wall to move inward with spontaneous inspiration (due to negative intrathoracic pressure) and outward with exhalation. Besides impaired chest wall function due to broken ribs, underlying lung parenchymal injuries are also significant leading to impaired gas exchange.

The cornerstones of rib fractures management are adequate pain control, good pulmonary hygiene by chest physiotherapy and incentive spirometry, and supplemental oxygenation. Few selected patients with isolated chest injuries, who have adequate pain control during incentive spirometry on oral medications and underlying pulmonary contusions are not significant, may be disposed to home directly from ED. Various scores such as CIBIL and SCARF are useful to assist this decision. Rest needs to be admitted for further monitoring and management.

Recently, surgical stabilization of rib fractures (SSRFs) is in vogue **(Fig. 7)**. The aim of rib fixation is to restore respiratory mechanics and improve lung volumes. This may not require fixation of all ribs or all fracture sites. The restoration of mechanics with rib fixation should be balanced by the knowledge that access to the ribs requires division of chest wall muscles leading to reduced forced vital capacity. The highest level of evidence exists on ventilated patients with flail chest. There is moderate quality evidence to support rib fixation for non-flail chest with severe displacement and with respiratory compromise **(Box 2)**. If indicated, it is advocated to perform SSRF within 48–72 hours.[10,11] Recently, 3D printing technology is also being utilized for planning and designing of customized implants in complex cases.

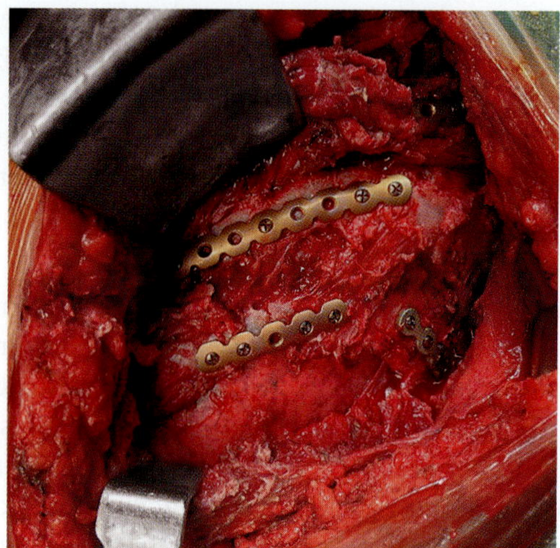

**Fig. 7:** Intraoperative picture of surgical stabilization of rib fractures (SSRFs).

**BOX 2:** Current indications for surgical stabilization of rib fractures (SSRFs).

- *SSRF should be considered in all flail chest (FC) patients*
- *SSRF should be considered in non-FC patients with rib fractures, in the presence of:*
  - Multiple (≥3) ipsilateral severely displaced rib fractures
  - Multiple (≥3) ipsilateral displaced rib fractures in ribs 3–10 in combination with respiratory failure despite mechanical ventilation or weaning failure or at least two pulmonary derangements in nonventilated patients despite locoregional anesthesia and multimodal analgesia:
    - Respiratory rate >20 breaths/min
    - Incentive spirometry <50% predicted
    - Numeric pain score (NPS) >5/10) and poor cough
  - A chest wall deformity that significantly affects lung function (i.e., implosion chest wall injuries, "stoved-in chest") or that shows mechanical instability on palpation
  - Severe pain nonresponsive to other treatments

## Pulmonary Contusion

Pulmonary contusion is defined as injury to the alveolar capillaries and extravasation of blood into the pulmonary parenchyma without its disruption. The interstitial hemorrhage result in surrounding edema and impairment of gaseous exchange as alveoli gets filled with fluid. This is the most common intrathoracic injury, and clinical presentation ranging from completely asymptomatic to severe acute respiratory distress syndrome (ARDS). In majority, pulmonary contusions are associated with ribs fracturs. Pediatric patients can develop pulmonary contusion without rib fractures, owing to flexible cartilaginous chest wall. Unlike aspiration pneumonitis and pneumonia, contusions are not confined to anatomical segments and lobes. A mismatch between ventilation and perfusion occurs, thereby creating an intrapulmonary shunt and segmental lung damage with loss of lung compliance. These pathophysiological effects can lead to hypoxemia and hypercapnia. Pulmonary contusions due to blunt mechanisms tend to worsen during first 48–96 hours following trauma. Pneumonia and ARDS are common complications in patients with significant contusions.

The management principle is to ensure adequate oxygenation. This is to be done by giving supplemental oxygen using noninvasive methods such as face mask, high frequency nasal cannula, continuous positive airway pressure (CPAP) mask, or invasive lung protective ventilation depending on the severity of contusions. Simultaneous use of adequate pain control and pulmonary hygiene is paramount. Recently, use of extracorporeal membrane oxygenation (ECMO) also showed promising results in patients with refractory ARDS.[12]

## Pain Management

Adequate analgesia is cornerstone in the management of patients with chest trauma. Rib fractures and underlying contusions are painful and restrict adequate lung expansion leading to atelectasis, mucus plugging, impaired gas exchange, and pneumonia. Initial analgesia should include regular paracetamol and nonsteroidal anti-inflammatory drugs (NSAIDs), pregabalin, etc. If pain control is not adequate using these drugs, transdermal drug delivery patches are also used, especially for opioids. Regional blocks in the form of paravertebral, erector spinae, serratus anterior, and epidural are very effective modality in patients not able to gain adequate pain control on medications. Adequate pain control is critical to assist patients in chest physiotherapy and performing incentive spirometry for good pulmonary hygiene. Few patients, not able to maintain oxygenation may need to be intubated. Recently, SSRF is increasingly being used, especially in flail chest patients. Use of SSRF has shown short-term and long-term benefits to flail chest patients.

## Blunt Cardiac Injury

Blunt cardiac injury (BCI) can present as a spectrum of pathologies ranging from clinically silent, transient arrythmias to deadly cardiac wall rupture due to blunt trauma to chest. Sternal fracture should raise high degree of suspicion for BCI and should be excluded. The right heart wall is most injured due to its position closest to anterior chest wall. Myocardial contusions are the most common manifestation. Rarely, valvular tears or rupture, septal tears, and coronary artery thrombosis or laceration are also seen. Clinically, it can range from chest wall tenderness to wall motion abnormalities, decreased contractility, arrythmia, or conduction abnormalities. Right bundle branch block is a common result of cardiac contusions. These injuries should typically resolve within 24 hours without intervention. But if associated features such as hypotension, pulmonary edema, malignant arrhythmia, or conduction disturbances are present, then it should raise an alarm for clinically significant contusion which needs prompt attention.

Blunt cardiac injury is a diagnosis of exclusion in a polytrauma patient. Most guidelines and literature suggest echocardiogram (ECG) with troponin I test which has highest specificity (85%) and is now rerecommended to rule myocardial injury. Adjunct use of echocardiography in clinically overt cases is advisable to diagnose any heart wall motion abnormality or valvular defects early. Patients with abnormal ECG or positive troponin I should be admitted for observation for at least 48 hours to monitor for dysrhythmias. Dysrhythmias and hypokinesis from myocardial contusion usually resolve within 24 hours. Structural injuries such as myocardial rupture, pericardium rupture, and traumatic valvular injuries require immediate operative repair and immediate surgery.

## Traumatic Aortic Injuries

Aortic injuries, resulting from blunt trauma, are the leading cause of immediate death. Pathologically, aortic injuries range from small tear, laceration, and occlusion to complete rupture. Most of the patients with complete tear will exsanguinate at scene. Patients who survive the initial injury have a high likelihood of survival if the disruption is identified and treated rapidly. The most common site of tears or rupture in the aorta is in the descending portion distal to the left subclavian artery at the ligamentum arteriosum. The clinical features are largely nonspecific and are of associated chest or other injuries. Possible signs include a pulse deficit in any area, particularly lower extremities or the left arm, hypotension, unexplained by other injuries, or hypertension of the upper extremities compared with the lower extremities. Chest X-ray findings suggestive of aortic injuries are widened mediastinum (>8 cm at the level of D4 vertebrae), obscured aortic knob, left apical pleural cap, tracheal deviation to the right, and elevation and rightward deviation of the right mainstem bronchus. Any abnormal finding should be confirmed by CECT scan. Sometimes, ECG-gated CT scan may be required for better characterization of the aortic lesions. In a patient with high-grade aortic injury, major focus is to keep the blood pressure <100 mm Hg and heart rate <100 per minutes till definitive treatment is planned. Short-acting β-blockers and calcium channel blockers are commonly used to achieve desired vitals. Management of aortic injuries consists of thoracic endovascular aortic repair (TEVAR) or surgical repair depending upon the severity in consultation with the cardiothoracic surgeon **(Fig. 8)**.[13]

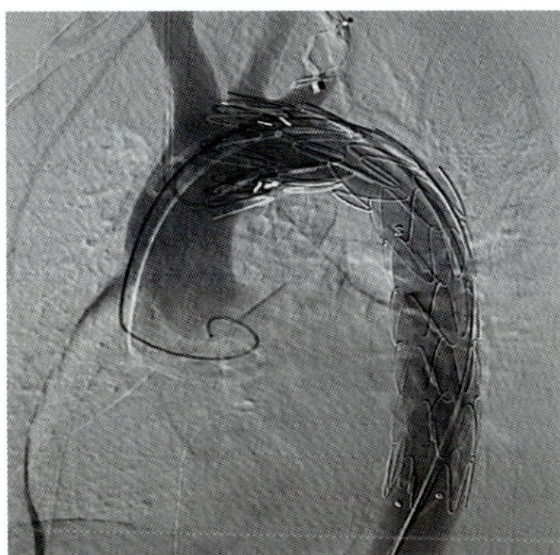

**Fig. 8:** Thoracic endovascular aortic repair (TEVAR) in a case of traumatic aortic injury.

## Traumatic Diaphragmatic Injury

Traumatic diaphragm injuries are present in approximately 0.5% of all trauma patients, with two-thirds of cases due to penetrating mechanisms. In case of penetrating injuries, diaphragmatic rupture needs to be suspected based on location of wounds and involvement of contiguous visceral injury on both sides of diaphragm. In most of the cases, there are no specific clinical and imaging findings on initial assessment. Over the time, due to constant negative intrapleural pressure, diaphragmatic herniation may occur and diagnosis will be made while evaluating the patient with nonspecific chest complaints. In few cases, where there is large diaphragmatic rent during acute injury, abdominal organs may herniate into pleural cavity. These patients may present with respiratory features and chest X-ray may show diaphragmatic hernia in form of presence of bowel loops into pleural cavity with gastric tube tip into pleural cavity during primary survey. CECT scan of torso, a secondary survey adjunct, has sensitivity of 70–80%. In cases with high index of suspicion, diagnostic laparoscopy may be contemplated. Blunt trauma mostly affects left side and typically results from high energy compression mechanisms, often accompanied by other thoracoabdominal injuries.

Management is based on two key principles: (1) The complete reduction of herniated organs into the abdominal cavity and (2) a watertight closure of the defect to prevent recurrence. Stable patients may undergo diagnostic laparoscopy, with subsequent laparoscopic repair or conversion to laparotomy depending on resources and surgeon's expertise. Limited evidence suggests that asymptomatic stable patients with right-sided penetrating wounds can be managed nonoperatively. Surgical repair is indicated in cases with large defects or bile leakage into pleural cavity.

### Blunt Esophageal Rupture

Traumatic esophageal injuries are rare, occurring in <1% of blunt and up to 10% of penetrating trauma cases. The cervical esophagus is commonly affected, followed by thoracic and abdominal esophagus. Clinical findings are often nonspecific. Thoracic esophageal injury may present with concomitant pneumothorax or hemothorax, and drainage from thoracostomy tube containing saliva or food particles necessitates urgent exploration. In missed cases, especially due to localized contamination into mediastinum, patients may present late with fever, erythema, swelling, or airway distress due to mediastinitis. Computed tomography (CT) scan is useful for localizing trajectory of penetrating injuries and assessing risk of esophageal injury. Combining esophagoscopy with CECT scan offers nearly 100% diagnostic accuracy. Management depends on the patient's condition, location, size, and extent of injury, with surgical repair being the preferred treatment option whenever possible. When primary repair is not feasible due to hemodynamic instability, severe contamination, delayed diagnosis or extensive damage, complete diversion (cervical esophagostomy) with feeding jejunostomy, along with debridement and drainage of distal esophagus are recommended. If the patient survives, definitive reconstruction with gastric pull-up or colonic interposition may be planned at a later stage.

Recent literature suggests that endoscopic interventions include endoscopic clipping, with 59–83% success, and covered esophageal stents may be contemplated in stable patients with minimal clinical impact or in surgically unsuitable patients.

## SPECIAL SCENARIOS

### Sternal Fracture

Sternal fracture occurs in 2% of patients with blunt trauma, most have associated with thoracic injuries. Sternal fractures can present with focal tenderness over the sternum or anterior chest wall ecchymosis. Chest X-ray lacks specificity, with 81–93% of fractures visualized on CT scan only A sternal fracture might be indirect evidence of underlying blunt cardiac injury that needs to be ruled out in all these patients. Sternal fractures are managed with multimodal analgesia, respiratory therapy, and early mobility. Operative fixation is used for unstable fractures, fracture displacement, respiratory insufficiency, and uncontrolled severe pain, but long-term data are lacking.

### Chylothorax

Post-traumatic thoracic duct injuries are rare injuries. These injuries present as drainage of chyle (milky white fluid) from ICD after initial hemorrhagic drainage. The diagnosis is clinical supplemented with biochemical analysis of drainage fluid. Depending upon amount of fluid drained, treatment options

| **TABLE 2:** *Denver's criteria:* Rib fracture admission algorithm. | |
|---|---|
| ***Parameter*** | ***Points*** |
| Respiratory rate (RR) >18 | 1 |
| Incentive spirometry <75% predicted | 1 |
| Numeric pain score >5 | 1 |
| Poor cough | 1 |
| Age >65 years | 1 |
| >3 fractures | 1 |

| **TABLE 3:** Sequential clinical assessment of respiratory function (SCARF) score. | |
|---|---|
| ***Parameter*** | ***Points*** |
| Numeric pain score >5 | 1 |
| Incentive spirometry <50% predicted | 1 |
| Respiratory rate >20 | 1 |
| Poor cough | 1 |

range from dietary changes to surgical ligation of thoracic duct. Recently, embolization of thoracic duct also being used in selective cases.[14]

*Isolated subcutaneous emphysema:* Isolated subcutaneous emphysema with no underlying rib fractures or hemopneumothorax in a hemodynamically stable patient may be managed with close monitoring without ICD insertion at a resourceful healthcare facility after CECT scan of torso.

*Isolated rib fractures:* Often dilemma is whether patient with isolated rib fractures can be managed as an outpatient or not. Certain objective criteria like Denver's criteria may be helpful in such situations. Patients having Denver's score >2 need to be admitted for observation **(Table 2)**. Recently, sequential clinical assessment of respiratory function (SCARF) score is proposed to assess the progress of patients with chest trauma **(Table 3)**.[15]

## CONCLUSION

Thoracic injuries are common form of injuries with wide spectrum of presentations and are responsible for high mortality in patients with polytrauma. Most of these injuries need vigilant evaluation and timely interventions. These interventions such as endotracheal intubation, needle thoracocentesis, ICD insertion, etc. are simple and lifesaving and may be performed by the primary care doctors working in ED. Patients with complex and severe chest injuries need expert surgical and interventional care. Recently, inclusion of various advanced imaging such as digital subtraction angiography (DSA), ECG-gated CT scan, and procedures such as VATS, SSRF, TEVAR, embolization, and vascular stenting in the armamentarium of trauma surgeons has increased their scope of managing patients with chest trauma. However, selection of a patient for such procedures is of utmost importance for a favorable outcome. In a resource-constraint setting, timely recognition and initial management of life-threatening injuries and subsequent transfer to a closest and appropriate facility are the key to success.

## REFERENCES


1. Initial Assessment: Primary survey. In: ATLS Course Student Manual: American College of Surgeons-Committee on Trauma. 2025; 11th Ed: 4-17.
2. Gupta B, Bagaria D, Kumar A, Perveen F. Successful airway management of traumatic complete tracheal transection. BMJ Case Rep. 2022;15(12):e251688.
3. Kumar A, Vaidyanathan R, Priyadarshini P, Bagaria D, Choudhary N, Alam J, et al. Clinical determinants for survival following emergency thoracotomy in trauma patients: An 8-year experience from a level 1 trauma centre. Chin J Traumatol. 2025;:S1008-1275(25)00062-8.
4. Figueroa JF, Karam BS, Gomez J, Milia D, Morris RS, Dodgion C, et al. The 35-mm rule to guide pneumothorax management: increases appropriate observation and decreases unnecessary chest tubes. J Trauma Acute Care Surg. 2022; 92(6):951-7.
5. Gilbert RW, Fontebasso AM, Park L, Tran A, Lampron J. The management of occult hemothorax in adults with thoracic trauma: A systematic review and meta-analysis. J Trauma Acute Care Surg. 2020;89(6):1225-32.
6. Kumar A, Gora D, Bagaria D, Priyadarshini P, Choudhary N, Priyadarshi A, et al. Outcomes of video-assisted thoracic surgery-guided early evacuation of traumatic hemothorax: A randomized pilot study at level I trauma center. J Emerg Trauma Shock. 2024;17(2):73-9.
7. Beeton G, Ngatuvai M, Breeding T, Andrade R, Zagales R, Khan A, et al. Outcomes of pigtail catheter placement versus chest tube placement in adult thoracic trauma patients: a systematic review and meta-analysis. Am Surg. 2023;89(6):2743-54.
8. Priyadarshi A, Gupta S, Priyadarshini P, Kumar A, Alam J, Bagaria D, et al. Role of low-pressure negative pleural suction in patients with thoracic trauma-a randomized controlled trial. Eur J Trauma Emerg Surg. 2024;50(5):2105-11.
9. Teyi T, James JD, Kumar V, Bagaria D, Kumar A, Choudhary N, et al. No role of antibiotics in patients with chest trauma requiring inter-costal drain: a pilot randomized controlled trial. Eur J Trauma Emerg Surg. 2023;49(2):1113-20.
10. Sermonesi G, Bertelli R, Pieracci FM, Balogh ZJ, Coimbra R, Galante JM, et al. Surgical stabilization of rib fractures (SSRF): the WSES and CWIS position paper. World J Emerg Surg. 2024;19(1):33.
11. James JD, Choudhary N, Bagaria D, Boddeda J, Kumar A, Priyadarshini P, et al. Benefits of rib fixation utilizing low-cost materials: a randomized pilot trial. J Surg Res. 2024;299:322-8.
12. Zhang Y, Zhang L, Huang X, Ma N, Wang P, Li L, et al. ECMO in adult patients with severe trauma: a systematic review and meta-analysis. Eur J Med Res. 2023;28(1):412.

13. Kumar A, Choudhary N, Priyadarshi P, Bagaria D, Alam J, Soni KD, et al. Kumar S Clinical Spectrum and Outcome Analysis of Blunt Thoracic Aortic Injuries: a 10-year Experience from a Level I Trauma Center. Ind J Surg. 2023; 85(Suppl 2):371-80.
14. Dar PMUD, Gamanagatti S, Priyadarshini P, Kumar S. Traumatic chylothorax: a dilemma to surgeons and interventionists. BMJ Case Rep. 2021;14(5):e238961.
15. Hardin KS, Leasia KN, Haenel J, Moore EE, Burlew CC, Pieracci FM. The Sequential Clinical Assessment of Respiratory Function (SCARF) score: a dynamic pulmonary physiologic score that predicts adverse outcomes in critically ill rib fracture patients. J Trauma Acute Care Surg. 2019;87(6):1260-8.

CHAPTER 10

# Management of Axilla in Breast Cancer

*Divya Dsilva, Toshita Jain, Dhaval Vasa, Shalaka Joshi*

## INTRODUCTION

Status of axillary lymph nodes (ALNs) is the most important prognostic factor in breast cancer and adjuvant treatment decisions are made based on the status of ALN. A complete axillary nodal clearance used to be the standard of care. However, surgery for the breast primary and axilla both have seen a significant trend toward de-escalation as systemic therapies expand. This is especially true in early breast cancer (EBC) (cT1/2, cN0/1). In this chapter, we describe the status of management of axilla in early as well as locally advanced breast cancers (LABCs), upfront, and postsystemic therapy.

Halsted's theory of orderly progression of disease reigned in the 20th century and an aggressive resection of the entire skin along with breast tissue and the entire fibrofatty and lymph node tissue of axilla was carried out for all patients, irrespective of nodal stage. However, only 40% of patients survived for 5 years despite aggressive surgery.[1] Bernard Fischer hypothesized breast cancer to be systemic at inception. Less radical surgery was tested in systematic randomized trials establishing the role of breast conservation surgery in suitable cases. Systemic therapy and radiation therapy were evolving simultaneously. Better understanding of tumor biology and molecular subtypes has led to treatment based on tumor biology and surgical de-escalation has been feasible. This has helped in reducing long-term sequelae of treatment as all patients with negative ALN do not require a complete axillary lymph node dissection (ALND).

## MANAGEMENT OF AXILLA IN EARLY BREAST CANCER—PER PRIMUM SURGERY

### cN0 and Sentinel Node Biopsy pN0

Surgical assessment of ALN is standard as clinical examination and subsequently, imaging modalities such as CT, PET, and MRI are inaccurate in axillary staging. Hence, 15–30% of times, a clinicoradiologically negative axilla may be false negative. The role of ALND has been scrutinized in this setting and sentinel node mapping and biopsy was successfully established for clinically node negative axilla. A "sentinel node" is the first echelon node to be involved with cancer as it is anatomically the first draining node from the tumor. Guiliano et al. demonstrated the feasibility of doing sentinel node biopsy (SNB) in breast cancer and that it can accurately predict the ALN status, in 1994.[2] Since then, several randomized trials have been conducted to establish the safety of SNB in EBC as compared to complete ALND. A false-negative rate (FNR) of 5–10% was found to be noninferior for long-term disease-free survival (DFS) and local or regional recurrence-free survival. The morbidity data also supported SNB over ALND as the short-term and long-term side effects of ALND such as seromas, paresthesia, shoulder mobility, and lymphedema were significantly lesser with SNB.

The first attempt to establish that axillary surgery is unnecessary in all patients was NSABP-B04 wherein patients with clinically negative axilla received no axillary surgery versus axillary radiation versus ALND with no difference in DFS.[3] This trial also postulated that axillary radiotherapy (RT) was equivalent to ALND. Although 40% of patients in the ALND arm had positive ALN further proving fallacy of clinical evaluation, also, only half of them had a regional recurrence. However, the trial is old and systemic therapy options were not well-developed then. Several trails subsequently proved the noninferiority of SNB over ALND in the cN0 setting, notably the NSABP-B32 and the ALMANAC trials. **Table 1** enumerates all the studies done in EBC establishing the safety of SNB and their advantages. Today, dual-tracer SNB is the standard of care in cN0 EBC. And if pN0, no further axillary treatment is indicated. Addition of indocyanine green fluorescence dye has further made dual tracer SNB feasible by eliminating the need of injection of radiocolloid and nuclear medicine facility.[4-7]

## Axillary Sampling

Nottingham 4 node sampling as a technique to stage axilla was described previously. Tanaka et al. in 2006 evaluated four nodes axillary sampling (4NAS) in management of EBC. This technique involved selectively excising four palpable lymph nodes, minimizing morbidity. With an FNR of 6.5%, 4NAS demonstrated high sensitivity (93.4%) and specificity (100%), offering a cost-effective and reliable alternative to axillary node clearance.[8] Parmar et al. evaluated the effectiveness of SNB and low-axillary sampling (LAS) in staging ALN in cN0 breast cancer patients. LAS was described as a distinct procedure with anatomical boundaries—superiorly the intercostobrachial nerve, inferiorly the angular vein, medially serratus first and second digitations, and laterally the lateral border of the latissimus dorsi muscle. It documented an FNR of 10.5% for LAS, comparable to 12.7% of SNB. Both techniques showed similar accuracy, with LAS offering advantages such as reduced surgical complexity and lower costs, 23% less expensive than SNB, making it particularly suitable for resource-limited settings. The vagueness of

**TABLE 1:** Studies evaluating the role of SNB in early breast cancer.

| *Trial* | *Year* | *Inclusion criteria* | *Sample size* | *SLN identification rate* | *False-negative rate* | *Disease-free survival* | *Lymphedema rate* | *Axillary recurrence rate* |
|---|---|---|---|---|---|---|---|---|
| Veronesi et al.[4] | 2003 | cT ≤2 cm<br>Undergoing BCS | 649 | 99% | 4.6% | 88% in ALND arm vs. 89.9% in SNB arm at 79 months median follow-up | - | 1.1% in SNB arm |
| ALMANAC[5] | 2006 | cN0 | 1,031 | 98% | Not reported | - | 5% in SNB group vs. 13% in ALND group at 12 months | 0.2% in SNB group vs. 0.8% in ALND group |
| SNAC[6] | 2009 | cT ≤3 cm<br>cN0 | 1,088 | 94% | 5.5% | - | 4.2% in SNB group vs. 6.9% in ALND group (increase in arm volume >15%) | - |
| NSABP-B32[7] | 2007 | cT ≤5 cm<br>cN0 | 5,611 | Not reported | 9.8% | 82.4% in ALND vs. 81.5% in ALND alone group at median follow-up of 7.9 years | 8% in SNB group vs. 14% in ALND group | <1% in both arms |

(ALND: axillary lymph node dissection; BCS: breast-conserving surgery; SLN: sentinel lymph node; SNB: sentinel node biopsy) the earlier described 4NAS was mitigated by this more anatomical technique. The findings supported LAS as a cost-effective and reliable alternative for axillary staging in breast cancer.[9]

## cN0 and Sentinel Node Biopsy pN0(i+)/pN1mi

With extensive step sectioning of the ALN, molecular techniques and immunohistochemistry (IHC), nodal assessment improved. NSABP-B32 study reported an additional nodal positivity of almost 15% when SNB negative ALN was sectioned vigorously.[10] Immunohistochemical evaluation of ALN was also carried out in some studies. A subsequent systematic review reported occult nodal positivity to be between 9 and 42% and this conferred poorer disease-free and overall survival (OS).[11] The American Joint Committee on Cancer incorporated (1) isolated tumor cells (ITCs) (<0.2 mm or <200 cells) (pN0i+), (2) micrometastases (0.2–2 mm) (pN1mi or >200 cells), and (3) macrometastases (>2 mm) (pN+) based on size of the metastatic focus. AJCC 8th edition does not upstage the disease for ITC but does upstage the nodal stage to pN1mi for micrometastatic disease.[12] As per ACOSOG Z0010, the presence of disseminated tumor cells (DTCs) in bone marrow or ITCs in ALN did not affect long-term outcomes and hence treatment does not change as per the presence of these.[13] An important question was whether the presence of ITCs or micrometastases in ALN warrant additional treatment like ALND and adjuvant systemic therapy. Studies using the SEER database have shown that micrometastatic disease has an intermediate prognosis compared to no lymph node involvement and macrometastatic disease.[14] Several trials both randomized and non-randomized studied the presence of micrometastatic disease in SNB and otherwise.

The IBCSG 23-01(International Breast Cancer Study Group) multicenter phase 3 randomized controlled trial evaluated the need for completion ALND exclusively for presence of micrometastatic disease in SNB. At 10-year follow-up, there was no significant difference in local, axillary recurrence, and DFS for patients who underwent SNB alone. There were significantly lower rates of lymphedema (13% in ALND vs. 4% in no ALND) and sensory neuropathy (19% in ALND vs. 13% in SNB alone group) at 10-year follow-up. Most patients had tumors <3 cm in size (92%), 90% had breast-conserving surgery (BCS), and 96% had systemic therapy.[15] The multicenter AATRM randomized trial also showed similar results ($n = 247$). On 5-year follow-up, there were similar disease recurrence rates in patients who underwent ALND versus observation.[16] No survival advantage was observed despite finding additional nodal metastases in 13% in the ALND group in both studies.

The MIRROR study in Netherlands divided 2,707 patients having ITCs and micrometastases into three groups—patients without lymph node metastases who did not receive systemic treatment (group 1, $n = 856$); patients with micrometastases/ITC in sentinel lymph node (SLN) and did not receive systemic therapy (group 2, $n = 856$) and patients with micrometastases/ITC who received systemic therapy (group 3, $n = 995$). This retrospective analysis showed poorer 5-year DFS of group 2 as compared to group 1 (76.5% vs. 85.7%; $p < 0.001$) with equal negative impact for ITCs and micrometastases. Systemic therapy did impact survival in patients with ITCs/micrometastases (group 2 vs. 3–76.5% vs. 86.2%, $p < 0.001$) with a 10% gain in DFS. The prognostic impact of micrometastases and ITCs was comparable. However, the results of this study were published in 2009, an era where chemotherapy was given only to those N0 patients in the trial whose 10-year predicted survival was <80% further debating the clinical significance of micrometastases and ITCs.[17]

The prospective SENOMIC (omission of axillary lymph node dissection in SENtinel NOde MICrometases) trial showed that event-free survival was excellent and higher than anticipated (96.3%) in patients with breast cancer and sentinel node micrometastases despite omission of ALND, at 3 years of follow-up. However, patients who had mastectomy without adjuvant RT had a significantly higher risk of recurrence than those who underwent BCS [hazard ratio (HR): 2.91, 1.25–6.75].[18]

ACOSOG Z0010 was a prospective observational study in which cT1-2, cN0 patients underwent bilateral iliac crest bone marrow aspiration and IHC on histologically negative nodes. Of these, 3,904 (76.3%) patients had histologically negative SLN. An additional 10.5% patients had IHC positive occult lymph node involvement, and bone marrow involvement was identified on IHC in 3% patients. It was shown that there was no difference in local, regional, or distant recurrences in those with IHC-detected nodal disease versus those without. On multivariable analysis, presence of bone marrow disease or IHC-positive nodes did not have an impact on OS. However, the presence of micrometastatic disease in bone marrow predicted a poorer OS whereas IHC-positive SNB did not affect it.[13] Routine use of IHC to detect micrometastases in histologically negative nodes is thus not warranted. They further prospectively randomized patients with 1–2 positive nodes (about 40% with micrometastatic nodes) to receive completion of ALND versus observation. At a median follow-up of 9.3 years, the 10-year OS was 86.3% in the sentinel lymph node dissection (SLND) alone group and 83.6% in the ALND group [HR: 0.85 (one-sided 95% confidence interval (CI): 0–1.16); noninferiority $p = 0.02$].[19]

The National Institute of Oncology, Budapest conducted a single-center randomized controlled trial (OTOASAR) of patients presenting with cN0 disease and cT size <3 cm and pSLN+ status to undergo completion ALND or regional nodal irradiation (RNI). Out of the 2,106 patients, 25% had positive SLN. Of the 526 patients with positive SLN, 474 were evaluable—244 had ALND (with an additional nodal positivity of 38.5%) and 230 RNI. 33.5% of patients in the RNI group and 7% in the ALND group had micrometastatic nodes.[20] At 97 months mean follow-up, axillary recurrence was 2% and 1.7% in the ALND and RNI arm respectively, which was the primary endpoint of the study. DFS and OS also were not significantly different. AMAROS—After Mapping of the Axilla: Radiotherapy or Surgery (EORTC 10981-22023 - A) trial studied the role of completion ALND versus axillary RT in SLN-positive patients with micro-/macrometastatic disease with the primary endpoint of axillary recurrence rates and secondary endpoints of morbidity—lymphedema. 25% of patients had micrometastatic disease. 12% patients who had ITCs were excluded from the study. They showed comparable control in axillary recurrence, DFS, and OS with either treatment modalities, however, showed significantly reduced rates of lymphedema with axillary RT (11% vs. 23%) at 5 years.[21] **Table 2** summarizes all the studies in the setting of micrometastatic axillary nodes.

### cN0 and SNB pN1

In most SLN trials, the additional non-SLN burden is between 30 and 40%. Conventionally, for macrometastatic lymph nodes in axilla, a complete ALND was considered necessary. Recent studies have explored the role of observation and axillary radiation or RNI in patients with 1–2 positive macrometastatic nodes. The SENOMAC study included patients with primary tumors, cT <5 cm, cN0, and 1–2 positive nodes with macrometastases on SNB; and were randomized to ALND versus observation. The 5-year axillary recurrence, DFS, and OS were comparable in the two arms.[22] SINODAR-ONE study also compared SNB alone versus ALND in patients with T1–T2 breast cancer and one or two positive SLN. The findings suggested that preserving axillary lymph nodes without full dissection did not compromise outcomes in selected patients, potentially reducing complications like lymphedema.[23] Additionally, a Japanese multi-institutional prospective cohort study examined outcomes in patients with 1–3 positive SLNs (including macrometastases). It was found that SNB alone, even in the presence of macrometastases, resulted in low regional node recurrence rates—around 2% at 5 years—comparable to those who underwent ALND.[24] **Table 2** summarizes all the axillary conservation strategies in the macrometastatic nodal setting.

## EARLY BREAST CANCER—OMITTING AXILLARY SURGERY WHEN C/RN0

Further de-escalation/omitting axillary surgery altogether was studied in the SOUND and INSEMA trials,[25,26] both of which proved the noninferiority of "no SNB" in patients with clinicoradiologically negative axilla at a nodal positivity rate of 15% in the control arm. In both studies, >95% patients were hormone receptor positive, human epidermal growth factor receptor 2 (HER2)

**TABLE 2:** Studies showing results of micro- or macrometastatic disease after SNB.

| *Sr. No.* | *Trial (year of publication)* | *Sample size* | *Inclusion criteria* | *Randomization* | *End points* | *Results* |
|---|---|---|---|---|---|---|
| ***Trials which studied micrometastatic disease in SLN*** | | | | | | |
| 1. | *IBCSG 23-01 (2007)*[15] | 934 | cT1-2; 1 or more sentinel nodes positive for metastases <2 mm size | 1:1 to ALND vs. no ALND | • DFS (primary)<br>• Locoregional recurrences and axillary failure rates<br>• Lymphedema | • *DFS:* 74.9% vs. 76.8%<br>• Similar local recurrences<br>• Lymphedema 13% vs. 4% |
| 2. | *AATRM 048/13/2000 (2013)*[16] | 247 | T size <3.5 cm, clinical N0 M0 with micrometastatic SN | 1:1 to complete ALND vs. no ALND | Disease recurrence rates | Similar disease recurrence rates 1% vs. 2.5% ($p = 0.348$) |
| 3. | *MIRROR study (2013)*[17] | 2,707 | • cT <1 cm (irrespective of grade)<br>• cT <3 cm (grades 1 and 2)<br>• cN0 | • Three groups<br>• Cohort study | DFS | *5-year DFS:*<br>• *Group 1:* 85.7%<br>• *Group 2:* 76.5%<br>• *Group 3:* 86.2% |
| 4. | *SENOMIC (2009)*[18] | 566 | Sentinel node micro-metastases with BCT/ mastectomy | Prospective Cohort trial | Event-free survival (EFS) | 3-year EFS = 96.2% |
| ***Trials which studied presence of micro- and macro-metastases in SLN and its further management options with outcomes*** | | | | | | |
| 5. | *ACOSOG Z0010 (2012)*[13] | 5,119 | T1-2 N0 M0 who had SLN positive at surgery | 3,904 (76.3%) had H&E negative SLN and rest had H&E negative IHC positive SLN | Clinicopathological factors associated with LRR | • Hormone receptor negative status ($p = 0.004$)<br>• Younger age ($p = 0.047$) associated with reduced LRR |

*Contd…*

*Contd...*

| Sr. No. | *Trial (year of publication)* | *Sample size* | *Inclusion criteria* | *Randomization* | *End points* | *Results* |
|---|---|---|---|---|---|---|
| ***Trials which studied presence of micro- and macro-metastases in SLN and its further management options with outcomes*** | | | | | | |
| 6. | *ACOSOG Z0011 (2010)*[19] | 891 | T1-2, clinically N0 patients with ≤2 SLN positive | 1:1 randomization to no ALND vs. ALND | • OS<br>• DFS<br>• Local recurrence | • No difference in 10-year OS (86.3% vs. 83.6%; HR: 0.93; $p = 0.72$)<br>• DFS (80.2% vs. 78.2%; HR: 0.9, $p = 0.51$)<br>• Local recurrence (83% vs. 81.2%; HR: 0.93, $p = 0.66$) |
| 7. | *AMAROS (2014)*[21] | 4,806 | cT1-2 N0 undergoing SNB | 1:1 randomized to ALND vs. axillary RT (1,425 patients with positive SLN) | • Axillary recurrence rate<br>• DFS<br>• OS<br>• Lymphedema rates | • 5-year axillary recurrence rates 0.43% vs. 1.19%<br>• *DFS:* 86.9 vs. 82.7% (HR: 1.18 95% CI: 0.93–1.51; $p = 0.18$)<br>• *OS:* 93.3% vs. 92.5% (HR: 1.17 95% CI: 0.85–1.62; $p = 0.34$)<br>• Lymphedema rates 23% vs. 11% |
| 8. | *OTOASOR (2017)*[20] | 2,106 | cT < 3 cm N0 | 1:1 randomization to ALND vs. RNI; 474 patients with positive SNB (244 vs. 230 patients) | • Axillary recurrence (primary)<br>• OS, DFS (secondary) | • 8-year follow-up<br>• *Axillary recurrence:* 2% vs. 1.9% ($p = 1.0$)<br>• *OS:* 77.9% vs. 84.8% ($p = 0.6$)<br>• *DFS:* 72.1% vs. 77.4% ($p = 0.51$) |

***Trials summarizing role of omission of ALND in presence of macrometastatic disease***

| *Trial* | *Inclusion criteria* | *Sample size* | *DFS* | *OS* | *Axillary recurrence rate* |
|---|---|---|---|---|---|
| *SENOMAC (2024)*[22] | • cT1-T3; cN0<br>• pN1 (1–2 LN) | 2,540 | 88.7% in ALND group vs. 89.7% in SNB group | 92% in ALND group vs. 92.9% in SNB group | 0.5% in ALND group vs. 0.4% in SNB group |
| *SINODAR ONE (2022)*[23] | • cT1-T2; cN0<br>• pN1 (1–2 LN) | 889 | 95.7% in ALND group vs. 94.1% in SNB group | 97.8% in ALND group vs. 98.9% in SNB group | <1% |

(ALND: axillary lymph node dissection; BCS: breast-conserving surgery; BCT: breast-conserving therapy; CI: confidence interval; DFS: disease-free survival; HR: hazard ratio; IHC: immunohistochemistry; LRR: locoregional recurrence; OS: overall survival; SLN: sentinel lymph node; SN: sentinel node; SNB: sentinel node biopsy)

**TABLE 3:** Axillary surgery omission trials.

| *Trial* | *Sample size* | *Eligibility* | *FNR* | *Results* |
|---|---|---|---|---|
| *SOUND*[25] | 1,463 | cT ≤2 cm; cN0; undergoing BCT followed by RT | 13.7% | • 5-year DDFS;<br>• *SNB group:* 97.7%<br>• *No axillary surgery group:* 98% |
| *INSEMA*[26] | 4,858 | cT ≤5 cm; cN0; undergoing BCS | Not reported | *iDFS:* 91.9% in surgery omission group vs. 91.7% in surgery group |
| *BOOG 2013-08 (Dutch)*[28] | 1,735 | cT ≤5 cm; cN0; undergoing BCT followed by RT | Not reported | 5-year and 10-year LRR (awaiting results) |
| *NAUTILUS*[29] | 1,734 | cT ≤5 cm; cN0; undergoing BCT followed by RT | Not reported | 5-year iDFS (awaiting results) |

(BCS: breast-conserving surgery; BCT: breast-conserving therapy; DDFS: distant disease-free survival; FNR: false-negative rate; iDFS: invasive disease-free survival; LRR: locoregional recurrence; SNB: sentinel node biopsy)

negative, and low-grade and median tumor size was <1.5 cm. There were very few pT2 patients. It is likely that a significant proportion of these patients would be screen detected with luminal-A cancers which are known to be of better biology. Both the trials also relied upon preoperative ultrasound and if necessary, guided fine needle aspiration cytology (FNAC) from the nodes to confirm N0 status. The accuracy and reliability of ultrasound is questionable in real-world setting.[27] **Table 3** summarizes the studies involving no SNB and axillary ultrasound in EBC.[28,29]

The combination of insights from these trials has shifted clinical practices significantly. Most institutions have adopted SNB as a standard approach for node negative and node positive tumors, minimizing the reliance on ALND. However, majority of patients included in these studies were of luminal subtype A and had low-grade T1 tumors. Some proportions of them are also likely to be screen detected, impalpable, and asymptomatic, representing a subset of breast cancer with good biology. Hence, generalized extrapolation in the Indian setting is not recommended. In a comparison of Indian node negative cohort with that of ACOSOG-Z11, the median pT size was >3 cm, rate of diagnosis of micrometastatic nodes was <1%, and an additional 35% nodes were positive after complete ALND.[30] Also, in a cohort of patients with positive axillary nodes, a median of 3 were positive, with level 3 involvement of >25%, and 40% patients had N2/3 nodal involvement.[31]

Although these studies support a growing trend toward less invasive axillary management, especially when combined with adjuvant therapies like RNI, more personalization of locoregional treatment may be necessary while making individual treatment plans. Axillary nodes remain important for staging, although treatment decisions are increasingly driven by tumor molecular subtype and overall risk assessment, rather than anatomical stage alone. In essence, the paradigm is shifting from a "one-size-fits-all" surgical approach to precision care—where the least invasive, most effective treatment is guided by both clinical and molecular profiles.

## POSTCHEMOTHERAPY APPROACH TO AXILLA

With the advent of risk adapted strategies and better choices of targeted and immunotherapy treatments, the utilization of preoperative systemic treatment in EBC has increased. If clinicoradiologically node negative before starting chemotherapy, SNB can be used in the postchemotherapy setting with acceptable FNR.[32]

Traditionally, ALND has been considered the standard of care for patients with prechemotherapy node-positive disease. The management of the axilla in EBC patients who have received neoadjuvant chemotherapy (NACT) has evolved significantly in the past two decades. With better systemic therapy, 40–75% of previously node positive patients have negative axilla postchemotherapy, with expected higher response rates in triple negative and HER2-positive tumors.[33] Less invasive approaches such as SNB, targeted axillary dissection (TAD), and LAS are being investigated in the postchemotherapy setting as well.

## PRECHEMOTHERAPY AND POSTCHEMOTHERAPY cN0

The MD Anderson Institute published the largest single institution study showing adequacy of postchemotherapy SNB in the subset of patients who were cN0 before chemotherapy. A total of 3,746 patients with cT1-3, cN0 breast cancer underwent SNB from 1994 to 2007. Of the patients, 575 (15.3%) underwent SNB after chemotherapy and 3,171 (84.7%) underwent surgery first. SLN identification rates were 97.4% in the NACT group and 98.7% in the surgery first group ($p = 0.017$). FNRs were similar between groups [5/84 (5.9%) in neoadjuvant vs. 22/542 (4.1%)] in the surgery first group ($p = 0.39$). Adjusting for clinical stage revealed no differences in local-regional recurrences, disease-free or OS between groups.[32] Xing et al.'s 2006 meta-analysis of 21 studies comprising 1,273 patients reported a pooled FNR of 12%, identification rate of 90%, and sensitivity of 88%.[34] Kelly et al.'s meta-analysis of over 1,700 patients post-NACT reported a lower FNR of 8%, with improved accuracy when dual tracers and same-day mapping were employed.[35] Hence, postchemotherapy SNB is feasible in patients who are prechemotherapy clinicoradiologically proven N0.[36]

## PRECHEMOTHERAPY cN1 AND POSTCHEMOTHERAPY cN0 and pN0

Multiple studies have tested SNB in the post-NACT setting. The ACOSOG Z1071 trial enrolled 756 patients with prechemotherapy biopsy-confirmed node-positive patients who became clinically node-negative after NACT. They found an FNR of 12.6% with SNB. The FNR improved to 6.8% with the retrieval of three or more SLNs using dual tracers.[37] However, the median number of harvested nodes was 3 and only 33% patients had 4 or more nodes retrieved in SNB. The SENTINA trial was a large, four-arm prospective, non-randomized European study that investigated SNB before and/or after NACT. In Arm-A, SNB was performed before NACT in cN0 patients; Arm-B involved a second SNB after NACT in those who had SNB before; Arm-C performed SNB only post-NACT in cN1 patients who converted to cN0; and Arm-D involved SNB in patients who remained node-positive after NACT. Arm C, the most clinically relevant for de-escalation, showed an FNR of 14.2%, which improved to 8.6% with dual tracer and removal of three or more SLNs.[38] The SN FNAC trial examined 417 patients with biopsy-proven axillary metastases who underwent SNB post-NACT. The overall FNR was 13%, but it dropped to below 5% when three or more SLNs were removed and ITCs were included in the analysis.[39] Similarly, the French GANEA 2 trial reported an identification rate of 95% and FNR of 11.7% in cN1 patients following NACT, with residual tumor size >5 mm and lympho-vascular invasion as key predictors of residual nodal disease.[39] Parmar et al. validated LAS as compared to dual-tracer SNB in a large cohort of predominantly locally advanced cN1 disease. LAS demonstrated superior outcomes with an FNR of 9.9% compared to 19.7% for SNB, particularly when three or more nodes were sampled, where the FNR dropped to 8.8%.[40]

### Targeted Axillary Dissection

Despite improvements in SNB, concerns remain regarding its accuracy post-NACT due to potential fibrosis or obliteration of previously involved nodes and inability to identify accurately the prechemotherapy positive node. This catalyzed interest in targeted axillary dissection (TAD), a hybrid technique combining SNB with the removal of a prechemotherapy-marked positive node. Caudle et al. (JCO 2016) pioneered this approach, demonstrating that TAD significantly reduced the FNR to 2% compared to 10.1% for SNB alone. In their study of 208 patients, the clipped node was successfully retrieved in most cases, enhancing staging reliability, however 22% of the clipped/marked node was not the sentinel node.[41]

The *MARI* (Marking the Axillary lymph node with Radioactive Iodine seed) trial used Iodine-125 seeds placed in biopsy-confirmed positive nodes before

NACT. In 174 patients, the FNR was reduced to 7% when selective removal of the marked node was combined with axillary imaging, although 35% of the sentinel node did not have the marked node.[42] Additional innovations include *carbon tattooing*, which involves intranodal carbon injection at the time of biopsy to facilitate accurate intraoperative identification. Choy et al. demonstrated that this technique yields an FNR of approximately 3.5% in small cohort studies, making it a viable option in centers lacking access to radioisotopes. 27% of the marked node was not concordant with the sentinel node.[43]

*Magseed (Endomag Ltd., UK)* is a small paramagnetic metallic seed (5 mm × 1 mm) that is deployed using an 18-gauge needle into the target lymph node under ultrasound or mammographic guidance, either before or after NACT. The Magseed is detected intraoperatively with the Sentimag probe, which senses magnetic signals with millimeter accuracy. This method allows precise localization even in deep tissues, is MRI-compatible, and poses no radiation exposure risk. Clinical studies have reported a retrieval success rate of over 95% and an FNR < 5% in patients undergoing TAD with Magseed localization. In 17% patients, the marked node was not a sentinel node.[44]

*SAVI SCOUT (Cianna Medical, USA)* is a radar-based reflector system. The reflector is a 12 mm by 1 mm electromagnetic transponder placed into the clipped lymph node using a needle deployment system. It is detected intraoperatively using an infrared light and microimpulse radar hand piece, which gives both distance and directional feedback, improving surgical precision. Unlike radioactive seeds, the reflector can be placed days to weeks before surgery. In a systematic review evaluates radar reflector localizations (RRLs) performance during TAD, assessing localization and retrieval rates, the concordance between marked lymph node biopsy (MLNB) and SNB, and the pathological complete response (pCR) in clinically node-positive patients post-NST was assessed. Four studies (252 TAD procedures) met the inclusion criteria, with a 99.6% (98.9–100) successful localization rate, 100% retrieval rate, and 81% (76–86) concordance rate between SNB and MLNB. The average duration from RRL deployment to surgery was 52 days (range:1–202). pCR was observed in 42%. SAVI SCOUT's benefits include no radiation exposure, minimal migration risk, and suitability for deep tissue localization without reliance on radioisotopes.[45]

The National Comprehensive Cancer Network (NCCN) recommends clip placement in biopsy-proven positive nodes before NACT. SNB post-NACT may be considered in cN1 patients who convert to cN0, provided dual tracers and ≥3 SLNs are retrieved. TAD is encouraged where feasible.[46] **Tables 4 and 5** summarize the studies involving SNB and TAD in the postchemotherapy setting.

**TABLE 4:** Key trials and studies in postchemotherapy management of axilla.

| *Trial* | *Population (cN+)* | *Procedure* | *FNR (%)* | *Remarks* |
|---|---|---|---|---|
| ACOSOG Z1071 (2013)[38] | 756 | SNB ± Clip | 12.6 | FNR reduced to 6.8% with clip removal |
| SENTINA (2013)[39] | 1,022 | SNB (post-NACT) | 14.2 | Improved with dual tracer, ≥3 SLNs |
| SN FNAC Study (2015)[39] | 417 | SNB post-FNAC proven | 13.0 | FNR dropped to <5% with ≥3 SLNs and ITC inclusion |
| GANEA 2 (2015)[40] | 289 | SNB | 11.7 | FNR higher in cN1 |
| TMH (India) (2020)[39] | 751 | LAS vs. SNB | 9.9 (LAS) | LAS superior to SNB |

(FNAC: fine needle aspiration cytology; FNR: false-negative rate; ITC: isolated tumor cell; LAS: low-axillary sampling; SLN: sentinel lymph node; SNB: sentinel node biopsy)

**TABLE 5:** Key trials and studies in targeted axillary dissection methods.

| *Trial/study* | *Population* | *Procedure* | *FNR (%)* | *Remarks* |
|---|---|---|---|---|
| Caudle (TAD)[42] | 208 | SNB + Clip | 2.0 | TAD significantly reduces FNR |
| MARI study[43] | 174 | Iodine seed marked node excision post-NACT | 7.0 | FNR improved by selective node removal |
| Carbon tattooing[44] | 28 | Carbon dye node marking | ~3.5 | High intraoperative visibility post-NACT |
| Magseed—meta-analysis[45] | 494 | Metallic seed marked node-excised using magnetic probe | 4.2 | Radiation free and low FNR |
| SAVI SCOUT meta-analysis[46] | 252 | Electromagnetic transponder placed into clipped node, identified using radar reflector localization | 4–5% | Radiation free, 100% retrieval rate, suitable for deep-tissue localization |

(FNR: false-negative rate; NACT: neoadjuvant chemotherapy; SNB: sentinel node biopsy; TAD: targeted axillary dissection)

## MANAGEMENT OF AXILLA IN ADVANCED DISEASE

### Locally Advanced Breast Cancer

Locally advanced breast cancer includes cT3-T4 and/or cN2-N3 tumors. Some centers consider cT3 and cN0-N1 as large operable breast cancer. Nearly 40–60% of patients present with LABC in lower middle-income developing countries.[47] These patients need metastatic workup in the form of PET scan or a combination of bone scan and contrast-enhanced CT scan of thorax, abdomen, and pelvis as 20–30% patients can have an occult metastasis and can upstage to oligometastatic or metastatic clinical stage.[48] Neoadjuvant treatment in the form of chemotherapy (or rarely hormonal therapy) has been the standard of care for LABC, which can eradicate nodal disease in up to 40–65% patients depending on the ER, PR, and HER2-neu status. The rationale for NACT is to downstage the disease, to make breast conservation surgery feasible and judge the effectiveness of preoperative systemic chemotherapy so that adjuvant treatment can be tailored according to the histopathology report.[49-53]

A complete ALND (level 1–3) is recommended for all LABC. Any conservative axillary surgery in LABC is not recommended outside the realms of a clinical trial. A retrospective dataset of 793 LABC patients who had post-NACT surgery showed that at least half of patients (58.7%) with cN1 and a third of patients (36.6%) with cN2 breast cancer developed clinical and pathological complete axillary response. These patients may be suitable candidates for axillary conservation post-NACT. A careful postchemotherapy assessment followed by a conservative axillary procedure may be an alternative to ALND and this needs to be studied in prospective clinical trials.[54] NCCN guidelines recommend axillary dissection of level 1 and 2 with dissection of level 3 nodes in cases of nodal involvement at level 3 or gross nodal involvement at level 2.[36] Axillary RT is not routinely recommended if a complete axillary clearance is performed. Indications of axillary RT include R1/R2 resection in the axilla due to nodal disease encasing critical neurovascular structures.[55]

### *cN3 Disease*

For patients presenting with advanced lymphadenopathy such as that involving internal mammary, supraclavicular or infraclavicular lymph nodes, management of lymph node basins is controversial. In India, 10–15% patients of nonmetastatic breast cancers present with clinicoradiologically N3 disease. NACT (as per molecular subtypes) is instituted first after ruling out distant metastases. A response assessment CT can help to decide optimal locoregional management. In the event of complete regression, RNI can cover the additional nodal basins. However, in the event of persistent lymphadenopathy, it is common practice to carry out an extended nodal basin clearance—either as internal mammary or supraclavicular lymph node dissection.[56] We have previously documented a 25–40% incidence of positive internal mammary nodes on surgical dissection.[57] Feasibility of internal mammary lymph node chain dissection with video-assisted thoracoscopic approach has been proven.[58] RNI usually follows surgery for extended lymph node basin. With appropriate treatment, long-term cure can be achieved for patients with cN3 nodal disease with an aggressive locoregional approach after initial systemic treatment.[59]

Despite individual seminal trials on RNI showing significant improvement in local/regional/distance control or DFS, the role of RNI still remained controversial due to its failure to impact OS. Hence, the Early Breast Cancer Trialists' Collaborative Group (EBCTCG) undertook an individual patient data meta-analysis of 14,324 women in 16 trials including over 13,000 patients. In the eight newer trials comprised of 12,167 patients and conducted during 1989–2008, regional node RT significantly reduced recurrence [relative risk (RR): 0.88, 0.81–0.95; $p = 0.0008$]. The benefit was largely seen in the reduction of distant recurrence as very few regional failures were reported. RT not only reduced breast cancer mortality (RR: 0.87, 0.80–0.94; $p = 0.001$) but also lead to significantly reduced all-cause mortality (RR: 0.90, 0.84–0.96; $p = 0.0022$). The largest benefit was seen in women with four or more axillary nodes positive and medial/central quadrant tumors.[60] However, majority of these trials were in EBC. The benefit of RNI in LABC is largely extrapolated from its studies in EBC.

### Oligometastatic Breast Cancer

Oligometastatic disease [oligometastatic breast cancer (OMBC)] is defined as presence of ≤5 metastases in three or less organ systems, all of which can be treated with curative therapy in the form of surgery, ablation, or local RT.[61] This subset of patients is different from that of high burden metastatic disease where locoregional treatment has fared poorer prognosis as seen in study by Badwe et al.[62] Selecting patients for curative intent treatments in OMBC is challenging, requiring consideration of factors such as lesion characteristics, patient health, and intervention feasibility. A personalized, multidisciplinary approach is essential for determining the optimal strategy based on individualized factors.[63] The patients with oligometastatic disease are treated with curative intent for locoregional disease as well as for each metastatic site. The standard of care for management of axilla in such cases is a complete ALND postneoadjuvant therapy. There is no evidence for conserving axilla in oligometastatic disease who present with positive nodes. However, individualization of treatment is considered in this stage.

## ONGOING STUDIES IN MANAGEMENT OF AXILLA IN THE UPFRONT AND POSTCHEMOTHERAPY SETTING

The *TAXIS trial (NCT03513614)* is an international phase III study in patients with node-positive breast cancer. It compares tailored axillary surgery followed by either ALND plus RT or axillary RT alone. The primary endpoint is DFS, with the aim of reducing morbidity such as lymphedema while maintaining oncologic safety.[64]

The *TADPOLE trial* is a UK multicenter pragmatic phase III study enrolling patients with 1–2 positive axillary nodes undergoing primary surgery. It compares TAD with axillary clearance. The main outcome is the rate of lymphedema at 12 months, reflecting the trial's emphasis on quality of life and recurrence control.[65]

The *ASLAN trial (NCT04993625)* is a prospective multicenter study from Korea focused on HER2-positive and triple-negative patients who achieve an excellent response to NACT. In this setting, SLN biopsy is omitted and patients proceed with BCS and RT. The primary endpoint is 5-year recurrence-free survival, testing whether axillary surgery can be safely avoided.[66]

Finally, the *OPTIMIST trial (NCT05505357)*, also from Korea, is a single-arm noninferiority study investigating the omission of breast surgery when pCR is predicted after neoadjuvant systemic therapy. Eligibility requires MRI and vacuum-assisted biopsy confirmation of pCR, and in selected patient's axillary surgery may also be omitted. The primary endpoint is 5-year DFS, pushing the boundaries of surgical omission in carefully selected patients.[67]

## CONCLUSION

*Early breast cancer:* Patients presenting with cN0 disease and planned for surgery first should undergo SNB. Sending sentinel nodes for frozen section analysis is optional and not mandatory. In the event of pN0, pN0(i+) and pN1mi nodes, no further ALND is recommended. If 1–2 sentinel nodes harbor macro- or micrometastatic disease, then axillary radiation can be planned instead of further ALND, especially if small sized and hormone receptor positive tumors in patients >50 years of age. However, in younger patients with adverse molecular subtypes, an ALND is a safer alternative. However, if >2 micro-/macrometastatic nodes are seen, then a complete ALND is often carried out.

*Locally advanced breast cancer:* A complete ALND (up to level 2 or 3) is necessary in LABC outside the realms of a clinical trial. *Surgery for cN3 disease* may need supraclavicular or internal mammary lymph node space clearance in the event of persistent nodes post-systemic therapy. This should be followed by RNI.

*Postchemotherapy axilla:* Management of the axilla post-NACT in EBC is rapidly shifting from ALND to less invasive modalities. SNB alone is acceptable in selected prechemotherapy cN0 patients. TAD with SNB reduces FNR and improves diagnostic accuracy in patients with positive prechemotherapy nodes. Use of dual tracers and retrieval of ≥3 SLNs improves FNR and accuracy of TAD. LAS is an effective alternative in resource-constrained settings to TAD + SNB in the postchemotherapy setting. Ongoing trials and their longer-term outcomes will further shape practice paradigms.

## REFERENCES


1. Halsted WS. I. The Results of Radical Operations for the Cure of Carcinoma of the Breast. Ann Surg. 1907;46(1):1-19.
2. Giuliano AE, Kirgan DM, Guenther JM, Morton DL. Lymphatic mapping and sentinel lymphadenectomy for breast cancer. Ann Surg. 1994;220(3):391-8; discussion 398-401.
3. Fisher B, Jeong JH, Anderson S, Bryant J, Fisher ER, Wolmark N. Radical versus total mastectomy: twenty-five-year follow-up of a randomized trial comparing radical mastectomy, total mastectomy, and total mastectomy followed by irradiation. N Engl J Med. 2002;347(8):567-75.
4. Veronesi U, Paganelli G, Viale G, Luini A, Zurrida S, Galimberti V, et al. Sentinel-lymph-node biopsy as a staging procedure in breast cancer: update of a randomised controlled study. Lancet Oncol. 2006;7(12):983-90.
5. Mansel RE, Fallowfield L, Kissin M, Goyal A, Newcombe RG, Dixon JM, et al. Randomized multicenter trial of sentinel node biopsy versus standard axillary treatment in operable breast cancer: the ALMANAC Trial. J Natl Cancer Inst. 2006;98(9):599-609.
6. Gill G. Sentinel-lymph-node-based management or routine axillary clearance? One-year outcomes of sentinel node biopsy versus axillary clearance (SNAC): a randomized controlled surgical trial. Ann Surg Oncol. 2008;16:266-75.
7. Krag DN, Anderson SJ, Julian TB, Brown AM, Harlow SP, Costantino JP, et al. Sentinel-lymph-node resection compared with conventional axillary-lymph-node dissection in clinically node-negative patients with breast cancer: overall survival findings from the NSABP B-32 randomised phase 3 trial. Lancet Oncol. 2010;11(10):927-33.
8. Tanaka K, Yamamoto D, Kanematsu S, Okugawa H, Kamiyama Y. A four node axillary sampling trial on breast cancer patients. Breast. 2006;15(2):203-9.
9. Parmar V, Hawaldar R, Nadkarni MS, Badwe RA. Low axillary sampling in clinically node-negative operable breast cancer. Natl Med J India. 2009;22(5):234-6.
10. Weaver DL, Le UP, Dupuis SL, Weaver KAE, Harlow SP, Ashikaga T, et al. Metastasis detection in sentinel lymph nodes: comparison of a limited widely spaced (NSABP protocol B-32) and a comprehensive narrowly spaced paraffin block sectioning strategy. J Clin Oncol. 2009;27(30):5313-21.
11. de Boer M, van Dijck JAAM, Bult P, Borm GF, Tjan-Heijnen VCG. Breast cancer prognosis and occult lymph node metastases, isolated tumor cells, and micrometastases: a meta-analysis. J Natl Cancer Inst. 2010;102(6):410-25.
12. Giuliano AE, Edge SB, Hortobagyi GN. Eighth Edition of the AJCC Cancer Staging Manual: Breast Cancer. Ann Surg Oncol. 2018;25(7):1783-5.
13. Hunt KK, Ballman KV, McCall LM, Boughey JC, Mittendorf EA, Cox CE, et al. Factors associated with local-regional recurrence after a negative sentinel node dissection: results of the ACOSOG Z0010 trial. Ann Surg. 2012;256(3):428-36.
14. Chen SL, Hoehne FM, Hiuliano AE. The prognostic significance of micrometastases in breast cancer: a SEER population based analysis. Ann Surg Oncol. 2007;14(12):3378-84.
15. Galimberti V, Cole BF, Zurrida S, Viale G, Luini A, Veronesi P, et al. International Breast Cancer Study Group Trial 23-01 investigators. Axillary dissection versus no axillary dissection in patients with sentinel-node micrometastases (IBCSG 23-01): a phase 3 randomised controlled trial. Lancet Oncol. 2013;14(4):297-305.

16. Solá M, Alberro JA, Fraile M, Santesteban P, Ramos M, Fabregas R, et al. Complete axillary lymph node dissection versus clinical follow-up in breast cancer patients with sentinel node micrometastasis: final results from the multicenter clinical trial AATRM 048/13/2000. Ann Surg Oncol. 2013;20(1):120-7.
17. Tjan-Heijnen VC, de Boer M. Minimal lymph node involvement and outcome of breast cancer. The results of the Dutch MIRROR study. Discov Med. 2009; 8(42):137-9.
18. Andersson Y, Bergkvist L, Frisell J, de Boniface J. Omitting completion axillary lymph node dissection after detection of sentinel node micrometastases in breast cancer: first results from the prospective SENOMIC trial. Br J Surg. 2021;108(9):1105-11.
19. Giuliano AE, McCall LM, Beitsch PD, Whitworth PW, Morrow M, Blumencranz PW, et al. ACOSOG Z0011: A randomized trial of axillary node dissection in women with clinical T1-2 N0 M0 breast cancer who have a positive sentinel node. J Clin Oncol. 2010;28:CRA506.
20. Sávolt Á, Péley G, Polgár C, Udvarhelyi N, Rubovszky G, Kovács E, et al. Eight-year follow up result of the OTOASOR trial: The Optimal Treatment of the Axilla - Surgery Or Radiotherapy after positive sentinel lymph node biopsy in early-stage breast cancer: A randomized, single centre, phase III, non-inferiority trial. Eur J Surg Oncol. 2017;43(4):672-9.
21. Donker M, van Tienhoven G, Straver ME, Meijnen P, van de Velde CJ, Mansel RE, et al. Radiotherapy or surgery of the axilla after a positive sentinel node in breast cancer (EORTC 10981-22023 AMAROS): a randomised, multicentre, open-label, phase 3 non-inferiority trial. Lancet Oncol. 2014;15(12):1303-10.
22. de Boniface J, Filtenborg Tvedskov T, Rydén L, Szulkin R, Reimer T, Kühn T, et al. Omitting Axillary Dissection in Breast Cancer with Sentinel-Node Metastases. N Engl J Med. 2024;390(13):1163-75.
23. Tinterri C, Gentile D, Gatzemeier W, Sagona A, Barbieri E, Testori A, et al. Preservation of axillary lymph nodes compared with complete dissection in T1–2 breast cancer patients presenting one or two metastatic sentinel lymph nodes: the SINODAR-ONE multicenter randomized clinical trial. Ann Surg Oncol. 2022;29(9):5732-44.
24. Yasojima H, Imoto S, Nagashima T, Onishi T, Takashima T, Kitada M, et al. Observational study of axilla treatment for breast cancer patients with 1 to 3 positive micrometastases or macrometastases in sentinel lymph nodes. J Clin Oncol. 2022;40:e12576.
25. Gentilini OD, Botteri E, Sangalli C, Galimberti V, Porpiglia M, Agresti R, et al. Sentinel lymph node biopsy vs no axillary surgery in patients with small breast cancer and negative results on ultrasonography of axillary lymph nodes. JAMA Oncol. 2023;9(11):1557.
26. Reimer T, Stachs A, Veselinovic K, Kühn T, Heil J, Polata S, et al. Axillary surgery in breast cancer—primary results of the INSEMA trial. N Engl J Med. 2025;392(11):1051-64.
27. Parmar V, Sanghvi Z, Joshi S, Nair N, Popat P, Kembhavi S, et al. Abstract PO3-03-03: Prospective non-randomized study to compare accuracy of clinical examination under anesthesia, axillary ultrasound and histo-pathological evaluation for axillary nodal staging in women with clinically N0 early breast cancer. Cancer Res. 2024;84(9_Suppl):PO3-03-03.

28. van Roozendaal LM, Vane MLG, van Dalen T, van der Hage JA, Strobbe LJA, Boersma LJ, et al. Clinically node negative breast cancer patients undergoing breast conserving therapy, sentinel lymph node procedure versus follow-up: a Dutch randomized controlled multicentre trial (BOOG 2013-08). BMC Cancer. 2017;17(1):459.
29. Jung JG, Ahn SH, Lee S, Kim EK, Ryu JM, Park S, et al. No axillary surgical treatment for lymph node-negative patients after ultrasonography (NAUTILUS): protocol of a prospective randomized clinical trial. BMC Cancer. 2022;22(1):189.
30. Reddy A, Nair NS, Mokal S, Parmar V, Shet T, Pathak R, et al. Can we avoid axillary lymph node dissection (ALND) in patients with 1-2 positive sentinel/low axillary lymph nodes (SLN/LAS+) in the Indian setting? Indian J Surg Oncol. 2021;12(2):272-8.
31. Noronha J, Joshi S, Hawaldar R, Nair N, Vanmali V, Parmar V, et al. Sterilization rate of the axilla after neoadjuvant chemotherapy: the scope for conservative surgery. JCO Glob Oncol. 2020;6:1184-91.
32. Hunt KK, Yi M, Mittendorf EA, Guerrero C, Babiera GV, Bedrosian I, et al. Sentinel lymph node surgery after neoadjuvant chemotherapy is accurate and reduces the need for axillary dissection in breast cancer patients. Ann Surg. 2009;250(4):558-66.
33. Samiei S, Simons JM, Engelen SME, Beets-Tan RGH, Classe JM, Smidt ML; EUBREAST Group. Axillary pathologic complete response after neoadjuvant systemic therapy by breast cancer subtype in patients with initially clinically node-positive disease: a systematic review and meta-analysis. JAMA Surg. 2021;156(6): e210891.
34. Xing Y, Foy M, Cox DD, Kuerer HM, Hunt KK, Cormier JN. Meta-analysis of sentinel lymph node biopsy after preoperative chemotherapy in patients with breast cancer. Br J Surg. 2006;93(5):539-46.
35. Kelly AM, Douek M, Cody HS. Sentinel lymph node biopsy after neoadjuvant chemotherapy for breast cancer: a systematic review and meta-analysis. Acad Radiol. 2009;16(5):551-63.
36. NCCN. (2025). NCCN Clinical Practice Guidelines in Oncology (NCCN Guidelines®) for Poland. Breast Cancer. Version 4.2025. [online] Available from https://kom.nio.gov.pl/uploads/attachments/e4464aa737d-04fe0bf8fe452bedb257580390/wytyczne-postepowania-diagnostyczno-terapeutycznego-w-raku-piersi-adaptacja-nccn-042025.pdf [Last accessed November, 2025].
37. Boughey JC, Suman VJ, Mittendorf EA, Ahrendt GM, Wilke LG, Taback B, et al. Sentinel lymph node surgery after neoadjuvant chemotherapy in patients with node-positive breast cancer: the ACOSOG Z1071 (Alliance) clinical trial. JAMA. 2013;310(14):1455-61.
38. Kuehn T, Bauerfeind I, Fehm T, Fleige B, Hausschild M, Helms G, et al. Sentinel-lymph-node biopsy in patients with breast cancer before and after neoadjuvant chemotherapy (SENTINA): a prospective, multicentre cohort study. Lancet Oncol. 2013;14(7):609-18.
39. Boileau JF, Poirier B, Basik M, Holloway CM, Gaboury L, Sideris L, et al. Sentinel node biopsy after neoadjuvant chemotherapy in biopsy-proven node-positive breast cancer: the SN FNAC study. J Clin Oncol. 2015;33(3):258-64.

40. Parmar V, Krishnamurthy A, Hawaldar R, et al. Low axillary sampling versus sentinel lymph node biopsy in node-positive breast cancer post neoadjuvant chemotherapy: a randomized controlled trial. JCO Glob Oncol. 2020;6:395-407.
41. Caudle AS, Yang WT, Krishnamurthy S, Mittendorf EA, Black DM, Gilcrease MZ, et al. Improved Axillary Evaluation Following Neoadjuvant Therapy for Patients With Node-Positive Breast Cancer Using Selective Evaluation of Clipped Nodes: Implementation of Targeted Axillary Dissection. J Clin Oncol. 2016;34(10):1072-8.
42. Donker M, Straver ME, Wesseling J, Loo CE, Schot M, Drukker CA, et al. Marking axillary lymph nodes with radioactive iodine seeds for axillary staging after neoadjuvant systemic treatment in breast cancer patients: the MARI procedure. Ann Surg. 2015;261(2):378-82.
43. Choy N, Lipson J, Porter C, Ozawa M, Kieryn A, Pal S, et al. Initial results with preoperative tattooing of biopsied axillary lymph nodes and correlation to sentinel lymph nodes in breast cancer patients. Ann Surg Oncol. 2015;22(2):377-82.
44. Alamoodi M, Wazir U, Sakr RA, Venkataraman J, Mokbel K. Evaluating magnetic seed localization in targeted axillary dissection for node-positive early breast cancer patients receiving neoadjuvant systemic therapy: a comprehensive review and pooled analysis. J Clin Med. 2024;13(10):2908.
45. Wazir U, Michell MJ, Alamoodi M, Mokbel K. Evaluating radar reflector localisation in targeted axillary dissection in patients undergoing neoadjuvant systemic therapy for node-positive early breast cancer: a systematic review and pooled analysis. Cancers (Basel). 2024;16(7):1345.
46. NCCN. (2025). Clinical Practice Guidelines in Oncology: Breast Cancer. Version 2.2025. [online] https://www.nccn.org/patients/guidelines/content/PDF/breastcancerscreening-patient.pdf [Last accessed November, 2025].
47. Manzoor S, Anwer M, Soomro S, Kumar D. Presentation, diagnosis and management of locally advanced breast cancer: Is it different in low/middle income countries? Pak J Med Sci. 2019;35(6):1554-7.
48. Ali B, Mubarik F, Zahid N, Sattar AK. Clinicopathologic features predictive of distant metastases in patients diagnosed with invasive breast cancer. JCO Glob Oncol. 2020;6:1346-51.
49. Gralow JR, Burstein HJ, Wood W, Hortobagyi GN, Gianni L, von Minckwitz G, et al. Preoperative therapy in invasive breast cancer: Pathologic assessment and systemic therapy issues in operable disease. J Clin Oncol. 2008;26:814-9.
50. Kaufmann M, Hortobagyi GN, Goldhirsch A, Scholl S, Makris A, Valagussa P, et al. Recommendations from an international expert panel on the use of neoadjuvant (primary) systemic treatment of operable breast cancer: An update. J Clin Oncol. 2006;24:1940-9.
51. Schwartz GF, Hortobagyi GN. Proceedings of the consensus conference on neoadjuvant chemotherapy in carcinoma of the breast, April 26-28, 2003, Philadelphia, Pennsylvania. Cancer. 2004;100:2512-32.
52. Mamtani A, Barrio AV, King TA, Van Zee KJ, Plitas G, Pilewskie M, et al. How often does neoadjuvant chemotherapy avoid axillary dissection in patients with histologically confirmed nodal metastases? Results of a prospective study. Ann Surg Oncol. 2016;23:3467-74.
53. Woeste MR, Bhutiani N, Donaldson M, McMasters KM, Ajkay N. Evaluating the effect of neoadjuvant chemotherapy on surgical outcomes after breast conserving surgery. J Surg Oncol. 2021;123:439-45.

54. Jarin N, Joshi S, Rohini H, Vaibhav V, Nair N, Parmar V, et al. Sterilization Rate of the Axilla after Neo-Adjuvant Chemotherapy - The Scope for Conservative Surgery of the Axilla. Eur J Surg Oncol. 2020;46;e59-e60.
55. Gradishar WJ, Moran MS, Abraham J, Aft R, Agnese D, Allison KH, et al. Breast Cancer, Version 3.2022, NCCN Clinical Practice Guidelines in Oncology. J Natl Compr Canc Netw. 2022;20(6):691-722.
56. Dsilva D, Joshi S, Officewala Z, Krishnamurthy R, Vanmali V, Kothari B, et al. Burden of clinico-radiological N3 lymphadenopathy in non-metastatic breast cancer – single centre experience. Breast. 2025;80:104016.
57. Joshi S, Vora T, Talole S, Hawaldar R, Budrukkar A, Badwe R. Retrospective audit of the yield of internal mammary lymph node dissection and literature review. Indian J Cancer. 2024;61(1):61-7.
58. Kawaguchi S, Tamura N, Suzuki S, Nishikawa A, Shibata A, Tanaka K, et al. Effectiveness of PET/CT and VATS for detecting and treating internal mammary lymph node metastasis: a case series. Jpn J Clin Oncol. 2023;53(7):562-71.
59. Dsilva D, Shenoy P, Ali B, Sanghvi Z, Joshi S, Vanmali V, et al. Ipsilateral supraclavicular lymphadenopathy in advanced, non-metastatic breast cancer – 8-year outcome analysis. Breast. 2025;80:104017.
60. Early Breast Cancer Trialists' Collaborative Group (EBCTCG). Radiotherapy to regional nodes in early breast cancer: An individual patient data meta-analysis of 14 324 women in 16 trials. Lancet Lond Engl. 2023;402:1991-2003.
61. Barberi V, Pietragalla A, Franceschini G, Marazzi F, Paris I, Cognetti F, et al. Oligometastatic Breast Cancer: How to Manage It? J Pers Med. 2021;11(6):532.
62. Badwe R, Hawaldar R, Nair N, Kaushik R, Parmar V, Siddique S, et al. Locoregional treatment versus no treatment of the primary tumour in metastatic breast cancer: An open-label randomised controlled trial. Lancet Oncol. 2015;16:1380-8.
63. Makhlin I, Fox K. Oligometastatic Breast Cancer: Is This a Curable Entity? A Contemporary Review of the Literature. Curr Oncol Rep. 2020;22:1-10.
64. Henke G, Knauer M, Ribi K, Hayoz S, Gérard MA, Ruhstaller T, et al. Tailored axillary surgery with or without axillary lymph node dissection followed by radiotherapy in patients with clinically node-positive breast cancer (TAXIS): study protocol for a multicenter, randomized phase-III trial. Trials. 2018;19(1):667.
65. Potter S, Mullan R, Cain H, St John ES, Barry P, Masannat Y, et al. Consensus process to agree upon surgical quality assurance processes within a pragmatic, multicentre randomised clinical trial comparing targeted axillary dissection and axillary node clearance: the TADPOLE-TOGETHER project. BMJ Open. 2025;15(6):e095774.
66. Ryu JM, Han W, Lee HB, Ahn SG, Kim HJ, Park HS, et al. Selective avoidance of sentinel lymph node biopsy after neoadjuvant chemotherapy in patients with HER-2 positive/triple negative breast cancer (ASLAN): prospective, multicenter, single-arm study. J Clin Oncol. 2023 Jun 1;41(16_suppl).
67. Lee HB, Kim HK, Ahn SG, Choi JS, Kim HJ, Lee JE, et al. Omission of breast surgery for breast cancer patients with pathologic complete response on MRI and vacuum-assisted biopsy after neoadjuvant systemic therapy: a multicenter, single-arm, non-inferiority trial (OPTIMIST). J Clin Oncol. 2025;43(15_suppl):TPS624.

CHAPTER 11

# Granulomatous Lobular Mastitis

*Tushar S Mishra, Shanto Shila Guha*

## INTRODUCTION

Granulomatous lobular mastitis (GLM) is a chronic inflammatory disease of the breast, predominantly affecting women of reproductive age. It was first identified by Kessler and Woloch as a distinct form of mastitis, initially described in a series of five patients who were referred to surgeons for potential surgical treatment of breast cancer. Two of these patients had previously received preoperative radiotherapy for a presumed diagnosis of breast cancer.[1] The status of the disease has largely remained unchanged, even after 50 years since it was first identified. Diagnoses are frequently missed, as cases are sometimes mistaken for simple recurrent breast abscesses or confused with breast carcinoma, due to the presence of a lump often with a high BIRADS (Breast Imaging-Reporting and Data System) score. While a high index of suspicion can lead to a diagnosis, it remains unclear until a core needle of biopsy is performed, often to rule out a malignancy or to determine the cause of recurrent abscesses.

Granulomatous lobular mastitis has been reported in almost all races, with no specific predisposition to any ethnic group. However, few studies have reported its association with non-white ethnic groups, such as Asian, Hispanic, and Middle Eastern descent. The estimated prevalence is 2.4 per 100,000 women between the ages of 20 and 40 years. The figures likely underestimate the true scope of the issue, as many cases remain undiagnosed or unreported. The recent observation of an increased incidence is more likely due to greater awareness of the condition or more frequent biopsies conducted for other closely related differential diagnoses. The exact etiology remains uncertain[2,3] and hence GLM is idiopathic. Although it is uncommon during pregnancy or lactation, it has a strong association with previous lactational history. GLM in nulliparous women is a rarity, where it may be associated with high levels of serum prolactin, which could either be drug-induced or due to a pituitary prolactinoma. Its association with breast cancer seems more coincidental than causal, with fewer than 10 cases reported in individuals with a prior history of GLM treatment.[4]

Randomized controlled trials and systematic reviews have not been strong enough to impact the uniformity of treatment; thus, the treatment is currently reliant upon consensus guidelines. Antibiotics, antitubercular treatment, multiple incisions and drainages, resection surgeries, systemic steroids (oral, topical, and intralesional), and other interventions have all been part of the surgeon's armamentarium, highlighting prevailing ignorance. Recently, artificial intelligence has also been employed to make progress in the proper line of treatment.[5-9]

The unwarranted cocktail of unclear etiology or pathognomonic clinical features, and nonspecific radiological findings has led to delays in diagnosis, resulting in poor outcomes that significantly impact the physical and mental health of the patient, as well as their quality of life.[10] This chapter aims to clarify many of the existing uncertainties, based on the best available quality evidence from the literature.

## NOMENCLATURE

Granulomatous mastitis has been variously named as cystic neutrophilic granulomatous mastitis, or idiopathic granulomatous mastitis. Owing to the location of the disease in the lobules, granulomatous mastitis is more appropriately labelled as GLM or idiopathic granulomatous lobular mastitis (IGLM), the most accepted terminologies.[5] Although some researchers suggest a primary and secondary variety, all GLM should be considered primary/idiopathic until a cause is conclusively identified. This dictum will avoid unnecessary empirical therapy with drugs such as antitubercular therapy.

## PATHOPHYSIOLOGY

The precise etiological mechanism of GLM is not yet understood. Lactational disorders, autoimmunity, breast trauma, and infection with Corynebacterium species are some of the commonly implicated causes **(Flowchart 1)**.

### Milk Stasis and Hyperprolactinemia

Milk stasis is supposedly a crucial factor in the development of this disease. Although the pathogenesis possibly begins with an episode of acute mastitis during pregnancy or lactation, GLM first occurs a few months to years after cessation of lactation, more commonly on the side that was less breastfed. The accumulation of glandular proteinaceous secretions (milk) causes ductal ectasia and later disruption. This interstitial extravasation triggers an inflammatory response and the formation of noncaseating granulomas, characteristic of GLM. Similarly, prolactinoma and any drug that causes hyperprolactinemia, such as D2 receptor antagonists (e.g., risperidone) and selective serotonin reuptake inhibitors (SSRI) (e.g., fluoxetine), can cause GLM.[11,12] Oral contraceptive pills (OCPs) are considered a potential etiological factor for GLM, as they cause increased breast luminal secretions. The strength of their relationship is between 0% and 42%.

**Flowchart 1:** Algorithm of pathophysiology of granulomatous mastitis.

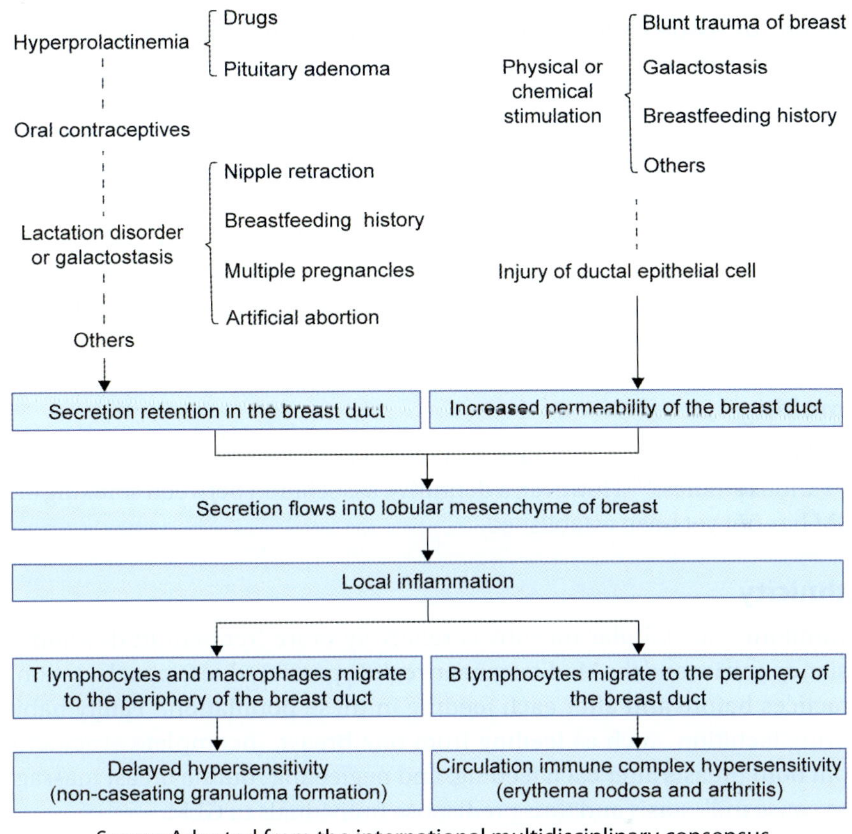


*Source:* Adopted from the international multidisciplinary consensus (2021 edition) by Yuan et al.[6]

## Autoimmunity

Granulomatous mastitis occasionally presents with additional extramammary symptoms, including erythema nodosum, inflammatory arthritis, arthralgias, and episcleritis, indicating the possibility of an immune-related disorder. Antigenic proteinaceous material leak when the lining of the congested duct is disrupted, resulting in the migration of lymphocytes and macrophages into the periductal areas, which leads to the formation of noncaseating granulomas. Conventional serological tests, such as ANA and rheumatoid factor, used for the diagnosis of other autoimmune disorders, however, are usually negative. The levels of interleukin (IL)-22/23, cytokines involved in autoimmune diseases, are sometimes elevated, supporting the autoimmune theory. The presence of Helper T cells, CD3, CD4, and CD8 lymphocytes throughout the lesion suggests the involvement of cell-mediated immunity in its pathogenesis, while CD79a lymphocyte positivity suggests that humoral immunity is also involved; however, stains for IgG and IgM usually are negative.[3,13]

## Infection

The pus or tissue culture in GLM is usually sterile. Although uncommon, Corynebacterium spp. is among the most isolated infectious agents reported in the literature.[14] The perilobular inflammatory response secondary to ductal content efflux gives rise to a special histologic type of GLM called cystic neutrophilic granulomatous mastitis (CNGM), characterized by a vacuole-like cavity formed by neutrophils and Gram-positive bacilli, along with the presence of diffuse granulomas in the cavity.[15] This variant of GLM is more likely to be antibiotic-sensitive. *Corynebacteria*, especially *Corynebacterium kroppenstedtii* and occasionally Staphylococcal *spp.*, have been isolated in CNGM by culture or by gene sequencing.[16]

## Smoking

Smoking has also been identified as a significant factor in the disease etiology by various studies.[3,17] However, a definitive association between smoking and IGM has not yet been established.

## Ethnicity

Granulomatous lobular mastitis is relatively more frequent in developing Asian countries and the Mediterranean region, possibly due to poor lactational practices before and after each feeding in these population.[6] Faulty habits during lactation, such as feeding from one breast, incomplete evacuation from both breasts after each feeding, and neglecting routine breast massage, can cause milk stasis and thus predispose individuals to GLM.

# CLINICAL FEATURES

Granulomatous lobular mastitis predominantly occurs in young to middle-aged women (in the third and fourth decades),[18] typically appearing within 1.5–5 years after the last delivery.[19] Most patients have a history of at least one live birth and breastfeeding.[20] The disease is rarely seen during pregnancy.[21] Despite the disease process being supposed to be due to milk stasis, the disease typically presents only a few months after cessation of lactation. The disease is more common unilaterally and affects the side on which the woman has less breastfed, supporting the milk stasis theory. However, the cause of unilateral involvement in patients who were equally breastfed on both sides is unknown. Poor breast hygiene before and after breastfeeding is another proposed theory for its development. GLM in males is extremely rare, with only 13 cases documented so far. A higher endogenous estrogen-to-androgen ratio has been suggested in some of them.[22]

Granulomatous lobular mastitis usually presents as a unilateral tender breast mass; however, both breasts can be rarely affected. The clinical manifestation can vary from a painless lump to a discharging sinus or scars. The most common symptom is a breast mass of varying sizes, of which

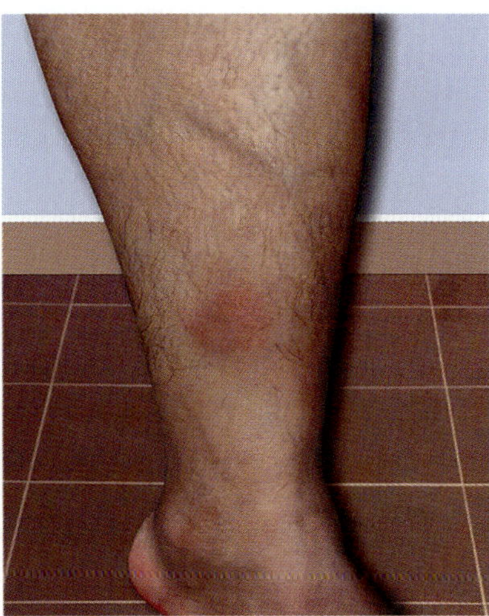

**Fig. 1:** Clinical photograph showing erythema nodosum in the left leg in a patient with granulomatous mastitis.

most (66%) are painful.[23] The disease typically manifests in the periphery of the breast, usually in one of the quadrants, with the areola spared, even in advanced stages of the disease. However, the disease can occasionally spread centripetally to involve the areola and can spread to more than one quadrant, involving the entire breast. Fistulae or sinuses involving one or more quadrants of the breast are the picture of the more advanced stage of the disease. Systemic features of inflammation, such as fever, are typically absent.[6] Erythema nodosum and oligo- or polyarthritis are among the extramammary features in patients with GLM, regardless of the stage of the disease[6] **(Fig. 1)**. A painless lump, which can be a feature of GLM associated with peau d'orange and nipple retraction with or without axillary lymphadenopathy,[12,16] closely mimicking inflammatory breast cancer. The duration of the disease may vary from weeks to months and can be self-limiting over several months.

## CLINICAL STAGES

Based on the presence of a mass and its size, skin change, presence of abscesses, sinuses, or fistula, GLM can be divided into four stages[6] **(Figs. 2A and B)**:

- *Self-limited stage:* Limited mass, <5 cm, with mild tenderness.
- *Congestive swelling stage:* Mass ≥5 cm; tenderness, skin hyperemia, and swelling.
- *Abscess formation stage:* Mass involving two quadrants, abscesses, tenderness, skin hyperemia, and swelling.
- *Complex refractory stage:* Mass involving three or four quadrants, multiple abscesses, sinus formation, fistula formation, and persistent wound infection.

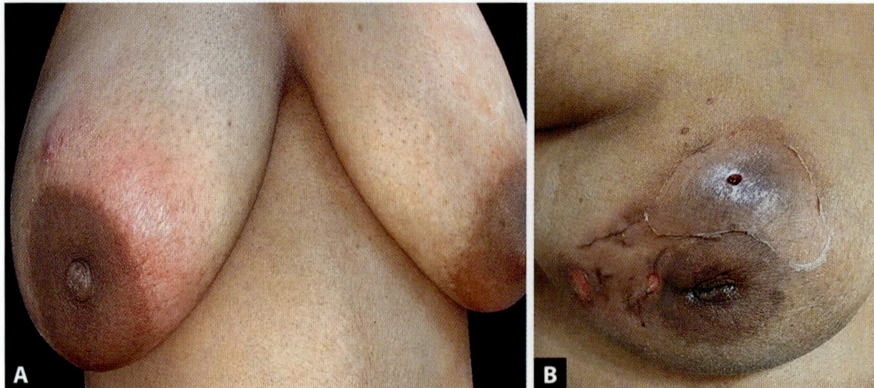


**Figs. 2A and B:** (A) Stage 2 disease in granulomatous lobular mastitis (GLM) involving the right central and upper inner quadrants; (B) Stage 4 disease in GLM involving the upper inner and upper outer quadrants of the right breast.

## DIAGNOSIS

The diagnosis of GLM can be challenging due to varied clinical findings overlapping with other breast diseases at presentation and nonspecific radiological features, which often overlapping with other diseases, including local infection to cancer. This leads to lower rates of early diagnosis and higher chances of false-positive radiological diagnosis of breast carcinoma.[24] Risk factors, including reproductive age, hormonal imbalance or contraceptive treatment, and a recent history of pregnancy or faulty lactational habits, should be sought. Histological evidence of noncaseating granulomas with multinucleated giant cells is supportive; however, repeated biopsies may be necessary to demonstrate this characteristic feature.[10] Systemic diseases, such as granulomatous inflammation, including Wegener's granulomatosis or sarcoidosis, may need to be excluded during the diagnostic workup.[10]

### Ultrasound

In line with triple assessment, a radiological assessment using ultrasound is first performed for GLM.[6] An irregular, lobulated, heterogeneous, hypoechoic mass with indistinct hyperechoic rims and internal vascularity, presence of tubular echoes, and multiple intercommunicating abscesses in the breast parenchyma[25] are the common findings on sonography. Even when a mass is not present, sonological evidence of parenchymal mixed echo pattern with deformity, multiple collections in the breast parenchyma with intercommunicating tracks, focal signs of mastitis with interstitial edema, may indicate GLM[26] **(Figs. 3A and B)**. The ultrasound can also find features of skin thickening, edema, obliteration of subcutaneous fat, intercommunicating abscesses, and sinus tracts leading to the skin. A US-guided biopsy is often

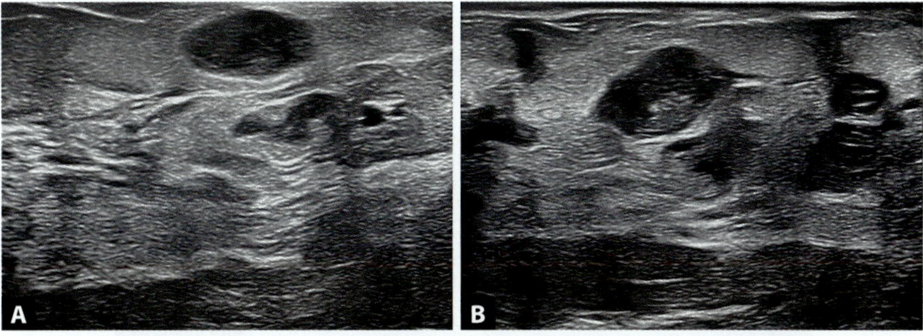


**Figs. 3A and B:** US images with irregular hypoechoic masses and a mixed internal echo pattern with intercommunicating abscesses and sinus tracts opening to the skin in a patient with GLM. (GLM: granulomatous lobular mastitis; US: ultrasound)

necessary from a representative area to assess the course of the disease, i.e., remission, progression, or cure.[6]

## MAMMOGRAPHY

An ill-defined mass with asymmetric diffuse density is the most common mammographic finding.[27] Other findings include diffusely increased density, associated parenchymal distortion, skin thickening, and benign-appearing axillary lymph node enlargement.[28] GLM may be associated with heterogeneous calcification **(Fig. 4)**, which can lead to a high BIRADS score, potentially reaching levels of IV or V. Consequently, mammographic findings are nonspecific, and carcinoma cannot always be definitively excluded.

### Magnetic Resonance Imaging

Although not routinely required for its diagnosis, MRI can be helpful in differentiating it from breast carcinoma.[6] Heterogeneously enhancing masses, segmental nonmass enhancement, signs of edema and inflammation, tumor-like lesions, as well as abscess-fistula formation in the parenchyma are hallmarks of GLM, which increase its diagnostic accuracy to 88.9%.[29] The accuracy of MRI-enhanced imaging in the diagnosis of GLM lesions is significantly higher than the accuracy of US with or without mammography combined.[29,30] It can also be used to track the course of the disease, indicating whether it is progressing or regressing, and in cases where treatment is purely conservative.[6]

### Laboratory Investigations

Laboratory examinations do not specifically contribute to the diagnosis of GLM. They are usually performed to rule out leukocytosis, a raised erythrocyte sedimentation rate, and for presence of any inflammatory markers, such as elevated C-reactive protein. Serum prolactin levels are

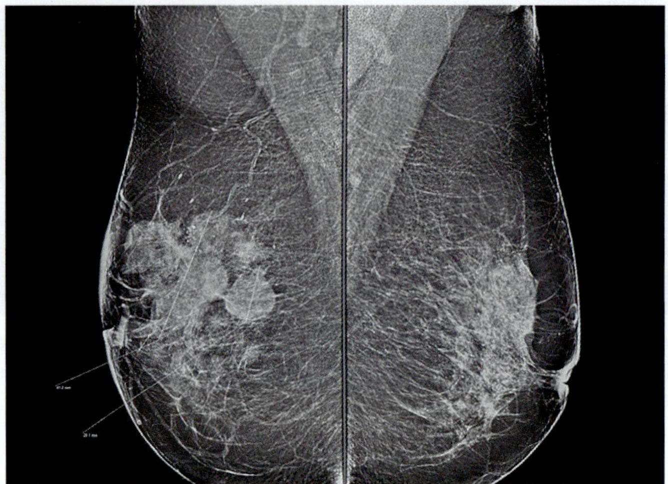

**Fig. 4:** Mammogram showing irregular asymmetric density with no calcification in the right breast.

used to assess any secondary cause of GLM. It is essential to emphasize that routine immunological tests, such as an antinuclear antibody (ANA) profile and rheumatoid factor, may be costly and often unnecessary in every case.[31] Serum prolactin should be measured routinely in all cases and, more importantly, in all nulliparous women with GLM to rule out hyperprolactinemia or up-regulated prolactin receptors or hypersensitivity to the normally circulating prolactin.[7] Deoxyribonucleic acid (DNA) test of *Mycobacterium tuberculosis* helps to distinguish tuberculous granulomatous mastitis and should be done in all cases to rule out tuberculous mastitis,[32] which is a separate disease entity, and so is its management.

## Histopathology

Histopathological examination is the most reliable diagnostic test for GLM and should be performed routinely before initiating therapy. Core-needle biopsy and vacuum-assisted biopsies score higher than fine needle aspiration cytology for diagnostic accuracy.[6] Noncaseating granulomas with epithelioid histiocytes, multinucleated giant cells, lymphocytes, and plasma cells, located in the center of the lobules, are typical of GLM **(Figs. 5A and B)**. Inflammation of GLM is usually confined to the breast lobules, seldom involving the main ducts.[33] The inflammatory processes are more perilobular than periductal. Organized microabscesses with neutrophilic ducts, tracts, damaged ducts, and loss of acinar structures in the parenchyma are typical signs of GLM.[11]

Gram stain, acid-fast stain, fungal stain, periodic acid-Schiff (PAS), and Gomori methenamine silver (GMS) are usually performed to exclude

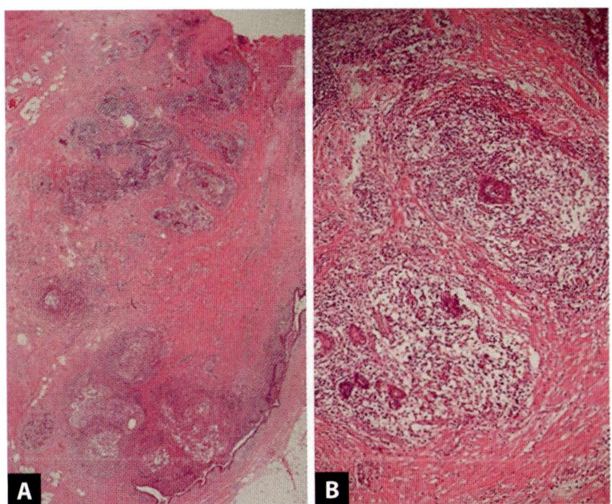


**Figs. 5A and B:** Histological findings in Gomori methenamine silver (GLM) include epithelioid histiocytes, multinucleated giant cells, lymphocytes, and plasma cells, located in the center of the lobules. (On Hematoxylin and Eosin stain.)

specific infectious granulomas. The absence of caseating necrosis excludes the diagnosis of tuberculosis. The lesion affecting lobules versus the duct also helps in differentiating the cause.

## DIFFERENTIAL DIAGNOSIS

### Duct Ectasia/Periductal Inflammation of the Breast

They present with nipple discharge and nipple retraction, secondary to ductal dilatation and shortening. Women of any age group can be affected, with the perimenopausal being more commonly affected. Unlike GLM, the disease manifests in the areolar region, showing eccentric development.[34] Sonography demonstrates ductal dilation with fine light spots inside, and flow signs when the duct is pressurized. Galactography can show dilated, tortuous, blocked, and deformed ducts.[6] On histopathology, the ducts are highly dilated, with thick walls containing lymphocytes, plasma cells, and neutrophilic infiltrates surrounding the dilated duct.[35]

### Zuska Disease/Subareolar Abscess

Nonlactating women are typically affected by this disease, presenting with recurrent swelling, abscesses, or lactiferous fistulas around the areola. Sonography demonstrates single or multiple hypoechoic or anechoic areas with blood flow signals. Squamous metaplasia of the lactiferous duct columnar epithelium at the base of the nipple, as seen on histopathology, is diagnostic of the disease.

### Breast Carcinoma

Granulomatous lobular mastitis often closely mimics breast cancer, although the latter is more frequent in perimenopausal and postmenopausal women with the presence of a hard, painless mass with irregular borders, and often with ipsilateral axillary lymphadenopathy. Both inflammatory breast carcinomas and GLM can present with overlapping signs of local skin inflammation-like manifestations, including redness, edema, a peau d'orange appearance, and sometimes increased surface temperature. Ill-defined lumps with sonological evidence, hypoechoic areas with unclear borders and blood flow signals, and mammographic findings of shadows with increased density, with irregular margins or with Burr sign, along with small and dense calcifications, suggest GLM. The definitive distinction between GLM and inflammatory breast cancer, however, can only be made by histopathology.

## ■ TREATMENT

There is no consensus regarding the treatment of GLM; it may vary from watchful waiting to the use of antibiotics, corticosteroids, immunosuppressants, or surgical treatment. Watchful waiting can be a valid treatment option for early-stage disease, typically Stage 1. However, symptom control with medication is recommended in these patients in the later stages, with surgery being the last resort in selected patients not responding to medical management.

### Etiologic Treatment

Patients with hyperprolactinemia due to pituitary adenoma should undergo adenoma resection. Low-dose corticosteroids have been found to be effective for postresection.[36] Patients with drug-induced hyperprolactinemia should be treated with drug substitution.[6] Bromocriptine has been found to be effective in patients with hyperprolactinemia.[37]

#### *Observation*

It is mostly recommended as first-line therapy in patients with limited and mild disease (usually Stage 1 disease), as half of the lesions of GLM resolve without any treatment or intervention over 6 months to 2 years. However, the diagnosis of GLM is mandatory before observation is advised for such patients. Supportive therapy is recommended to manage symptoms, enhance quality of life, and offer reassurance.

### Antibiotic Therapy

In the case of infectious GLM, antibiotic therapy should be administered based on the drug-susceptibility results.[6] However, in the absence of any organism, isolated quinolones, clarithromycin, clindamycin, and azithromycin have been administered empirically over variable durations, sometimes for months.[38,39] Most infections in GLM are polymicrobial in nature. Rifampicin (300 mg twice daily for a period of 6–9 months) has been proven to be effective in all stages of disease, irrespective of whether *Corynebacterium* infection is positive or negative.[40] Antibiotics are commonly administered empirically prior to the histopathological diagnosis of GLM; however, antibiotic therapy has been demonstrated to be ineffective for noninfectious GLM treatment since it is a sterile condition.[39]

## Systemic Corticosteroids

There is good evidence to prove the efficacy of systemic steroids (prednisolone) in minimizing both the extent and the need for surgery.[41] The endpoint of steroid therapy is a complete clinical response (CCR), which is defined as skin changes completely ameliorated, including the disappearance of inflammatory signs, inactivity or closure of fistulas, and disappearance of lumps.[42] The corticosteroid therapy should be titrated to the minimum effective dose and duration for obtaining CCR.[6] However, Montazer et al. have reported high success rates with lower recurrence and reduced need for surgery using high doses of prednisolone.[43] The therapy is usually started with 30–40 mg of prednisone daily and later tapered to 20 mg daily in a two to 4-week period. It is further tapered more gradually over a period of 3–6 months. Corticosteroid usage might be limited in pregnant, diabetic, or lactating women. Prolonged use of glucocorticoids may lead to unwanted side effects, including weight gain, osteoporosis, hirsutism, skin changes, abnormal fat deposition, and worsening infections.[44] Recent reports of topical application of steroids are emerging and have shown similar clinical and radiological response as systemic therapy with significantly reduced systemic side effects. The topical therapy of steroids can achieve a complete response with symptoms including skin erosion, fistula, and parenchymal lesions. The response with topical therapy has also been reported in patients with a relapse of the disease.[45,46]

## Intralesional Corticosteroids

Intralesional corticosteroid (triamcinolone) injection has demonstrated efficacy in patients with skin manifestations, including fistulas, skin erosions, and ulcers.[18,46] Intralesional triamcinolone has also been found effective for breast masses with breast abscesses or sinuses, where repeated US-guided aspiration of the pus with normal saline wash of the abscess cavity, followed by injection of 40 mg triamcinolone acetonide into the abscess cavity through the aspiration needle, has been effective.[47] Perilesional steroid injections are also efficacious in fibroglandular areas without abscess formation.[48] Intralesional therapy combined with topical therapy has also been found effective in GLM patients.

## Methotrexate

Methotrexate (MTX), when used in conjunction with corticosteroids, works synergistically, thereby being effective in disease control even at lower corticosteroid dosages.[49] Hence, MTX may be considered early in patients who are resistant to corticosteroids or when the patient is having side effects, or when there is disease upstaging or relapse after temporary disease control.[6] The dosage of MTX is 5–15 mg/week for 6–24 months. Patients receiving MTX should be given two doses of folic acid per week before MTX use.[6] MTX significantly lowers the recurrence rate when combined with corticosteroids. There are studies documenting MTX's efficacy in preventing disease relapse, lessening corticosteroid dose, and inducing disease remission.[41,49] MTX has been found to have the lowest recurrence rate among all medical treatment options.[41] However, its usage is associated with various side effects that need constant observation during therapy, such as impairment of liver and renal function, bone marrow suppression, interstitial pneumonia, folic acid deficiency, and gastrointestinal reactions.[49,50] The authors have also used cyclosporin along with steroids with good results in cases resistant to steroid therapy alone.

## Surgical Drainage

The recurrence rate of GLM after drainage is 65%. Hence, US-guided aspiration of the abscess with drain placement is preferred over surgical drainage.[41] The authors opt for repeated aspirations, with single or multiple tube drains placed through stab incisions instead of a liberal incision **(Fig. 6)**.

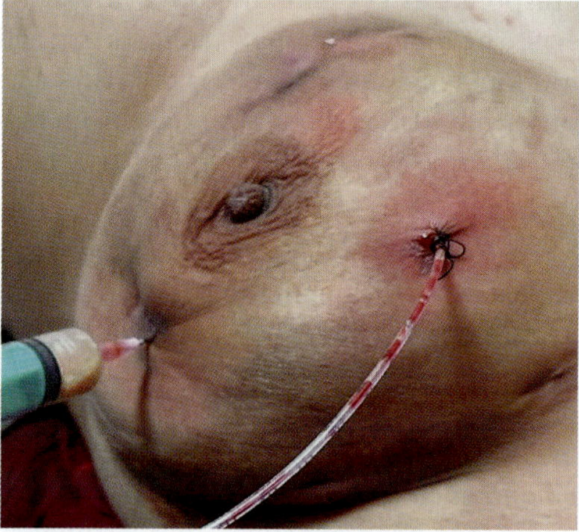

**Fig. 6:** Aspiration of an abscess in the breast with a wide-bore needle and placement of a mini suction drainage, with good results, thus avoiding unsightly scars, thereby cosmetically more acceptable.

**Flowchart 2:** Algorithm of clinical management of GLM based on clinical stage.

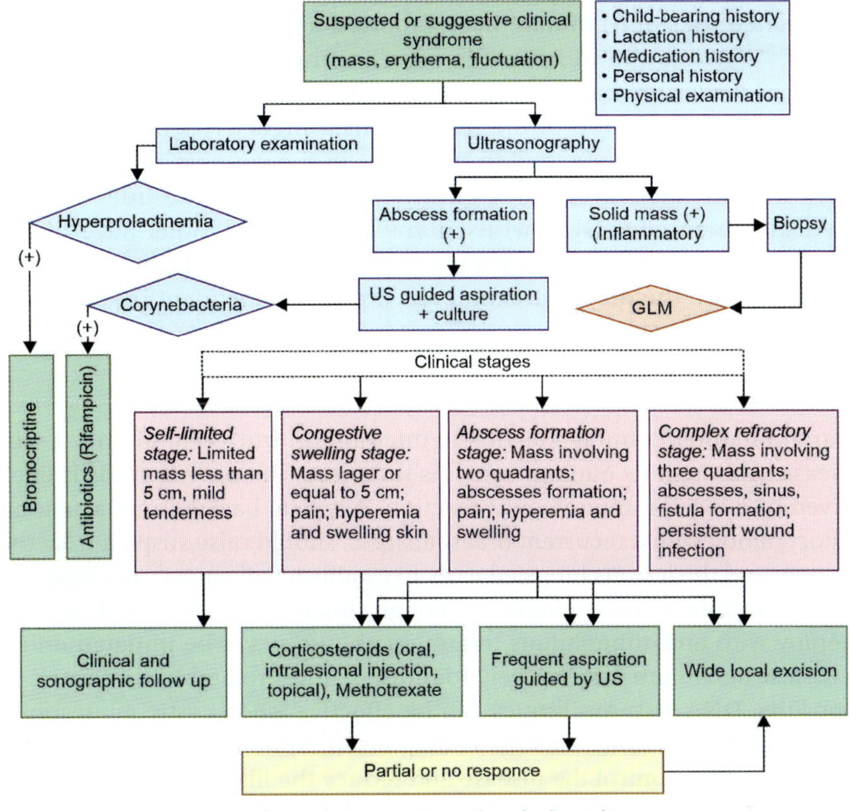


*Source:* Adopted from the international multidisciplinary consensus (2021 edition) by Yuan et al.[6]

Since the likelihood of the disease spreading to another quadrants is fair, incision and drainage procedures offer more of a symptomatic treatment rather than a curative one.

## Surgical Wide Local Excision

Wide local excision can be beneficial for complex and refractory cases when the area of involvement is limited and there are sinus tracts rather than abscesses. The authors, however, have not found it necessary in their experience of managing over 60 cases. A significant reason against wide local excision (WLE) is the potential for the disease to recur in another area of the same or a different quadrant.

Although treatment algorithms **(Flowchart 2)** have been proposed in consensus guidelines, which authors tend to agree with, they advise restraint in the use of surgery in case of one or two recurrences on or after steroid therapy. Hence, this may be kept as a last resort after exhausting all combinations of medical management for at least 6–12 months.

## RECURRENCE OR RELAPSE

Recurrence risks of GLM have been reported to range between 15.4% and 24.8%.[6,51,52] While the treatment is usually continued until all symptoms and signs have regressed, premature discontinuation of medications before the complete resolution of the mass spells a higher risk of recurrence.[6] The treatment durations tend to be longer in the younger patients, when there is associated pregnancy or when Corynebacterial infection has been documented.[52] GLM with cutaneous manifestations have higher odds of recurrence.[51] Patients presenting with higher prolactin levels after treatment than the pre-treatment levels are an independent risk factor for recurrence.[53]

## CONCLUSION

Granulomatous Lobular Mastitis is uncommon but certainly not a rare disease. Although its etiology remains unknown, the pathogenesis is likely driven by a local immunological reaction. A typical background lactational history, along with a recurrent breast abscess, should raise suspicion for this disease, and the lesions biopsied early to establish a diagnosis. It is essential to rule out infectious etiologies, although this is often not found. Specific therapy with anti-tuberculous treatment should never be initiated unless acid–fast bacilli are conclusively identified, and preferably confirmed by a positive DNA test. Antibiotics can be effective when cystic neutrophilic type of granulomatous mastitis is diagnosed. Systemic steroids initiated early can better control the disease and reduce the likelihood of recurrence when compared to antibiotics alone, especially when the culture is negative. Although concomitant immunosuppressants have shown positive results in some studies, their use is generally reserved for more resistant forms of the disease or in patients who experience side effects from steroids. One or two recurrences should not warrant resection procedures; such interventions should be reserved for more complex and progressive disease that does not respond to optimal medical therapy.

## REFERENCES

1. Kessler E, Wolloch Y. Granulomatous mastitis: a lesion clinically simulating carcinoma. Am J Clin Pathol. 1972;58(6):642-6.
2. Deng JQ, Yu L, Yang Y, Feng XJ, Sun J, Liu J, et al. Steroids administered after vacuum-assisted biopsy in the management of idiopathic granulomatous mastitis. J Clin Pathol. 2017;70(10):827-31.
3. Ozel L, Unal A, Unal E, Kara M, Erdoğdu E, Krand O, et al. Granulomatous mastitis: is it an autoimmune disease? Diagnostic and therapeutic dilemmas. Surg Today. 2012;42(8):729-33.
4. Akbari Rad M, Sheybani F, Gharib M, Aghel E, Emadzadeh M, Mottaghi M. Coexistence of lobular granulomatous mastitis and breast cancer: Case report and case-based literature review. Int J Surg Case Rep. 2025;133:111628.

5. Yin Y, Liu X, Meng Q, Han X, Zhang H, Lv Y. Idiopathic Granulomatous Mastitis: Etiology, Clinical Manifestation, Diagnosis and Treatment. J Investig Surg Off J Acad Surg Res. 2022;35(3):709-20.
6. Yuan QQ, Xiao SX, Farouk O, Du YT, Sheybani F, Tan QT, et al. Management of granulomatous lobular mastitis: an international multidisciplinary consensus (2021 edition). Mil Med Res. 2022;26(9):20.
7. Zhou F, Yu LX, Ma ZB, Yu ZG. Granulomatous lobular mastitis. Chronic Dis Transl Med. 2016;2(1):17-21.
8. Kayadibi Y, Saracoglu MS, Kurt SA, Deger E, Boy FNS, Ucar N, et al. Differentiation of Malignancy and Idiopathic Granulomatous Mastitis Presenting as Non-mass Lesions on MRI: Radiological, Clinical, Radiomics, and Clinical-Radiomics Models. Acad Radiol. 2024;31(9):3511-23.
9. Wang P, Sun JZ, Fang HY, Yang DJ, Ren GS. Optimal Timing for Corticosteroid Therapy in Idiopathic Granulomatous Mastitis: A Retrospective Analysis Highlighting Early Intervention Efficacy. J Inflamm Res. 2024;17:9617-24.
10. Bashir MU, Ramcharan A, Alothman S, Beaugris S, Khan SA, Sbeih MA, et al. The enigma of granulomatous mastitis: A series. Breast Dis. 2017;37(1):17-20.
11. Lin CH, Hsu CW, Tsao TY, Chou J. Idiopathic granulomatous mastitis associated with risperidone-induced hyperprolactinemia. Diagn Pathol. 2012;5:7:2.
12. Bellavia M, Damiano G, Palumbo VD, Spinelli G, Tomasello G, Marrazzo A, et al. Granulomatous Mastitis during Chronic Antidepressant Therapy: Is It Possible a Conservative Therapeutic Approach? J Breast Cancer. 2012;15(3):371-2.
13. Wang X, He X, Liu J, Zhang H, Wan H, Luo J, et al. Immune pathogenesis of idiopathic granulomatous mastitis: from etiology toward therapeutic approaches. Front Immunol. 2024;15:1295759.
14. Shojaeian F, Haghighat S, Abbasvandi F, Houshdar Tehrani A, Najar Najafi N, Zandi A, et al. Refractory and Recurrent Idiopathic Granulomatous Mastitis Treatment: Adaptive, Randomized Clinical Trial. J Am Coll Surg. 2024; 238(6):1153-65.
15. Omranipour R, Mohammadi SF, Samimi P. Idiopathic Granulomatous Lobular Mastitis – Report of 43 Cases from Iran; Introducing a Preliminary Clinical Practice Guideline. Breast Care. 2013;8(6):439-43.
16. Kutsuna S, Mezaki K, Nagamatsu M, Kunimatsu J, Yamamoto K, Fujiya Y, et al. Two Cases of Granulomatous Mastitis Caused by Corynebacterium kroppenstedtii Infection in Nulliparous Young Women with Hyperprolactinemia. Intern Med Tokyo Jpn. 2015;54(14):1815-8.
17. Oran EŞ, Gürdal SÖ, Yankol Y, Öznur M, Calay Z, Tunacı M, et al. Management of idiopathic granulomatous mastitis diagnosed by core biopsy: a retrospective multicenter study. Breast J. 2013;19(4):411-8.
18. Altintoprak F, Kivilcim T, Ozkan OV. Aetiology of idiopathic granulomatous mastitis. World J Clin Cases WJCC. 2014;2(12):852-8.
19. Kessler E, Wolloch Y. Granulomatous Mastitis: A Lesion Clinically Simulating Carcinoma. Am J Clin Pathol. 1972;58(6):642-6.
20. Azlina AF, Ariza Z, Arni T, Hisham AN. Chronic Granulomatous Mastitis: Diagnostic and Therapeutic Considerations. World J Surg. 2003;27(5):515-8.
21. Li SB, Xiong Y, Han XR, Liu ZY, Lv XL, Ning P. Pregnancy Associated Granulomatous Mastitis: Clinical Characteristics, Management, and Outcome. Breastfeed Med Off J Acad Breastfeed Med. 2021;16(9):759-64.

22. Yaghan RJ, Ayoub NM, Shenawi HM, Yaghan LR. Idiopathic granulomatous mastitis in the male population: A clinical analysis of 13 reported cases. Breast J. 2020;26(7):1481-2.
23. Martinez-Ramos D, Simon-Monterde L, Suelves-Piqueres C, Queralt-Martin R, Granel-Villach L, Laguna-Sastre JM, et al. Idiopathic granulomatous mastitis: A systematic review of 3060 patients. Breast J. 2019;25(6):1245-50.
24. Yaghan RJ, Ayoub NM, Hamouri S, Al-Mohtaseb A, Gharaibeh M, Yaghan L, et al. The Role of Establishing a Multidisciplinary Team for Idiopathic Granulomatous Mastitis in Improving Patient Outcomes and Spreading Awareness about Recent Disease Trends. Int J Breast Cancer. 2020;2020:5243958.
25. Pluguez-Turull CW, Nanyes JE, Quintero CJ, Alizai H, Mais DD, Kist KA, et al. Idiopathic Granulomatous Mastitis: Manifestations at Multimodality Imaging and Pitfalls. Radiogr Rev Publ Radiol Soc N Am Inc. 2018;38(2):330-56.
26. Kok KYY, Telisinghe PU. Granulomatous mastitis: presentation, treatment and outcome in 43 patients. Surg J R Coll Surg Edinb Irel. 2010;8(4):197-201.
27. Gurleyik G, Aktekin A, Aker F, Karagulle H, Saglamc A. Medical and Surgical Treatment of Idiopathic Granulomatous Lobular Mastitis: A Benign Inflammatory Disease Mimicking Invasive Carcinoma. J Breast Cancer. 2012;15(1):119-23.
28. Lee JH, Oh KK, Kim E K, Kwack KS, Jung WH, Lee HK. Radiologic and Clinical Features of Idiopathic Granulomatous Lobular Mastitis Mimicking Advanced Breast Cancer. Yonsei Med J. 2006 ;47(1):78-84.
29. Al-Khawari HAT, Al-Manfouhi HA, Madda JP, Kovacs A, Sheikh M, Roberts O. Radiologic features of granulomatous mastitis. Breast J. 2011;17(6):645-50.
30. Zhang L, Hu J, Guys N et al. Diffusion-weighted imaging in relation to morphology on dynamic contrast enhancement MRI: the diagnostic value of characterizing non-puerperal mastitis. Eur Radiol 2018;28:992-9.
31. Salesi M, Karimifar M, Salimi F, Mahzouni P. A case of granulomatous mastitis with erythema nodosum and arthritis. Rheumatol Int. 2011;31(8):1093-5.
32. Ben Abid F, Abdel Rahman S Al Soub H. A case report of TB versus idiopathic granulomatous mastitis with erythema nodosum, reactive arthritis, cough, and headache. Aging Male Off J Int Soc Study Aging Male. 2020;23(5):411-4.
33. Cui L, Sun C, Guo J, Zhang X, Liu S. Pathological manifestations of granulomatous lobular mastitis. Frontiers in Medicine. 2024; 11:1326587.
34. Liu L, Zhou F, Wang P, Yu L, Ma Z, Li Y, et al. Periductal Mastitis: An Inflammatory Disease Related to Bacterial Infection and Consequent Immune Responses? Mediators Inflamm. 2017;2017:5309081.
35. Jiao Y, Chang K, Jiang Y, Zhang J. Identification of periductal mastitis and granulomatous lobular mastitis: a literature review. Ann Transl Med. 2023;11(3):158.
36. Nikolaev A, Blake CN, Carlson DL. Association between Hyperprolactinemia and Granulomatous Mastitis. Breast J. 2016;22(2):224-31.
37. Aghajanzadeh M, Hassanzadeh R, Alizadeh Sefat S, Alavi A, Hemmati H, Esmaeili Delshad MS, et al. Granulomatous mastitis: Presentations, diagnosis, treatment and outcome in 206 patients from the north of Iran. Breast Edinb Scotl. 2015;24(4):456-60.
38. Tan QT, Tay SP, Gudi MA, Nadkarni NV, Lim SH, Chuwa EWL. Granulomatous Mastitis and Factors Associated with Recurrence: An 11-Year Single-Centre Study of 113 Patients in Singapore. World J Surg. 2019;43(7):1737-45.
39. Joseph KA, Luu X, Mor A. Granulomatous mastitis: a New York public hospital experience. Ann Surg Oncol. 2014;21(13):4159-63.

40. Farouk O, Abdelkhalek M, Abdallah A, Shata A, Senbel A, Attia E, et al. Rifampicin for Idiopathic Granulomatous Lobular Mastitis: A Promising Alternative for Treatment. World J Surg. 2017;41(5):1313-21.
41. Sarmadian R, Safi F, Sarmadian H, Shokrpour M, Almasi-Hashiani A. Treatment modalities for granulomatous mastitis, seeking the most appropriate treatment with the least recurrence rate: a systematic review and meta-analysis. Eur J Med Res. 2024;29(1):164.
42. Lei X, Chen K, Zhu L, Song E, Su F, Li S. Treatments for Idiopathic Granulomatous Mastitis: Systematic Review and Meta-Analysis. Breastfeed Med. 2017;12(7):415-21.
43. Montazer M, Dadashzadeh M, Mousavi Toomatari SE. Comparison of the Outcome of Low Dose and High-Dose Corticosteroid in the Treatment of Idiopathic Granulomatous Mastitis. Asian Pac J Cancer Prev APJCP. 2020;21(4):993-6.
44. Yaghan R, Hamouri S, Ayoub NM, Yaghan L, Mazahreh T. A Proposal of a Clinically Based Classification for Idiopathic Granulomatous Mastitis. Asian Pac J Cancer Prev APJCP. 2019;20(3):929-34.
45. Altintoprak F, Kivilcim T, Yalkin O, Uzunoglu Y, Kahyaoglu Z, Dilek ON. Topical Steroids Are Effective in the Treatment of Idiopathic Granulomatous Mastitis. World J Surg. 2015;39(11):2718-23.
46. Çetin K, Sıkar HE, Göret NE, Rona G, Barışık NÖ, Küçük HF, et al. Comparison of Topical, Systemic, and Combined Therapy with Steroids on Idiopathic Granulomatous Mastitis: A Prospective Randomized Study. World J Surg. 2019;43(11):2865-73.
47. Xiao M, Li S, Tong S. Clinical analysis of treatment with granulomatous lobular mastitis by ultrasonography-guided abscess puncture aspiration or drainage combined with local application of triamcinolone acetonide for 46 cases. Chinese Archives of General Surgery (Electronic Edition). 2019;13(01):30.
48. Korkut E, Akcay MN, Karadeniz E, Subasi ID, Gursan N. Granulomatous Mastitis: A Ten-Year Experience at a University Hospital. Eurasian J Med. 2015;47(3):165-73.
49. Akbulut S, Yilmaz D, Bakir S. Methotrexate in the management of idiopathic granulomatous mastitis: review of 108 published cases and report of four cases. Breast J. 2011;17(6):661-8.
50. Haddad M, Sheybani F, Arian M, Gharib M. Methotrexate-based regimen as initial treatment of patients with idiopathic granulomatous mastitis. Breast J. 2020;26(2):325-7.
51. Azizi A, Prasath V, Canner J, Gharib M, Sadat Fattahi A, Naser Forghani M, et al. Idiopathic granulomatous mastitis: Management and predictors of recurrence in 474 patients. Breast J. 2020;26(7):1358-62.
52. Tsai MJ, Huang WC, Wang JT, Wang MY, Lee YH, Lin SW, et al. Factors associated with treatment duration and recurrence rate of complicated mastitis. J Microbiol Immunol Infect Wei Mian Yu Gan Ran Za Zhi. 2020;53(6):875-81.
53. Huang Y, Wu H. A retrospective analysis of recurrence risk factors for granulomatous lobular mastitis in 130 patients: more attention should be paid to prolactin level. Ann Palliat Med. 2021;10(3):2824-31.

CHAPTER 12

# Urolithiasis

*Sameer Trivedi, Aviral Srivastava*

## INTRODUCTION

Urinary stone disease, i.e., urolithiasis, affects 12–20% of the global population, with a rising incidence and a high recurrence risk (up to 50%) that places a greater financial burden on global healthcare.[1,2] In India, prevalence is 12–15%, particularly high in the "stone belt" regions including Maharashtra, Gujarat, Rajasthan, Punjab, Haryana, Delhi, and northeastern states.[2] Its etiology is multifactorial, linked with age, male sex, family history, obesity, diabetes, genetic predisposition, diet, and geography.[1,2] Common presenting features are renal colic symptoms, which can be incidentally detected or cause complications such as hydronephrosis, pyonephrosis, renal dysfunction, or rarely xanthogranulomatous pyelonephritis.[1-3]

While the basic principles remain the same—viz., detailed history, appropriate laboratory and imaging studies, precise diagnosis, complete clearance, and recurrence prevention—there has been a paradigm shift in urolithiasis management, driven by technological innovations and refined clinical strategies. Advances in high-resolution imaging, enhanced endourological instrumentation, and widespread adoption of laser technologies [thulium fiber and holmium:yttrium aluminum garnet (Holmium:YAG)] have enabled efficient stone fragmentation and reduced operative times. Minimally invasive interventions like retrograde intrarenal surgery (RIRS) and miniaturized percutaneous nephrolithotomy (mini-PCNL) have reduced patient morbidity and shortened recovery times, thus broadening treatment options even for complex stone burdens. In parallel, individualized metabolic evaluation, risk stratification, and preventive strategies have gained traction. Emerging tools, such as artificial intelligence-assisted diagnostics and predictive algorithms, also hold promise for optimizing patient outcomes. This chapter presents an overview of the latest advancements in urolithiasis management that have enhanced procedural efficacy, safety, and patient-centered outcomes.

## CLASSIFICATION

Though several variations exist, urinary stones are primarily categorized by chemical composition **(Table 1)**.

**TABLE 1:** Classification of urinary stones.[1,3]

| *Etiological classification* | *Classification by location* | *Classification by X-ray characteristics* | *Classification by chemical composition* |
|---|---|---|---|
| • *Noninfection stones:*<br>– Calcium oxalate<br>– Calcium phosphate<br>– Uric acid<br>– Ammonium urate<br>• *Infection stones:*<br>– Magnesium ammonium phosphate<br>– Carbonated apatite<br>– Ammonium urate<br>• *Genetic causes:*<br>– Cystine<br>– Xanthine<br>– 2,8-dihydroxyadenine | *According to anatomical position:* Upper, middle, or lower calyx; renal pelvis; proximal or distal ureter; and urinary bladder | Depends on mineral composition. Noncontrast-enhanced computed tomography (NCCT) can further classify stones according to density, inner structure, and composition<br>• *Radiopaque:*<br>– Calcium oxalate dihydrate<br>– Calcium oxalate monohydrate<br>– Calcium phosphate<br>• *Poor radiopaque:*<br>– Magnesium ammonium phosphate<br>– Cystine<br>– Calcium phosphate<br>• *Radiolucent:*<br>– Uric acid<br>– Ammonium urate<br>– Xanthine<br>– 2,8-dihydroxyadenine<br>– Drug-stones | • *Calcium stones:*<br>– Calcium oxalate<br>– Calcium phosphate<br>• Uric acid stones<br>• Struvite stones<br>• Cystine stones |

## PATHOPHYSIOLOGY

Urolithiasis arises when urinary solutes in supersaturated urine precipitate into crystalline aggregates, progressing to stone formation. Predisposing factors include urinary stasis from anatomical anomalies, low urine volume, dietary influences, urinary tract infections, drug exposure, and, rarely, genetic defects.[3-5] Pathogenesis often heralds with Randall's plaques—suburothelial calcium phosphate deposits at the papillae-collecting duct interface—which enlarge, disrupt urothelium, and extend into the renal pelvis, providing a nidus for crystal adherence in a supersaturated milieu **(Fig. 1)**. Endogenous supersaturation inhibitors such as citrate, glycosaminoglycans, nephrocalcin, Tamm-Horsfall protein, uropontin, and water normally prevent crystal aggregation; their inadequacy in supersaturated urine facilitates stone growth. Inadequate fluid intake and reduced urine output are the most common causes behind urolithiasis. Among metabolic contributors, hypercalciuria, hyperoxaluria, hyperuricosuria, and hypocitraturia are predominant.[1,3]

The etiopathogenesis of renal calculi varies with stone composition[1,3-6] **(Figs. 2A to H)**. Calcium-based stones account for 75–85% of cases, predominantly calcium oxalate (monohydrate or dihydrate) and less often calcium phosphate. They arise from metabolic abnormalities such as hyperparathyroidism, renal tubular acidosis (RTA), renal calcium leak, hyperoxaluria, hypomagnesemia, or hypocitraturia. Calcium oxalate stones exist as monohydrate (COM)—hard, smooth, dark brown stones—or dihydrate (COD)—lighter, brittle stones with jagged projections.

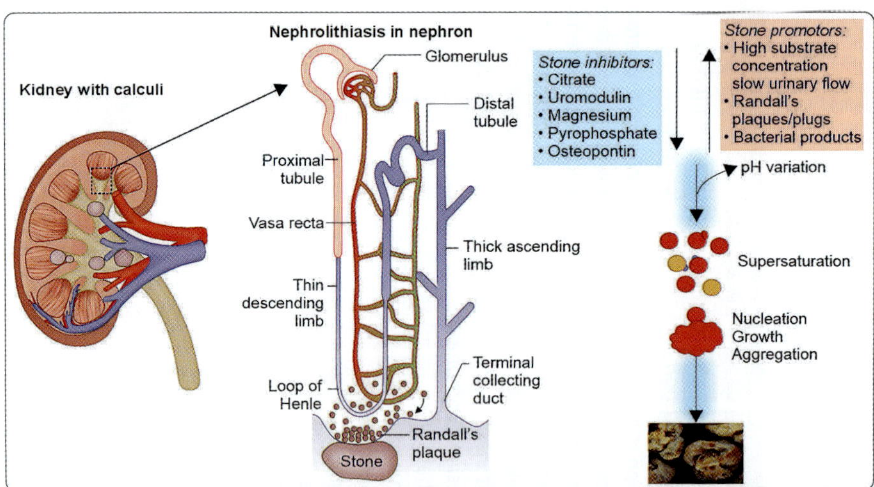


**Fig. 1:** Pathophysiology of urolithiasis—development of Randal's plaque in the nephron and subsequent renal stone formation through imbalance of inhibitors and promoters.[5] *Source:* Schott C, Pourtousi A, Connaughton DM. Monogenic causation of pediatric nephrolithiasis. Front Urol. 2022;2:1075711.

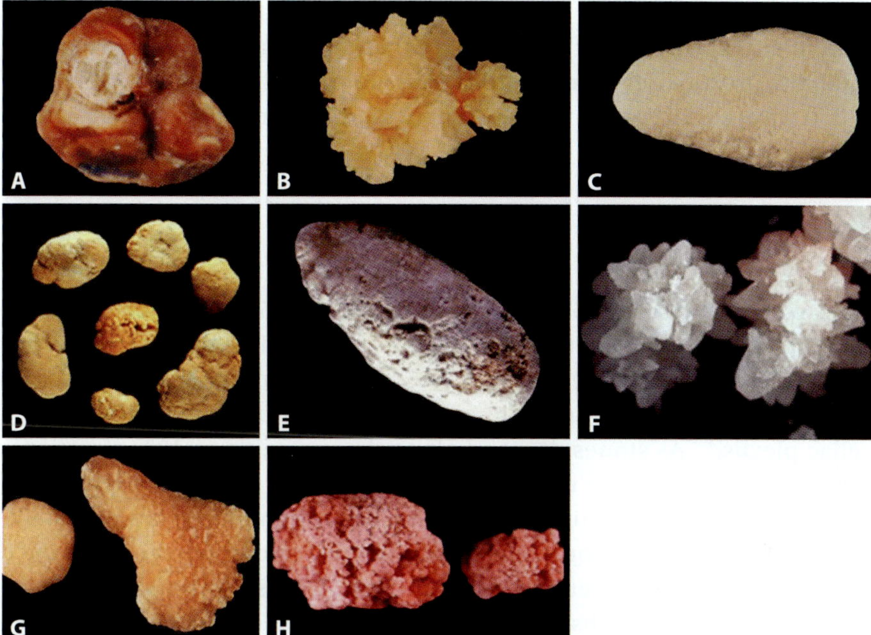


**Figs. 2A to H:** Calculi subtypes. (A) Calcium oxalate monohydrate; (B) Calcium oxalate dihydrate; (C) Calcium phosphate; (D) Uric acid; (E) Ammonium urate; (F) Struvite; (G) Cystine; (H) Drug (indinavir).[6]

*Source:* Adopted and modified from Courbebaisse M, Travers S, Bouderlique E, Michon-Colin A, Daudon M, De Mul A, Poli L, Baron S, Prot-Bertoye C. Hydration for adult patients with nephrolithiasis: specificities and current recommendations. Nutrients. 2023;15(23):4885.

Microscopically, calcium oxalate crystals display diverse morphologies, including envelope, oval, spindle, octahedral, or dumbbell forms.[3-5] Calcium phosphate calculi, composed of carbonate apatite (hydroxyapatite) or brushite (calcium hydrogen phosphate), develop in alkaline urine, often associated with RTA and hyperparathyroidism. These are white to yellowish and microscopically appear as plates, needles, rosettes, or stellate clusters, depending on mineral type.[3-5]

The other major stone types include uric acid (8–10%), struvite (calcium magnesium ammonium phosphate, 7–8%), and cystine stones (1–2%).[1,3] Uric acid stones typically form in persistently acidic urine (pH < 5.5) and are linked to a purine-rich diet (fish, legumes, and meat), gout, and malignancy with high cell turnover. They are radiolucent, yellow to reddish-brown, and exhibit rhomboid, plate-like, or rosette-shaped crystals under microscopy. Struvite stones result from infection with urease-producing gram-negative organisms, such as *Proteus*, *Klebsiella*, or *Pseudomonas*. Forming in alkaline urine, they frequently develop into staghorn calculi and appear chalky white or grey, brittle, and smooth-surfaced, with characteristic coffin-lid crystals microscopically.[4] Cystine stones, though rare, arise from inherited defects in tubular reabsorption of cystine and other dibasic amino acids. Their low solubility predisposes them to stone formation. Grossly amber to yellowish with a waxy surface, cystine stones show the classic microscopic hexagonal crystals.

## EVALUATION

### Symptoms and Signs[1,3-6]

Flank pain remains the most frequent symptom (35–55%), described as sharp, stabbing pain radiating to the groin, testicle, or labia. Renal colic episode has a sudden onset, intensifies within 15–45 minutes, and then steadies, often accompanied by nausea or vomiting from renal capsule stretch irritating the celiac plexus.[3-5] As stones descend along the ureter, up to 10% of patients experience pain shifting toward the groin or lower abdomen. Hematuria, usually microscopic, results from mucosal irritation by crystals or calculi. Irritative voiding symptoms, such as frequency and urgency, occur once the stone reaches the ureterovesical junction. A subset of patients remains asymptomatic, unless obstruction or infection develops within the kidney, ureteropelvic junction, or ureter.[3-5]

Serious complications include pyonephrosis, presenting with fever, chills, or sepsis, a urological emergency requiring urgent drainage, either via double-J stent or percutaneous nephrostomy. In hemodynamically unstable patients or those with large stone burdens, percutaneous drainage is preferred to prevent progression to urosepsis, shock, or death.[3-5]

### Comprehensive Assessment

History is vital for guiding evaluation and management, with focus on:[1,3-6]

- *Medical history:* Identification of systemic or metabolic conditions that predispose to stone formation **(Table 2)**.
- *Family history:* Inquiry into early-onset stones or inherited disorders like cystinuria and idiopathic hypercalciuria.
- *Dietary history:* Assessment of fluid intake, sodium and protein consumption, calcium sources (e.g., dairy), and oxalate-rich foods such as nuts, whole grains, dates, chocolate, and spinach.
- *Medication Review:* Evaluation for drugs that increase stone risk or directly form calculi **(Table 3)**.

Physical examination may reveal costovertebral angle tenderness, hypoactive bowel sounds, and tenderness in the testicular or pubic area.

## DIAGNOSTIC IMAGING

The choice of imaging modality depends on the clinical scenario and the suspected location of the stone—renal or ureteric—as guided by patient

**TABLE 2:** High-risk stone formers.[1]

| *Category* | *Clinical criteria/risk indicators* |
|---|---|
| Recurrent or complex stone disease | • Multiple or bilateral renal calculi<br>• Recurrent episodes of nephrolithiasis |
| Genetic or early-onset stone formation | • Onset of kidney stones before 18 years of age<br>• Positive family history of renal calculi<br>• Inherited metabolic conditions (e.g., cystinuria and primary hyperoxaluria)<br>• Known or suspected hereditary stone disorders |
| Stone types linked with metabolic disorders | • Pure calcium phosphate stones<br>• Uric acid, cystine, struvite, or magnesium ammonium phosphate stones |
| Systemic medical conditions associated with stones | • Hyperparathyroidism<br>• Sarcoidosis<br>• Inflammatory or malabsorptive bowel disease (e.g., IBD, chronic pancreatitis, and chronic diarrhea)<br>• History of gastrointestinal surgeries (e.g., colectomy, ileostomy, small bowel resection, Roux-en-Y bypass)<br>• Cystic fibrosis<br>• Metabolic syndrome—obesity, T2DM, dyslipidemia, and hypertension<br>• Gout<br>• Spinal cord injury<br>• Neurogenic bladder<br>• Chronic or recurrent UTIs<br>• Osteoporosis<br>• Renal tubular acidosis<br>• Polycystic kidney disease |
| Structural abnormalities of the urinary tract | Anomalies that obstruct urinary drainage, e.g., medullary sponge kidney, ureteral strictures, horseshoe kidney |
| Risk of stone-related complications | • Single functioning kidney (congenital or acquired)<br>• CKD<br>• Past episodes of complicated stone disease (e.g., AKI, urosepsis, and prolonged hospitalization) |
| High-stakes professional risk | Occupations where sudden obstruction is high-risk, e.g., pregnancy, pilots, police, military, and firefighters |

(AKI: acute kidney injury; CKD: chronic kidney disease; IBD: inflammatory bowel disease; T2DM: type 2 diabetes mellitus; UTIs: urinary tract infections)

history. Urgent imaging is warranted in cases of solitary kidney, associated fever, or diagnostic uncertainty.

- *Ultrasound (USG) kidney, ureter, and bladder (KUB)* is the primary imaging tool because it is safe, reproducible, inexpensive, and radiation-free. Stones appear in the renal pelvicalyceal system as bright (echogenic)

**TABLE 3:** Drugs associated with kidney stones.[1]

| *Medications increasing stone risk (via metabolic alteration)* | *Drugs that directly crystallize or form stones* |
|---|---|
| • *Hypercalciuria (↑ urinary calcium → calcium stones)*<br>– High-dose calcium or vitamin D supplements<br>– Loop diuretics (e.g., furosemide)<br>– Long-term glucocorticoids<br>• *Hypocitraturia and alkaline urine (→ calcium phosphate stones)*<br>– Carbonic anhydrase inhibitors (e.g., acetazolamide, topiramate, and zonisamide)<br>• *Hyperoxaluria (↑ urinary oxalate → calcium oxalate stones)*<br>– Repeated antibiotic use (alters gut flora)<br>– Excessive vitamin C intake<br>• *Hyperuricosuria (→ uric acid/calcium oxalate stones)*<br>– Uricosuric agents (e.g., probenecid and losartan)<br>• *Increased urinary ammonium (→ ammonium urate stones)*<br>– Chronic laxative misuse | • *Antiviral:*<br>– Indinavir<br>– Atazanavir<br>– Nelfinavir<br>– Tenofovir disoproxil fumarate<br>– Raltegravir<br>– Efavirenz<br>• *Antibiotics:*<br>– Sulfadiazine<br>– Sulfamethoxazole<br>– Ciprofloxacin<br>– Amoxicillin<br>– Ampicillin<br>– Ceftriaxone<br>• *Others:*<br>– Triamterene<br>– Sulfasalazine<br>– Allopurinol<br>– Guaifenesin/ephedrine<br>– Magnesium trisilicate |

areas with posterior acoustic shadowing. Often preferred during pregnancy and for assessing urinary obstruction and hydronephrosis, it can also identify noncalcified stones like uric acid calculi if their size exceeds 4 mm, though it misses smaller or distal ureteric stones due to interference from bowel gas. It has a sensitivity of 45% and specificity of 94% for ureteral stones and a sensitivity of 45% and specificity of 88% for renal stones.[3,4] The resistive index value [(peak systolic velocity-end-diastolic velocity)/peak systolic velocity], measured using Doppler USG, above 0.7 can suggest ureteral obstruction, while a lower index may predict a higher likelihood of spontaneous passage.[3-4,7]

- *X-ray KUB* has diagnostic sensitivity and specificity ranging from 44% to 77%. It can be used for screening but may not detect small calculi (≤2 mm), those obscured by intestinal gas, or radiolucent/noncalcified stones. Despite these limitations, it can serve as a baseline for follow-up imaging. Combined with USG KUB, it offers a radiation-sparing and cost-effective alternative to computed tomography (CT) to identify calcified and certain noncalcified stones in limited resources[3,4] **(Figs. 3A to D)**.
- *Noncontrast-enhanced abdominal and pelvic computed tomography (NCCT)–KUB* has become standard-of-care for diagnosing acute flank pain, offering superior accuracy (90–97% sensitivity and specificity)

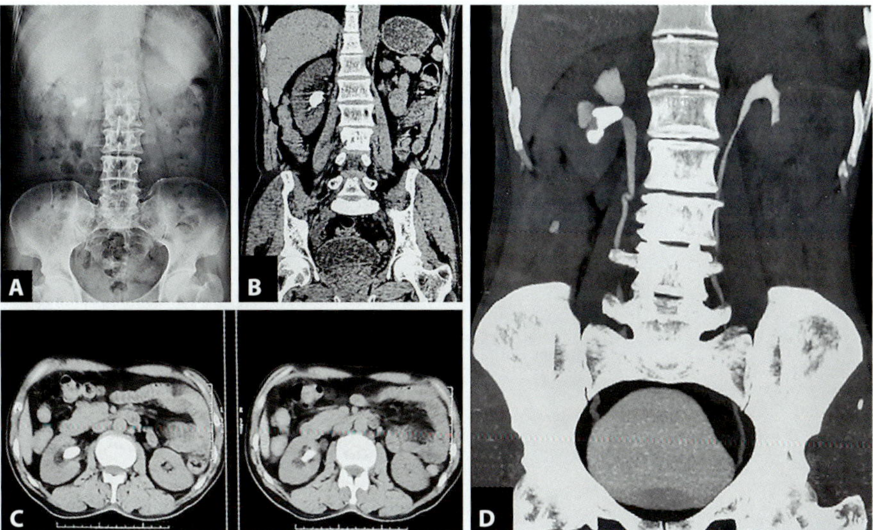


**Figs. 3A to D:** Right renal pelvic calculus seen on: (A) Plain X-ray KUB; (B) NCCT; (C) Contrast-enhanced CT scan; (D) CT urography. (CT: computed tomography; KUB: kidney, ureter, and bladder; NCCT: noncontrast computed tomography)

compared to intravenous urography (IVU) and ultrasound **(Figs. 3A to D)**. It enables a comprehensive assessment of renal parenchyma and pelvicalyceal anatomy to determine stone location, size, number, and density/composition (based on Hounsfield units, i.e., HU), including radiolucent stones missed over plain X-rays (uric acid and xanthine). Low-attenuation stones (<800 HU) include uric acid (400–600 HU), struvite (550–700 HU), and cystine (650–800 HU). High-attenuation stones (>800 HU) comprise carbonate apatite (850–1050 HU), calcium oxalate dihydrate (1,100–1,200 HU), calcium oxalate monohydrate (1,200–1,400 HU), and brushite (1,500 1,800 HU). NCCT, however, lacks information on renal function and may miss indinavir/drug stones. It is considered the modality of choice for distal ureteric calculi evaluation. Low-dose NCCT, described to reduce radiation risk, has 86-90% sensitivity for detecting ureteral stones < 3 mm and 92–94% for calculi > 3 mm.[1-4,7,8]

- *Computed tomography urography (CTU):* The imaging modality choice for nephrolithiasis assessment (98–100% sensitivity, 95–100% specificity), it uses multidetector computed tomography (MDCT) to evaluate the entire urinary tract, detecting radiolucent and radiopaque stones, obstruction, hydronephrosis, and anatomical anomalies. It typically includes three phases: Noncontrast phase—for detection of calculi, Nephrographic phase (80–100 seconds after contrast)—for contrast uptake and renal parenchyma evaluation, and Excretory phase (8–15 minutes after contrast)—to assess renal function and drainage

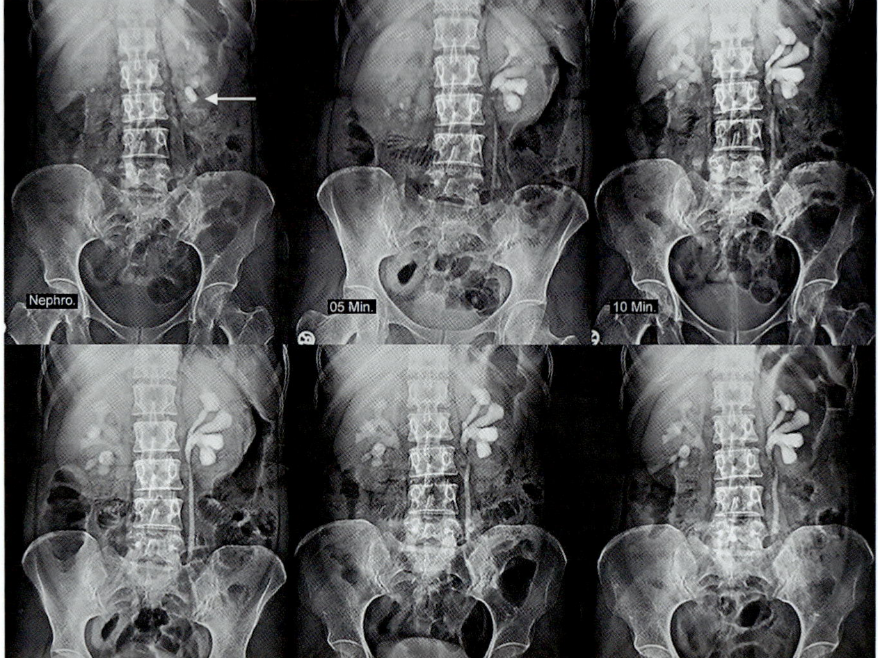


**Fig. 4:** Intravenous pyelogram (IVP) depicting a 2.5 cm radiopaque calculus in the left lower calyx (arrow), 5–15-minute images depict contrast opacification of the collecting system and ureters, 45 minutes to 3 hours images show delayed contrast progression into the bladder.

**(Fig. 4)**. It offers advantage over NCCT in functional assessment, 3D reconstruction and precise localization of pathology, but has higher radiation exposure, cost, and contrast-induced nephrotoxicity risk.[3,8-10]

- Intravenous urogram (IVU)—though largely replaced by CT, IVU remains useful in select cases for functional assessment, assessing the degree of obstruction and anatomical detail **(Fig. 4)**, especially in resource-limited settings.[1,3]

## BIOCHEMICAL ANALYSIS

The extent of biochemical evaluation depends on the risk of stone recurrence and the patients' interests. For first-time stone formers, urinalysis, urine culture, and basic metabolic panels should be obtained.

- *Basic metabolic panel (Serum analysis)*—includes renal function test (creatinine, uric acid), serum electrolytes (potassium, sodium, calcium, phosphorus, and magnesium), blood cell count, and serum C-reactive protein (CRP). Serum parathyroid hormone (PTH) is needed in suspected primary hyperparathyroidism.

- *Urine analysis*—dipstick test for RBCs, pus cells, nitrites, pH, casts, proteins, urine microscopy, and urine culture.

  For high-risk stone formers **(Table 2)** and interested first-time stone formers, a thorough evaluation is warranted, including the following tests:
- Basic metabolic panel (serum analysis)
- Urinalysis
- *24-hour urine analysis*—essential for stone risk assessment, measuring urine volume, creatinine, pH, and key solutes (sodium, potassium, magnesium, chloride, sulphate, phosphate, ammonium, calcium, citrate, oxalate, uric acid, and cystine if suspected), while calculating relative supersaturation of stone-forming substances. The sample is collected over a full day on a habitual diet, starting after discarding the first morning void and ending with the next day's first void. Follow-up testing at 8–16 weeks postintervention helps assess therapy response, with annual monitoring once biochemical targets are achieved to ensure long-term control and recurrence prevention.[1,3]
- *Stone analysis*—plays a crucial role in guiding appropriate intervention, identifying underlying metabolic disorders, and formulating preventive medical strategies to reduce recurrence.[3-5] Guidelines recommend that stone composition should be assessed in all first-time stone formers, if feasible.[1-3] Repeat analysis is warranted in certain clinical contexts, such as recurrence despite medical preventive therapy, early recurrence after interventional therapy with complete stone clearance, or late recurrence after a prolonged stone-free period. The most reliable methods for stone analysis are X-ray diffraction (XRD) and Fourier transform infrared spectroscopy (FTIR).[1-3] X-ray diffraction (XRD) uses monochromatic X-rays to generate a diffraction pattern unique to crystal structure, while FTIR records molecular absorption spectra of stone **(Figs. 5A and B)** compared with reference libraries.[3,11] Both techniques offer high precision for pure stone identification, but are limited in mixed compositions: XRD cannot detect noncrystalline substances, whereas FTIR is faster and cheaper but unreliable with minor components in mixed stones. Microcomputed tomography (MicroCT) is an emerging, nondestructive technique that preserves stone microarchitecture (unlike XRD or FTIR), provides high-resolution three-dimensional (3D) imaging, and reliably detects heterogeneous compositions and microfractures.[1-3,11] However, its clinical use is restricted by cost and required expertise.

## Management

The treatment of urolithiasis is based on many parameters, such as size, number, location, and constitution of stones, as well as anatomy of the pelvicalyceal system, and hence it is individualized.

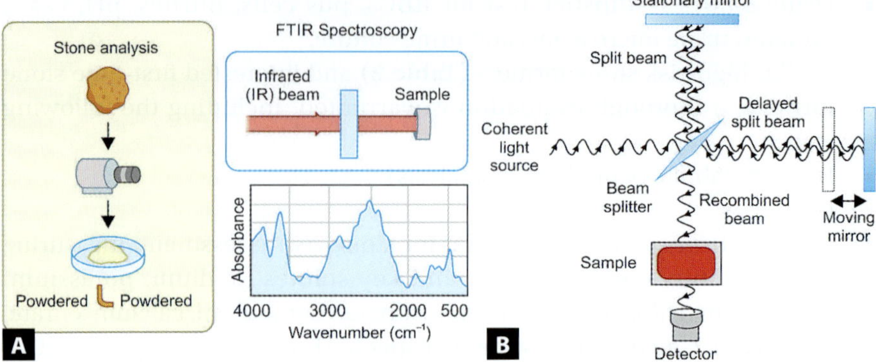


**Figs. 5A and B:** Principle and application of Fourier-transform infrared spectroscopy (FTIR) in kidney stone analysis; (B) Mathematical transformation of interferogram (via Fourier Transform) generates infrared absorption spectrum.
*Source:* https://www.biorender.com/

## *Acute Episode Management*

- *Management of renal colic:* Paracetamol and NSAIDs are preferred for initial pain management due to faster onset, safety, and efficacy over opioids, while also reducing ureteral inflammation and aiding stone expulsion.[3] Risks include cardiovascular events, gastrointestinal (GI) bleeding, and renal impairment in low glomerular filtration rate (GFR), requiring dose adjustment. Combining NSAIDs with antispasmodics offers no added benefit.[3] Persistent pain or complications (infection and obstruction) warrant interventions such as ureteral stenting, percutaneous nephrostomy, or stone extraction.[1,3]
- *Management of sepsis and/or anuria in obstructed kidney(s):* Unilateral/bilateral stone-related obstruction with infection/sepsis or anuria is a urological emergency requiring urgent decompression to prevent life-threatening complications. Emergency drainage is achieved via ureteral stent or percutaneous nephrostomy, while definitive stone removal is delayed until infection resolves. Management includes broad-spectrum IV antibiotics adjusted to culture results, along with supportive care—IV fluids, hemodynamic monitoring, and intensive care unit (ICU) for admission in urosepsis or septic shock.

## Conservative Management

- *Conservative treatment/observation:* Spontaneous ureteric stone passage depends on size, number, location, and composition. Smaller and distal ureteral stones pass more often, with reported rates of 49–70% for upper/mid and 68–83% for distal stones.[1,3] Approximately 75% of calculi ≤5 mm and 62% ≥5 mm pass spontaneously, typically within 17–20 days (range 6–29). Passage may occur with calcium oxalate, phosphate, uric acid, and cystine stones, but is rare with struvite or staghorn calculi.

- *Medical expulsive therapy (MET) and pharmacologic management:* MET is a noninvasive option reserved for stable patients with ureteral stones not requiring immediate intervention, especially distal calculi ≥5 mm less likely to pass spontaneously. It works by relaxing the ureteral smooth muscle, reducing oedema/spasm, and aiding stone movement towards the bladder. Common agents include alpha-blockers (e.g., tamsulosin), calcium channel blockers, and phosphodiesterase type 5 (PDE5) inhibitors. Treatment lasts 4–6 weeks with monitoring for infection, persistent symptoms, or renal function decline, which necessitates stopping MET and considering surgical intervention.

Oral dissolution therapy using alkalinization alone may be effective in dissolving renal uric acid calculi. For patients with uric acid stones, particularly located in the distal ureter, combining urinary alkalinization (e.g., potassium citrate to increase urine pH > 6.5) with MET can significantly improve spontaneous passage.

## Definitive Management

Key indications for surgical management of urolithiasis include anuria/severe oliguria requiring urgent drainage, large stones >10 mm with unlikely spontaneous expulsion, infected obstruction needing decompression with delayed clearance, obstruction in a solitary kidney, persistent symptoms despite analgesia, bilateral ureteral obstruction, urosepsis, and worsening renal function or parenchymal loss. Other specific indications for removal of ureteral stones are stones with low likelihood of spontaneous passage or failure to pass within 4–6 weeks, and persistent obstruction. Other specific indications for renal stones include high-risk patients for stone formation or social/professional concerns.[1-3]

Procedure selection for stone removal should be individualized based on stone characteristics—size, location, and composition—and patient-specific factors (body build, urinary tract anatomy, bleeding tendencies, associated comorbidities) to optimize outcomes.[3,12] UTIs must be screened and treated before intervention to reduce complications: single-dose antibiotic prophylaxis lowers postoperative fever risk, while high-risk patients or those with prior UTIs benefit from a longer 7–10-day course.[3,12] **Table 4** shows a summary of surgical management in urolithiasis.

### *Extracorporeal Shock Wave Lithotripsy*

Introduced in the 1980s, extracorporeal shockwave lithotripsy (ESWL) is a noninvasive treatment that uses externally applied shockwaves for calculi fragmentation. Selection depends on stone size, location, density,

**TABLE 4:** Summary of surgical management of urolithiasis (adapted and modified from EAU 2025 and AUA 2024 guidelines).[1,16]

| *Stone* | *Preferred surgical procedure* |
|---|---|
| *Ureteral stones:* | |
| Uncomplicated ureteral stone ≤10 mm | Trial of MET with pain control (NSAIDS > opioids) for up to 4–6 weeks with reassessment of pain control, renal function, and stone passage |
| Proximal ureteral stone <10 mm | ESWL or URS |
| Proximal ureteral stone >10 mm, mid or distal ureteral stone (any size) | URS/RIRS > SWL |
| *Renal stones:* | |
| Asymptomatic renal stone <15 mm | Conservative therapy with follow-up imaging at 6 months, then annually |
| Symptomatic nonlower pole renal stone ≤10 mm | SWL or RIRS > PCNL |
| Symptomatic nonlower pole renal stone 10–20 mm | SWL/RIRS/PCNL |
| Symptomatic nonlower pole renal stone >20 mm | PCNL > SWL/RIRS |
| Symptomatic lower pole renal stone ≤10 mm | SWL or URS/RIRS |
| Symptomatic lower pole renal stone >10 mm (unfavorable for SWL) | RIRS or PCNL > SWL |
| Symptomatic lower pole renal stone >10 mm | SWL/RIRS/PCNL |
| Staghorn stones | PCNL |
| Negligible renal function | Nephrectomy for recurrent infection or pain |

(ESWL: extracorporeal shock wave lithotripsy; MET: medical expulsive therapy; NSAIDs: nonsteroidal anti-inflammatory drugs; PCNL: percutaneous nephrolithotomy; RIRS: retrograde intrarenal surgery; SWL: shock wave lithotripsy; URS: ureteroscopy)

composition, and patient factors. ESWL is first-line therapy for nonstaghorn stones ≤2 cm in the kidney or upper ureter. Stones with Hounsfield Unit (HU) ≤1,000 have higher fragmentation, while dense stones (calcium oxalate monohydrate, cystine, calcium phosphate) are more resistant.[1-3] Obesity (skin-to-stone distance >10 cm) and anatomical abnormalities (calyceal diverticula, malrotated/horseshoe kidneys, narrow infundibula, long calyces, unfavorable angles) limit success.[1-3] It can be performed under local anesthesia or IV sedation, suitable for patients unfit for general anesthesia. Shockwaves (90–120/min) focus on the stone, fragmenting it by combining biomechanical forces: cavitation (bubble collapse creates high-velocity jets), cleavage (internal stresses form microcracks parallel or perpendicular to wave direction), fatigue fracture (repetitive stress at weak points), shear stress, spallation (internal fractures by interacting reflected and incoming waves), squeezing (differential transmission between stone and fluid), and superfocusing (local concentration initiates microfractures).[1-4]

Lithotripters are classified by their shockwave generation method: electrohydraulic, electromagnetic, and piezoelectric—each offering comparable efficacy in achieving stone clearance **(Figs. 6A to D)**.[3,12-14] Electrohydraulic lithotripters generate shockwaves via underwater spark discharge focused by an ellipsoidal reflector. They are effective for large/dense stones but cause moderate discomfort, have variable energy, and lower durability due to frequent electrode wear. Electromagnetic lithotripters use a vibrating metallic membrane with an acoustic lens/parabolic reflector for focusing, and deliver consistent energy, moderate efficacy for large stones, lower discomfort, and high durability, though precise targeting is required. Piezoelectric lithotripters employ vibrating ceramic crystals with direct crystal focusing, providing consistent energy, minimal discomfort, and excellent durability, but lower energy output, making them less effective for large/dense stones. *Emerging technologies* include *Break Wave Lithotripsy (BWL)*, which uses focused ultrasound—rather than shockwaves—for stone fragmentation. It requires minimal or no anesthesia and avoids ionizing radiation, but is limited in cases where ultrasound imaging is suboptimal. *Ultrasonic propulsion* is another adjunctive method using transcutaneous ultrasound to reposition stones, aiding passage or pretreatment alignment, but not a standalone alternative to ESWL.[13,14]

Contraindications include pregnancy, uncontrolled UTIs, severe skeletal malformations or obesity hindering targeting, arterial aneurysm near the

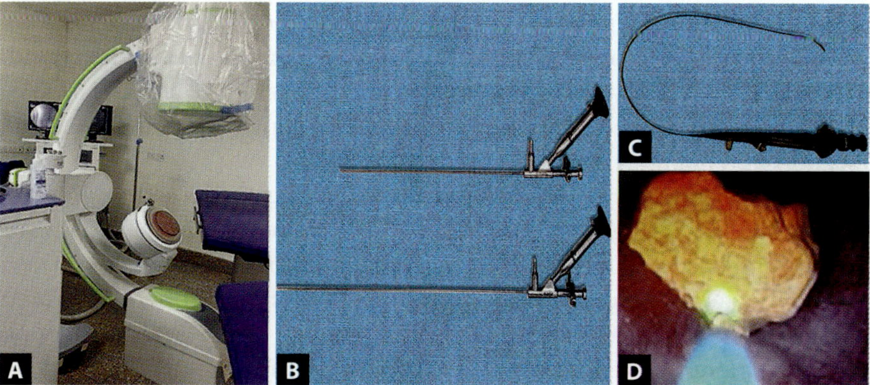

**Figs. 6A to D:** (A) Dornier's electromagnetic shock wave lithotripter; (B) Pediatric and adult semi-rigid ureteroscope; (C) Flexible ureteroscope; (D) Thulium fiber laser retrograde intrarenal surgery (RIRS).

stone, distal ureteral or UPJ obstruction, and uncorrected coagulopathy.[1-3] Complications occur in 5–10% of cases, with major events (<1%) being rare.[2-3] Fragment-related issues include steinstrasse (1–4%), hematuria (10–17%), pain (8–12%), residual fragment regrowth (21–59%), and renal colic (2–4%). Other complications include bacteriuria (7–23%), fever (1–2%), sepsis (0.1–0.15%), renal hematoma (0.2–1%), and dysrhythmias (11–59%).

### *Ureterorenoscopy (Antegrade—Ureteroscopic Lithotripsy and Retrograde—Retrograde Intrarenal Surgery)*

Ureteroscopy has applications in both diagnostic and therapeutic interventions in urolithiasis, with rigid/semirigid scopes preferred for the distal ureter and flexible scopes for the upper ureter, pelvis, and calyces. It can be done retrograde via the urethra or antegrade via percutaneous nephrostomy access. Though more invasive than ESWL, it offers higher success and lower retreatment rates.[3]

### *Ureteroscopic Lithotripsy*

Ureteroscopic lithotripsy is preferred over ESWL/PCNL for mid/distal ureteral stones, suspected cystine or uric acid stones unsuitable for ESWL, residual fragments after ESWL/PCNL, sandwich therapy (staged ureteroscopy with or without ESWL for patients unfit for PCNL), distal obstruction, ESWL contraindications, or failure (after two sessions).[15]

### *Retrograde Intrarenal Surgery*

Retrograde intrarenal surgery uses flexible ureteroscopes with modern optics and lasers to access and treat intrarenal calculi, making it a minimally invasive alternative to PCNL or ESWL for stones ≤ 2 cm.[16] Indications include renal stones ≤ 2 cm (especially lower pole or difficult anatomical locations), failed or recurrent stones after ESWL, bleeding risk/anticoagulation, anatomical anomalies, pediatric/obese patients, and multiple or bilateral stones. Stone-free rates (SFR) are 85–95% for ≤1 cm stones, 70–90% for 1–2 cm, and 60–80% for >2 cm (often needing multiple sessions), depending on stone size, location, and operator expertise.

Modern ureteroscopes are broadly categorized into semirigid and flexible types. Semirigid ureteroscopes (7–12 Fr sheath with 3–6 Fr single/dual channels) are mainly used for distal ureteral stones, offering lower cost, durability, larger channels, easier handling, and shorter operative times. Flexible ureteroscopes, essential for RIRS, provide 270–275° tip deflection (vs. <10° in semirigid), allowing access to the entire collecting system **(Figs. 7A to D)**. Digital imaging (CCD/CMOS) has replaced fiberoptics, improving image quality, durability, and maneuverability. Ureteral access sheaths aid flexible URS by enabling repeated exchanges, reducing trauma,

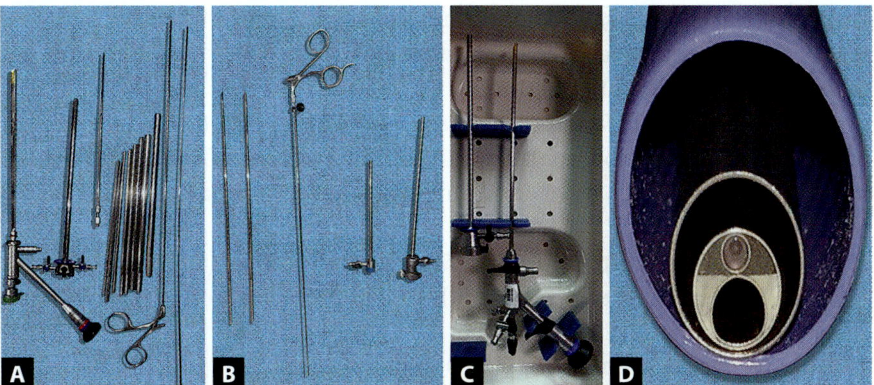


**Figs. 7A to D:** (A) PCNL instruments including 24 Fr nephroscope, 26 Fr sheath, Alken cannula, Alken metallic telescopic dilators, stone grasping alligator forceps, central rod (left to right); (B) Instruments in mini-PCNL including metallic dilators, stone forceps, metallic sheath (left to right); (C) 15 Fr mini-PCNL nephroscope with 16 Fr sheath; and (D) Close-up view of a PCNL nephroscope—showing central optical channel (top half) containing camera or fiberoptic lens, instrument channel (bottom half), and irrigation channel (surrounding space) for continuous irrigation and removal of debris.

and improving irrigation. Disposable ureteroscopes suit emergencies but have lower optical quality than digital systems.[1-4,15,16]

Lasers are highly effective for fragmenting all types of urinary stones. Since 1992, Holmium:YAG has been the gold standard, offering versatile power/frequency settings; thermal risks can be minimized with sensors, chilled irrigation, modified sheaths, and limiting power (<40 W). Thulium fiber lasers (TFL) introduced in 2018 are more efficient, use ~10% of Ho:YAG power, operate at higher frequencies (up to 2000 Hz), use smaller fibers, and provide faster fragmentation with less retropulsion and thermal injury. In URS/RIRS, dusting uses Ho:YAG (0.2–0.5 J, 20–50 Hz) or TFL (0.025–0.15 J, 100–1,500 Hz) for fine fragmentation, while fragmentation employs Ho:YAG (0.6–1.2 J, 8–15 Hz) or TFL (0.3–0.6 J, 20–100 Hz) to create larger fragments. Pulse-modulated Moses Technology further improves energy delivery by splitting laser pulses into two distinct sub-pulses—the first pulse creates a vapour bubble in the fluid medium, and the second pulse is delivered through the bubble directly to the stone surface with minimal energy loss, hence enhanced efficacy and reduced retropulsion.[17-19]

In RIRS, innovations include a low-friction hydrophilic-coated Ureteral Access Sheath (UAS), which reduces ureteral trauma and intrarenal pressure. Pressure-regulated systems, such as ThermoCool and irrigation control devices, help maintain low intrapelvic pressures, reducing sepsis risk. The Image-Guided Navigation with integrated 3D imaging—augmented reality (AR) for stone localization in complex or hidden calyces is promising.[18] FANS RIRS (Flexible and Navigable Suction Ureteral Access Sheath Retrograde

Intrarenal Surgery) advancement using a special sheath with suction to help stone removal improves visibility, increases stone-free rates, and reduces complications and reinterventions.[19]

Active, untreated UTIs are absolute, while uncorrected coagulopathy or ongoing anticoagulation are relative contraindications of URS.[1-3] RIRS/URS has a 9–25% overall complication rate, mostly minor; major (Clavien ≥III) occur in 2–4%:[1-4,15]

- *Intraoperative:* Mucosal injury (5–11%), perforation (0.5–3%), bleeding (<1%), stone migration (2–10%), instrument failure (<1%), avulsion (<0.1%).
- *Postoperative:* Hematuria (2–10%), flank pain (5–15%), UTI (3–8%), fever (2–7%), sepsis (0.3–3%), residual fragments (10–25%), stent-related symptoms (20–60%).
- Long-term: strictures (1–4%), VUR (<2%).

## Percutaneous Nephrolithotomy

Percutaneous nephrolithotomy is the primary treatment for renal calculi, achieving up to 95% stone-free rates and recommended for staghorn, calyceal diverticular, large (>2 cm), and lower pole stones.[3,15] It provides superior clearance compared to ESWL with similar recurrence and complication rates **(Figs. 7A to D)**.[4]

- Renal access during PCNL can be achieved via fluoroscopic or ultrasound guidance, depending on calyceal anatomy and the surgeon's familiarity. Ultrasound-guided procedures avoid radiation, lower visceral injury risk, and are safe in pregnancy but require expertise and may still need fluoroscopy for dilatation. Fluoroscopy offers precise posterior calyx puncture using bull's eye or triangulation techniques, but with higher radiation and no real-time feedback.[3] An emerging alternative is endoscopic-guided renal access, which utilizes a flexible ureteroscope to identify optimal calyx under direct vision, and further dilatation is performed under endoscopic or fluoroscopic which improves targeting and reduces secondary procedures.[19] Image-guided 3D CT-based navigation systems (e.g., Medrobotics Flex Robotic System) fuse real-time fluoroscopy with CT reconstruction of renal anatomy for improved precision.[20]
- *Advancements in PCNL* have led to the development of less invasive modifications such as *mini-PCNL, ultramini PCNL,* and *micro-PCNL,* aimed at reducing morbidity while maintaining high stone-free rates (SFR). Mini-PCNL (uses 14–20 Fr sheath, 8–16 Fr nephroscope) achieves SFR of 92–100% with lower transfusion rates (1–2%), reduced bleeding, and faster recovery; it is useful for 1–2.5 cm stones, though larger stones require longer operative time. Ultramini PCNL (11–13 Fr tract) offers

85–92% SFR with less pain and parenchymal preservation, suitable for stones <2 cm. Micro-PCNL (Microperc—4.8 Fr, 16-G needle, 0.9 mm microendoscope with laser) achieves 85–90% SFR for stones ≤ 1.5 cm via a single puncture, though fragments cannot be retrieved. Standard PCNL (24–30 Fr) remains optimal for large or staghorn calculi, achieving 92–100% SFR but with higher transfusion risk (3–6%).

Contraindications of PCNL are untreated UTI, ongoing anticoagulation, tumor in the access tract, suspected malignant renal tumor, and pregnancy.1-3 The overall rate of complications in PCNL is 20–25%, with major complications in 2–4%.[1,16,21]

- *Intraoperative:* Transfusion (6–8%), angioembolization requirement (0.5–1%), adjacent organ injury (0.5–1%), pelvicalyceal perforation (1–7%), and access loss (1–3%).
- *Postoperative:* Fever (10–20%), UTI (3–7%), urosepsis (0.5–4%), hematuria (5–12%), residual stones (10–15%), leakage (3–5%), pleural issues (0.5–2%), renal pelvis/infundibular injury (1–2%), and vascular fistula/pseudoaneurysm (<1%).
- *Long-term:* Partial renal function loss (<1%), strictures (1–3%), and rare chronic pain/scarring (<1%).

*Supine PCNL*, a PCNL technique modification first described by Valdivia (1987), allows simultaneous retrograde access with ureteroscopy, improved anesthesia management, and improved ergonomics, especially in obese or high-risk patients. The Galdakao-modified Valdivia position further enhances access.[22] Advantages offered are no need for repositioning, easier airway/cardiac monitoring, simultaneous antegrade–retrograde access (ECIRS), better ergonomics with less radiation, lower intrarenal pressure reducing sepsis risk, and safer in obese/cardiopulmonary patients. Disadvantages are limited upper calyx access, unfamiliar orientation with a higher learning curve, technically harder tract dilation with reduced kidney mobility for tract alignment and reduced working space from abdominal compression.[22]

*Endoscopic combined intrarenal surgery (ECIRS)* integrates antegrade (PCNL) and retrograde (RIRS) approaches for managing complex stones (large, staghorn, calyceal, or abnormal anatomy). Using both a nephroscope and a flexible ureteroscope simultaneously, it provides a panoramic view and enables single-session clearance to overcome limitations of conventional PCNL or RIRS alone.[3,23] Benefits include higher stone-free rates, fewer tracts, less trauma, lower pressure/sepsis risk, reduced bleeding, and shorter hospital stays. Drawbacks are longer operative time, need for dual expertise/equipment, and a steep learning curve.[23]

*Robot-assisted PCNL* incorporates robotics into renal access, tract dilation, and nephroscopy to enhance precision, ergonomics, safety, and reduce radiation. Percutaneous robotic-assisted nephrolithotomy (PRAN) uses image-guided robotic arms (e.g., ANT-X, ROSA, and Auris Monarch) for accurate puncture and instrument guidance. Robot-assisted flexible nephroscopy (e.g., Roboflex Avicenna) enables remote-controlled, precise flexible nephroscopy for stable, trauma-free laser lithotripsy. Electromagnetic systems (e.g., iSuite PCNL) add motor-driven punctures with real-time feedback.[24] Despite high cost and limited availability, these technologies are emerging in advanced endourology.

*Artificial intelligence (AI)-driven predictive tools* utilize preoperative anatomical details and stone characteristics to predict stone-free rates and potential complications. They integrate with machine learning, aiding tract planning, robotic guidance, and needle navigation—achieving up to 90% accuracy and improving precision while reducing risks. *3D printing* technology creates patient-specific kidney models using CT imaging for planning and training, while mixed reality platforms integrating AI and 3D imaging are advancing personalized, precision-based PCNL.[25]

## GENERAL AND SPECIFIC MEDICAL MANAGEMENT FOR PATIENTS WITH UROLITHIASIS AND RECURRENCE PREVENTION

Some risk factors (*e.g.,* low urine volume, hypocitraturia, high sodium intake, and high animal protein intake) are shared among different types of stones. General dietary measures targeting these risk factors can be recommended for stone prevention **(Table 5)**. Results from a 24-hour urine collection can further guide specific recommendations in high-risk groups[1,3,7-9] **(Table 6)**.

Beyond general dietary guidelines, specific beverage choices can influence stone risk. While water remains the cornerstone of prevention, orange juice,

**TABLE 5:** General dietary measures for all stone formers.[1,15]

| *Dietary Intervention* | *Targets* |
|---|---|
| Increase fluid intake to 2.5–3 L/day | Achieve 2–2.5 L/day urine output |
| Limit sodium intake to <100 mEq/day (2.3 g) | Reduce urinary calcium excretion |
| Moderate animal protein (0.8–1.0 g/kg/day) | Control hypercalciuria, hyperuricosuria, hyperphosphaturia, and low urine pH |
| Maintain calcium intake at 1,000–1,200 mg/day | Decrease intestinal oxalate absorption |
| Increase intake of fruits, vegetables, and dietary fiber | Boost urinary citrate and alkalinize urine |

*Sources: 1.* Andreas et al. European Association of Urology Guidelines on the Diagnosis and Treatment of Urolithiasis Skolarikos. European Urology. Volume 88, Issue 1, 64-75.

2. Assimos D, Krambeck A, Miller NL, Monga M, Murad MH, Nelson CP, et al. Surgical Management of Stones: American Urological Association/Endourological Society Guideline, PART I. J Urol. 2016;196(4):1153-60.

**TABLE 6:** 24-hour urine stone risk profile interpretation.[1,15]

| *Urine parameter* | *Reference range* | *Risk factor for stone types* | *Salient points* |
|---|---|---|---|
| ***Volume*** | ***>2–2.5 L/day*** | ***All*** | ***Low urine volume contributory for urolithiasis*** |
| Creatinine | • *Male:* 20–25 mg/kg/day<br>• *Female:* 15–20 mg/kg/day | — | |
| pH | 5.7–6.3 | • *High pH:* Calcium phosphate, struvite<br>• *Low pH:* Uric acid, cystine | • *High:* Distal RTA and UTI<br>• *Low:* High animal protein intake, chronic diarrhea |
| Calcium | • *Male:* <300 mg/day<br>• *Female:* <250 mg/day<br>• *Either sex:* <4 mg/kg/day | Calcium oxalate, calcium phosphate | Hypercalciuria increases stone risk |
| Oxalate | <45 mg/day | Calcium oxalate | >100 mg/day suggests primary hyperoxaluria; enteric absorption may be a cause |
| Citrate | >320 mg/day | Calcium oxalate and calcium phosphate | Hypocitraturia is a risk factor |
| Uric acid | <700 mg/day | Calcium oxalate and uric acid | Linked to a high purine diet or endogenous overproduction |
| Phosphorus | <1,100 mg/day | Calcium phosphate | Elevated in high protein intake |
| Sodium | <200 mmol/day | Calcium oxalate and calcium phosphate | Increases urinary calcium excretion |
| Chloride | <200 mmol/day | Calcium oxalate and calcium phosphate | |
| Sulphate | <40 mmol/day | Calcium oxalate and calcium phosphate, and uric acid | Correlates with animal protein intake |
| Ammonium | <40 mmol/day | — | Elevated in high acid load |
| Potassium | >40 mmol/day | — | Low levels suggest reduced intake or GI losses |

*Contd...*

*Contd...*

| *Urine parameter* | *Reference range* | *Risk factor for stone types* | *Salient points* |
|---|---|---|---|
| *Volume* | *>2–2.5 L/day* | *All* | *Low urine volume contributary for urolithiasis* |
| Magnesium | >80 mg/day | — | |
| Cystine | <40 mg/day | Cystine stone | |

(GI: gastrointestinal; RTA: renal tubular acidosis; UTI: urinary tract infection)

*Sources: 1.* Andreas et al. European Association of Urology Guidelines on the Diagnosis and Treatment of Urolithiasis Skolarikos. European Urology. Volume 88, Issue 1, 64-75.
2. Assimos D, Krambeck A, Miller NL, Monga M, Murad MH, Nelson CP, et al. Surgical Management of Stones: American Urological Association/Endourological Society Guideline, PART I. J Urol. 2016;196(4):1153-60.

lemonade, tea, coffee (both regular and decaf), and alcohol have shown potential benefits in reducing stone formation—though results are sometimes inconsistent. In contrast, cola and grapefruit juice are associated with a higher risk of nephrolithiasis. Restricting dietary calcium is not advised, as it can increase intestinal oxalate absorption, thereby enhancing the risk of calcium oxalate stone formation.[1,3] Additionally, calcium restriction may result in negative calcium balance and bone loss. A balanced intake of 1,000–1,200 mg/day of dietary calcium is recommended. Fruits and vegetables also offer protective effects beyond their citrate and potassium content. In individuals with low urinary citrate, reintroducing fruits and vegetables improves urine volume, pH, and magnesium, and reduces supersaturation of calcium oxalate and uric acid—factors contributing to reduced stone recurrence.[1-5]

## CONCLUSION

Management of urolithiasis has evolved with advances in diagnostic imaging, stone analysis, surgical techniques, and metabolic evaluation. While conventional modalities like ESWL, URS, and PCNL have remained cornerstones of surgical management, recent advances have refined precision, safety, and outcomes. Miniaturized PCNL techniques (mini-PCNL, ultramini, and micro-PCNL) reduce morbidity while maintaining high stone-free rates. New-generation laser technologies offer enhanced fragmentation and reduced retropulsion. Novel modalities like ultrasonic propulsion and break-wave lithotripsy are promising noninvasive alternatives. ECIRS offers ergonomic benefits over traditional approaches, especially in complex stone burdens and high-risk patients. Artificial intelligence-based prediction models now leverage preoperative data to anticipate stone-free rates and complications, aiding in real-time surgical decision-making. On the preventive front, nutritional counselling, metabolic evaluation, and individualized preventive strategies remain integral for long-term recurrence prevention. Micro-CT and infrared spectroscopy have revolutionized stone analysis by allowing detailed compositional assessment. With rapidly evolving tools and a multidisciplinary approach, modern urolithiasis management is becoming more patient-centric, less invasive, and significantly more effective in both treatment and prevention.

## REFERENCES


1. Andreas et al. European Association of Urology Guidelines on the Diagnosis and Treatment of Urolithiasis Skolarikos. European Urology. Volume 88, Issue 1, 64-75.
2. Singh S, Gupta S, Mishra T, Banerjee BD, Sharma T, Mishra TS. Risk factors of incident kidney stones in Indian adults: a hospital-based cross-sectional study. Cureus. 2023;15(2):e35558.
3. Thakore P, Liang TH. Urolithiasis. In: StatPearls [Internet]. Treasure Island (FL): StatPearls Publishing; 2025.
4. Song L, Maalouf NM. Nephrolithiasis. In: Feingold KR, Ahmed SF, Anawalt B, Blackman MR, Boyce A, Chrousos G, et al. (Eds). Endotext. South Dartmouth (MA): MDText.com, Inc.; 2000.
5. Schott C, Pourtousi A, Connaughton DM. Monogenic causation of pediatric nephrolithiasis. Front Urol. 2022;2:1075711.
6. Courbebaisse M, Travers S, Bouderlique E, Michon-Colin A, Daudon M, De Mul A, Poli L, Baron S, Prot-Bertoye C. Hydration for adult patients with nephrolithiasis: specificities and current recommendations. Nutrients. 2023;15(23):4885.
7. Grivas N, Thomas K, Drake T, Donaldson J, Neisius A, Petřík A, et al. Imaging modalities and treatment of paediatric upper tract urolithiasis: a systematic review and update on behalf of the EAU urolithiasis guidelines panel. J Pediatr Urol. 2020;16(5):612-24.
8. Batura D, Hashemzehi T, Gayed W. Should contrast CT urography replace non-contrast CT as an investigation for ureteric colic in the emergency department in those aged 65 and over? Emerg Radiol. 2018;25(6):621-6.
9. Silverman SG, Leyendecker JR, Amis Jr ES. What is the current role of CT urography and MR urography in the evaluation of the urinary tract? Radiology. 2009;250(2):309-23.
10. Akbar SA, Mortele KJ, Baeyens K, Kekelidze M, Silverman SG. Multidetector CT urography: techniques, clinical applications, and pitfalls. Semin Ultrasound CT MR. 2004;25(1):41-54.
11. Mandel NS, Mandel IC, Kolbach Mandel AM. Accurate stone analysis: the impact on disease diagnosis and treatment. Urolithiasis. 2017: 45(1): 3-9.
12. Yu J, Guo B, Yu J, Chen T, Han X, Niu Q, et al. Antibiotic prophylaxis in perioperative period of percutaneous nephrolithotomy: a systematic review and meta-analysis of comparative studies. World J Urol. 2020;38(7):1685-700.
13. Wang W, Peng L, Di X, Gao X, Wei X. Does previous unsuccessful shockwave lithotripsy influence the outcomes of ureteroscopy? -a systematic review and meta-analysis. Transl Androl Urol. 2021;10(5):2122-32.

14. Hall MK, Thiel J, Dunmire B, Samson PC, Kessler R, Sunaryo P, et al. First Series Using Ultrasonic Propulsion and Burst Wave Lithotripsy to Treat Ureteral Stones. The Journal of urology. 2022;208(5):1075-82.
15. Assimos D, Krambeck A, Miller NL, Monga M, Murad MH, Nelson CP, et al. Surgical Management of Stones: American Urological Association/ Endourological Society Guideline, PART I. J Urol. 2016;196(4):1153-60.
16. Salvadó JA, Cabello JM, Moreno S, Cabello R, Olivares R, Velasco A. Endoscopic treatment of lower pole stones: is a disposable ureteroscope preferable? Results of a prospective case-control study. Central Eur J Urol. 2019;72(3):280-4.
17. Kallidonis, Panagiotis, and Athanasios Vagionis. The future of laser technology in kidney stones. Current opinion in urology. 2022;32(4):411-4.
18. Coninck VD, Defraigne C, Traxer O. Watt determines the temperature during laser lithotripsy. World journal of urology. 2022;40(5):1257-8.
19. Isac W, Rizkala E, Liu X, Noble M, Monga M. Endoscopic-guided versus fluoroscopic-guided renal access for percutaneous nephrolithotomy: a comparative analysis. Urology. 2013;81(2):251-6.
20. Wright A, Rukin N, Smith D, Rosette JDL, Somani BK. 'Mini, ultra, micro'-nomenclature and cost of these new minimally invasive percutaneous nephrolithotomy (PCNL) techniques. Ther Adv Urol. 2016;8(2):142-6.
21. Fuller A, Razvi H, Denstedt JD, Nott L, Pearle M, Cauda F, et al. The CROES percutaneous nephrolithotomy global study: the influence of body mass index on outcome. J Urol. 2012;188(1):138-44.
22. Keller EX, Coninck VDE, Proietti S, Talso M, Emiliani E, Ploumidis A, et al. Prone versus supine percutaneous nephrolithotomy: a systematic review and meta-analysis of current literature. Minerva Urol Nephrol. 2021;73(1):50-8.
23. Zhu W, Huang Z, Zeng G. Miniaturization in percutaneous nephrolithotomy: What is new? Asian J Urol. 2023;10 (3):275-80.
24. Abid R, Hussein AA, Guru KA. Artificial Intelligence in Urology: Current Status and Future Perspectives. Urol Clin North Am. 2024;51(1):117-30.
25. Gauhar V, Giulioni C, Gadzhiev N, Stefano VD, Teoh JYC, Tiong HY, et al. An Update of in Vivo Application of Artificial Intelligence and Robotics for Percutaneous Nephrolithotripsy: Results from a Systematic Review. Curr Urol Rep. 2023;24(6):271-80.

CHAPTER 13

# Endovascular Treatment of Peripheral Vascular Disease

*Apurva Srivastava, Nikhil Chaudhari*

## INTRODUCTION

Peripheral vascular disease (PVD), also known as peripheral arterial disease (PAD), is a major global health concern, affecting over 200 million individuals worldwide. Driven primarily by atherosclerosis, PVD leads to the narrowing or occlusion of peripheral arteries, most commonly in the lower extremities, causing symptoms ranging from intermittent claudication to chronic limb-threatening ischemia (CLTI) and acute limb ischemia (ALI). For surgical postgraduates, mastering endovascular treatments in the catheterization laboratory (cath lab) is critical, as these minimally invasive procedures have become the cornerstone of PVD management. These techniques, performed under fluoroscopic guidance, leverage advanced imaging and catheter-based technologies to restore blood flow with reduced morbidity compared to traditional open surgery. This chapter provides a comprehensive, detailed exploration of cath lab-based endovascular treatments for PVD, covering classification systems, procedural techniques, devices, clinical evidence, emerging technologies such as atherectomy devices and bioresorbable stents, and future directions. The goal is to acquaint trainees with the knowledge and skills to excel in this rapidly evolving field of vascular surgery.

## DEFINITION AND EPIDEMIOLOGY

Peripheral vascular disease encompasses a spectrum of atherosclerotic conditions that impair blood flow in noncoronary arteries, predominantly affecting the lower limbs. Clinical manifestations include asymptomatic disease, intermittent claudication (pain with walking relieved by rest), CLTI characterized by rest pain or tissue loss, and ALI, a medical emergency requiring immediate intervention. The global prevalence of PVD has risen by 23.5% since 2010, with an estimated 6.5 million individuals aged 40 years and older affected in the United States alone. Key risk factors include diabetes mellitus, smoking, hypertension, and hyperlipidemia, with diabetes contributing to a particularly aggressive disease course due to its association with calcified lesions and infrapopliteal (IP) segment involvement.

PVD disproportionately affects older adults, with prevalence increasing with age, and is a leading cause of limb loss and cardiovascular morbidity worldwide.

## PATHOPHYSIOLOGY

Atherosclerosis in PVD results from plaque accumulation in arterial walls, reducing lumen diameter and impairing blood flow. Chronic lesions may progress to chronic total occlusions (CTOs), while acute thrombus formation can precipitate ALI. Microvascular dysfunction, particularly in diabetic patients, exacerbates tissue ischemia, complicating treatment. Understanding these mechanisms is essential for selecting appropriate cath lab interventions tailored to lesion characteristics and patient comorbidities. Mainly, PAD is divided into anatomical regions as per the involvement of the segments, which are the aortoiliac segment, infrainguinal segment, and infragenicular segment/infrapopliteal segment. In the lower extremities, the femoropopliteal (FP) and IP segments are most commonly affected.

## ROLE OF A VASCULAR CATHETERIZATION LABORATORY

A Vascular cath lab serves as the primary setting for endovascular interventions, offering a controlled environment for real-time imaging and catheter-based therapies. Fluoroscopy, augmented by advanced modalities like intravascular ultrasound (IVUS) and carbon dioxide angiography, enables precise visualization of arterial anatomy. Contrary to open surgery, endovascular procedures do not involve incisions or cut-downs as they are performed through needle hole access achieved into the femoral or brachial arteries, which are later sealed by compression or percutaneous closure devices. The patient can be mobilized on the first postoperative day and discharged from the hospital. Hence, endovascular procedures reduce perioperative morbidity, shorten hospital stays, and are suitable for high-risk patients with comorbidities such as coronary artery disease or chronic kidney disease (CKD). The integration of novel devices and imaging techniques continues to expand the scope of endovascular therapy, making it the preferred approach for many PVD patients.

## HYBRID VASCULAR CATHETERIZATION LABORATORY

A hybrid vascular catheterization laboratory (cath lab) is a state-of-the-art surgical suite that combines advanced imaging technology with a sterile operating room environment **(Fig. 1)**. It is designed to support both minimally invasive endovascular procedures and open surgical interventions, enabling seamless integration of diagnostic, interventional, and surgical techniques. This setup is particularly valuable for complex procedures, such as aortic aneurysm repairs, peripheral artery interventions, and hybrid revascularization.

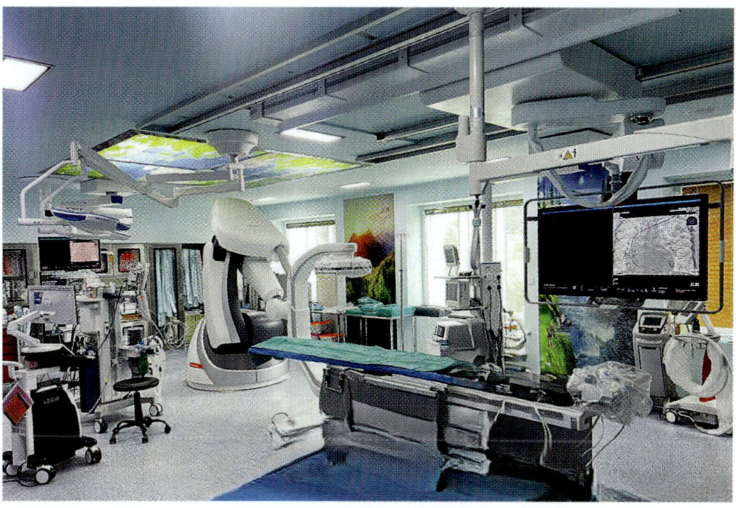

**Fig. 1:** Hybrid vascular catheterization laboratory.
*Courtesy:* With due permission from Sir Ganga Ram Hospital, Delhi.

## KEY FEATURES

- *Advanced imaging:* Equipped with high-resolution fluoroscopy, three-dimensional (3D) imaging, and real-time navigation systems to guide catheter-based interventions with precision.
- *Sterile environment:* Meets operating room standards, allowing immediate transition to open surgery if needed.
- *Versatility:* Multiple access for complex multi-level occlusive PADs enabling simultaneous open and endovascular approaches.

## BENEFITS FOR TRAINEES

- *Skill development:* Gain hands-on experience in catheter-based techniques, imaging interpretation, and open surgical skills in one setting.
- *Efficiency training:* Learn to manage complex cases requiring both endovascular and surgical approaches, reducing procedure time and patient risk.
- *Decision-making:* Develop critical thinking for real-time transitions between minimally invasive and open procedures based on patient needs.

## PRACTICAL CONSIDERATIONS

- *Workflow familiarity:* Understand the hybrid laboratory's layout, including imaging controls, sterile field maintenance, and equipment positioning.
- *Radiation safety:* Master protocols to minimize radiation exposure for patients and staff during fluoroscopy-guided procedures.

- *Team coordination:* Practice effective communication with the multidisciplinary team to ensure smooth procedure execution.

The hybrid vascular cath lab represents the future of vascular surgery, offering a unique opportunity to perform both endovascular and open techniques in a single, advanced environment. Proficiency in this setting prepares surgeons for the evolving demands of modern vascular care.[1]

## CLASSIFICATION SYSTEMS FOR PERIPHERAL VASCULAR DISEASE

Classification systems are critical for assessing disease severity, guiding treatment decisions, and predicting outcomes in the cath lab.

### Wound, Ischemia, and Foot Infection Classification

The Society for Vascular Surgery's WIfI classification system stratifies CLTI based on three components **(Table 1)**:

- *Wound:* Evaluates the size, depth, and extent of tissue loss (e.g., ulcers or gangrene).
- *Ischemia:* Quantified using noninvasive tests such as the ankle-brachial index (ABI), toe-brachial index (TBI), or transcutaneous oxygen pressure ($TcPO_2$). ABI values < 0.4 indicate severe ischemia.
- *Foot infection:* Assesses the presence and severity of infection, ranging from none to severe.

WIfI assign a score (0–3) to each component, generating a composite stage (1–4) that predicts amputation risk and guides intervention urgency. For example, a Stage 4 limb (severe wound, ischemia, and infection) often requires aggressive endovascular or hybrid revascularization to prevent major amputation.[2]

## GLOBAL LIMB ANATOMIC STAGING SYSTEM

Introduced in the 2019 Global Vascular Guidelines, the Global Anatomic Staging System (GLASS) evaluates anatomic complexity to inform endovascular feasibility:

- *Femoropopliteal (FP) segment:* Assesses lesion length, degree of calcification, and occlusion type (e.g., stenotic vs. CTO). Long, calcified CTOs are classified as high complexity (Stage III).
- *IP segment:* Evaluates vessel patency, runoff quality, and the presence of pedal arch disease.[2]

Global Anatomic Staging System stages (I–III) guide treatment selection, with Stage I lesions amenable to simple angioplasty and Stage III lesions requiring advanced techniques like atherectomy or percutaneous bypass. Combining WIfI and GLASS provides a comprehensive framework for tailoring cath lab strategies to both clinical and anatomic factors **(Fig. 2)**.

**TABLE 1:** WIfI Classification of Society for Vascular Surgery.[27]

| | *Wound (W)* | | *Ischemia (I)* | | *Foot infection (fi)* |
|---|---|---|---|---|---|
| Grade | Ulcer | Gangrene | Ankle-brachial index<br>Ankle systolic pressure | Toe pressure or transcutaneous oximetry | Clinical manifestation |
| 0 | None | None | ≥0.80<br>>100 mm Hg | ≥60 mm Hg | No symptoms or signs of infection |
| 1 | Small, shallow | None | 40–59 mm Hg | 40–59 mm Hg | Infection indicated by ≥ 2 of the following:<br>• Local swelling or induration<br>• Erythema 0.5 – 2.0 cm around ulcer<br>• Local tenderness or pain<br>• Purulent discharge (thick, opaque to white, or sanguineous) |
| 2 | Deep with exposed bone, joint, or tendon | Limited to digits | 30–39 mm Hg | 30–39 mm Hg | Infection as described above with:<br>• Erythema > 2 cm around ulcer<br>• Involving structures deeper than skin and subcutaneous tissues (e.g., Abscess, osteomyelitis, septic arthritis, fasciitis)<br>• No signs of systemic inflammatory response (see below) |
| 3 | Extensive, deep, and involving forefoot and/or midfoot with or without calcaneal involvement | Extensive and involving forefoot and/or midfoot Full thickness heel necrosis with or without calcaneal involvement | <30 mm Hg | <30 mm Hg | Infection as described above with ≥2 signs of systemic inflammatory response syndrome:<br>• Temperature >38°C or <36°C<br>• Heart rate >90/min<br>• Respiratory rate >20/min or $PaCO_2$ <32 mm Hg<br>• White blood cell count >12,000/μL or <4000/μL or 10% immature forms |

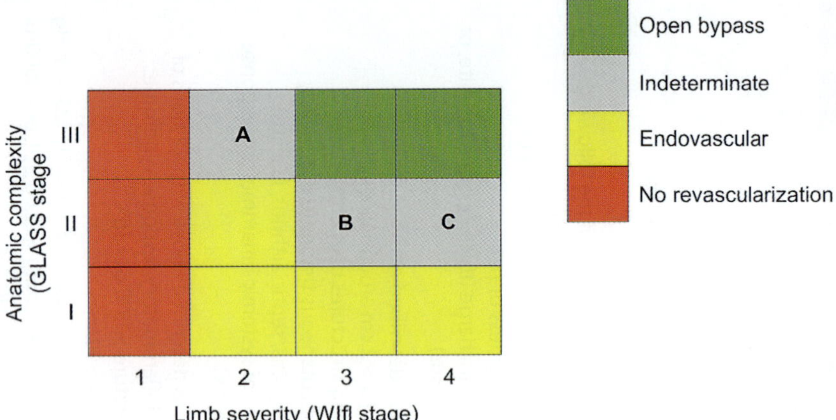


**Fig. 2:** Global Vascular Guidelines (GVG) Guidelines—Global Limb Anatomic Staging System (GLASS) and Limb severity for planning.[27]

## Trans-Atlantic Inter-Society Consensus II Classification

The Trans-Atlantic Inter-Society Consensus (TASC II) classification, though less commonly used today, categorizes lesions (A–D) based on complexity.[3] Type A lesions are short and focal, ideal for endovascular treatment, while Type D lesions, such as long CTOs, may require surgical bypass or hybrid approaches. TASC II remains relevant for understanding historical trial data and comparing treatment outcomes **(Fig. 3)**.

# OVERVIEW OF ENDOVASCULAR TREATMENT FOR PERIPHERAL VASCULAR DISEASE

Endovascular treatment has transformed PVD management by offering minimally invasive alternatives to open surgery. Performed in the cath lab, these procedures address a spectrum of lesions, from focal stenoses to complex CTOs, using radio-opaque guide wires, catheters, and specialized devices under fluoroscopic guidance. The evolution of device technology, including drug-coated balloons (DCBs), drug-eluting stents (DES), and novel approaches like atherectomy and thromboaspiration devices, has expanded the applicability of endovascular therapy.

## Advantages

- *Reduced morbidity and mortality:* Endovascular procedures have lower complication rates than open surgery, as they do not involve surgical incisions and are performed by needle hole access to arteries.
- *Shorter recovery times:* Most patients resume normal activities within days, compared to weeks or months for surgical bypass.

Type A lesions
- Unilateral or bilateral stenoses of CIA
- Unilateral or bilateral single short (≤3 cm) stenosis of EIA

Type B lesions:
- Short (≤3 cm) stenosis of the infrarenal aorta
- Unilateral CIA occlusion
- Single or multiple stenosis totaling 3–10 cm involving the EIA not extending into the CFA
- Unilateral EIA occlusion not involving the origins of internal iliac or CFA

Type C lesions:
- Bilateral CIA occlusions
- Bilateral EIA stenosis 3–10 cm long not extending into the CFA
- Unilateral EIA stenosis extending into the CFA
- Unilateral EIA occlusion that involves the origins of and/or CFA
- Heavily calcified unilateral EIA occlusion with or without involvement of origins of internal iliac and/or CFA

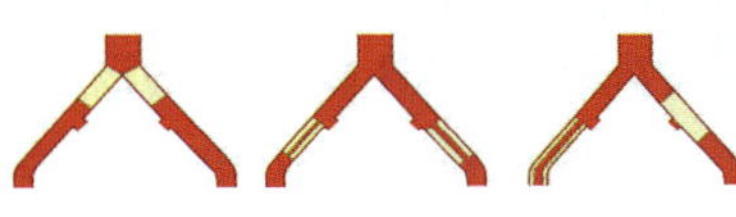

Type D lesions:
- Intra-renal aortoiliac occlusion
- Diffuse disease involving the aorta and both iliac arteries requiring treatment
- Diffuse multiple stenosis involving the unilateral CIA, EIA, CFA
- Unilateral occlusions of both CIA and EIA
- Bilateral occlusions of EIA
- Iliac stenoses in patients with abdominal aortic aneurysm (AAA) requiring treatment and not amenable to endograft placement or other lesions requiring open aortic or iliac surgery

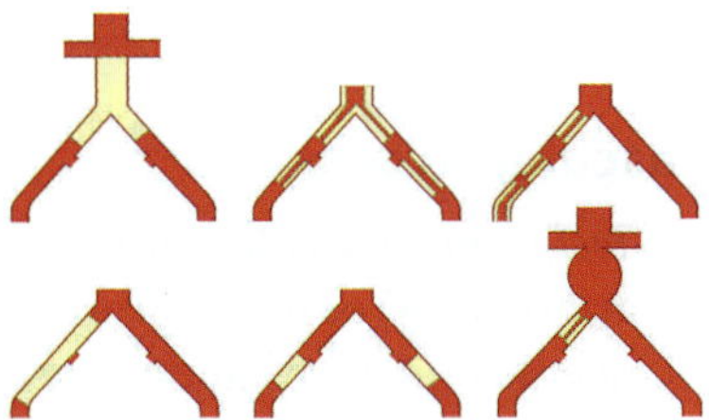

**Fig. 3:** TASC classification of aortoiliac disease.[3] (CFA: common femoral artery; EIA: external iliac artery; TASC: TransAtlantic Inter-Society Consensus)

- *Versatility:* Applicable to a wide range of lesion types (e.g., stenotic, occlusive, and calcified) and patient populations, including those unfit for surgery.
- *Repeatability:* Endovascular interventions can be repeated for restenosis or disease progression, preserving future surgical treatment options when required.

## Challenges

- *Restenosis:* Neointimal hyperplasia within arteries leads to restenosis in 20–50% of cases within 1–2 years, particularly in FP and IP segments.
- *Calcified lesions:* Severe calcification resists balloon dilation and increases procedural complexity.
- *CTOs:* Require advanced crossing techniques, such as subintimal recanalization or retrograde approaches.
- *Contrast nephrotoxicity:* Iodinated contrast used in angiography poses risks for patients with CKD, necessitating alternatives, such as $CO_2$ angiography.

## Patient Selection

Appropriate patient selection is critical for optimizing outcomes. Endovascular therapy is favored for patients with claudication, early-stage CLTI, or comorbidities precluding surgery. However, surgical bypass may be preferred for young patients with long life expectancy and complex TASC D lesions. Multidisciplinary evaluation, incorporating WIfI, GLASS, and patient comorbidities, ensures tailored treatment plans.[2]

# ENDOVASCULAR PROCEDURES FOR PERIPHERAL VASCULAR DISEASE

A variety of endovascular procedures can be performed in a vascular cath, each tailored to specific lesion characteristics and clinical scenarios. The following sections detail these techniques, emphasizing their technical execution, devices, and applications.

## Vascular Access

- *Technique:* Vascular access is typically achieved via the common femoral artery (CFA) or brachial artery (BA) using Seldinger's technique, involving needle puncture, guide wire insertion, and sheath placement. Ultrasound guidance is advisable as it reduces complications such as hematomas or pseudoaneurysms. Alternative access sites, such as radial or pedal arteries, are used for challenging anatomies or retrograde approaches **(Figs. 4A to E)**.
- *Devices:* 18-G puncture needle with 0.035-inch guide wire/micropuncture kits for pedal access (21-gauge needle, 0.018-inch guide wire), 4–6 Fr

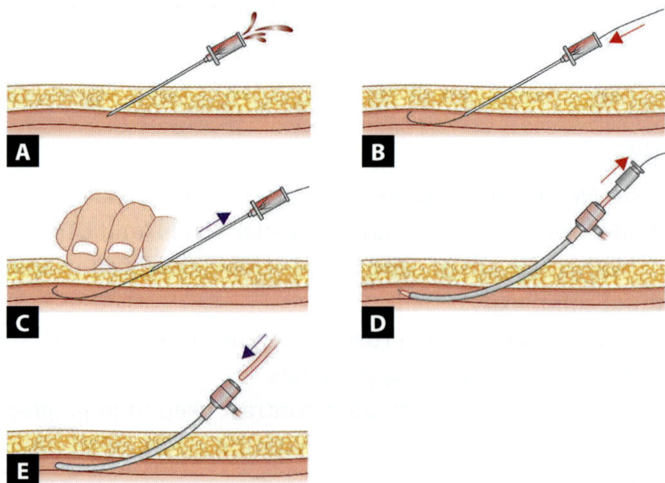


**Figs. 4A to E:** Vascular access sheath insertion technique using needle and guidewire.

vascular sheaths, and vascular closure devices (e.g., Perclose ProGlide™ and Angio-seal™).

- *Applications:* Provides a conduit for diagnostic and therapeutic devices, ensuring safe and effective intervention.
- *Complications:* Access site complications (e.g., bleeding, dissection, and pseudoaneurysm) occur in 2–5% of cases but are minimized with ultrasound and closure devices.

## Diagnostic Angiography

- *Technique:* A contrast agent is injected through a catheter to visualize arterial anatomy under fluoroscopy, delineating lesion location, length, severity, and distal runoff. Digital subtraction angiography (DSA) enhances image clarity by removing background structures, including bones **(Fig. 5)**.
- *Devices:* Pigtail tip or straight tip catheters (4–5 Fr), nonionic contrast agents (e.g., iohexol), and $CO_2$ delivery systems for patients with CKD.
- *Applications:* Essential for preprocedural planning, intraoperative guidance, and postprocedural assessment of patency.
- *Outcomes:* High diagnostic accuracy, with sensitivity and specificity > 95% for detecting significant stenoses.

## Carbon Dioxide Angiography

- *Technique:* $CO_2$ angiography uses carbon dioxide gas as a contrast agent, delivered via a specialized system to visualize arterial anatomy. $CO_2$ is injected through a catheter, displacing blood to create a negative contrast

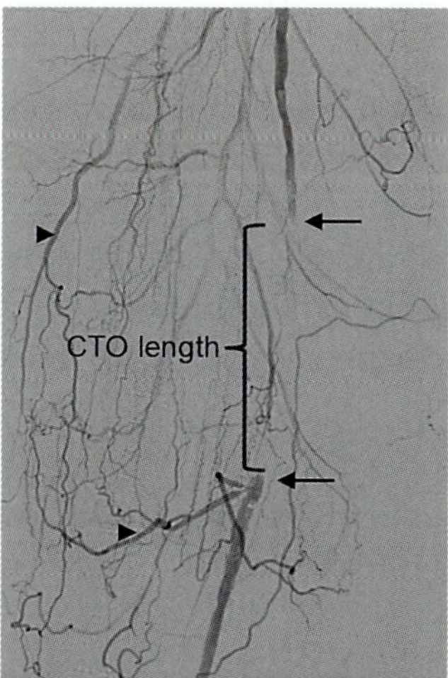


**Fig. 5:** Chronic total occlusion (CTO) of the femoral artery on digital subtraction angiography.

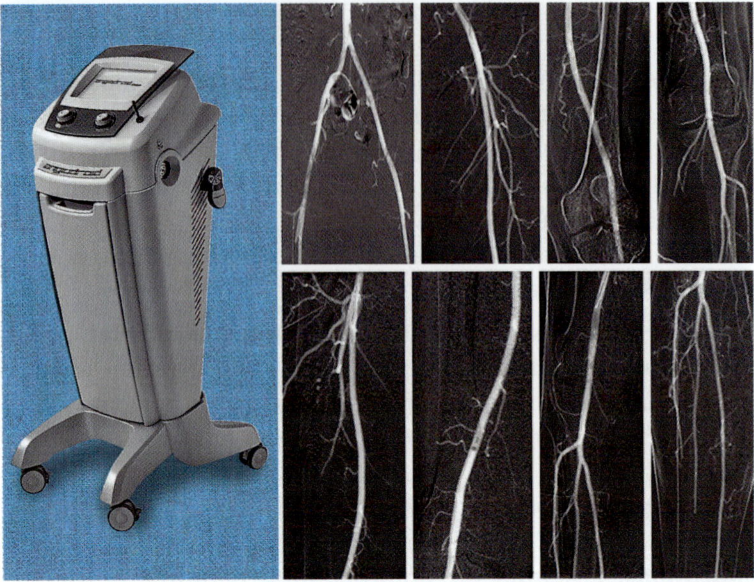

**Fig. 6:** Angiodroid™ automated $CO_2$ injector and $CO_2$ angiography images.

image under fluoroscopy. The gas is rapidly absorbed, reducing the risk of nephrotoxicity **(Fig. 6)**.

- *Devices:* Dedicated $CO_2$ delivery systems (e.g., Angiodroid™) with precise pressure and volume control to prevent air embolism or tissue ischemia.
- *Applications:* Ideal for patients with CKD or contrast allergies, particularly for aortoiliac and femoropopliteal segment interventions. $CO_2$ angiography is less effective for IP vessels due to poor visualization of small-caliber arteries.
- *Outcomes:* Studies report >90% diagnostic accuracy in aortoiliac disease, with procedural success rates comparable to iodinated contrast. Limitations include potential discomfort from $CO_2$ injection and the need for specialized training.[4,5]
- *Complications:* Rare but include transient abdominal pain, air trapping in cerebral or pulmonary circulation (if delivery is mismanaged), and poor image quality in obese patients.

## Balloon Angioplasty

Balloon angioplasty remains a foundational endovascular technique, mechanically dilating stenotic or occluded arteries to restore blood flow.

### Plain Old Balloon Angioplasty

- *Technique:* A balloon catheter is advanced over a 0.014- or 0.035″ guide wire to the lesion, inflated to 6–12 atm for 2–3 minutes to laterally compress plaque, following which it is deflated and removed. Prolonged inflation (>3 minutes) may be done in selected cases.

- *Device examples:* Noncompliant balloons (e.g., Atlas™) for high-pressure dilation; semi-compliant balloons (e.g., Armada™) for flexible sizing.[6]
- *Applications:* Best suited for short (<5 cm), noncalcified FP or IP lesions in claudicants or early CLTI.
- *Outcomes:* Primary patency rates of 40–50% at 12 months, with higher restenosis in longer or calcified lesions.
- *Challenges:* Elastic recoil, dissection, and restenosis limit efficacy in complex diseases.

### *Drug-coated Balloon Angioplasty*

- *Technique:* DCBs deliver antiproliferative drugs (e.g., paclitaxel and sirolimus) to the vessel wall during inflation, inhibiting postprocedure neointimal hyperplasia. The balloon is inflated for 2–3 minutes to ensure drug transfer **(Fig. 7)**.
- *Device examples:* In.Pact Admiral™ (Paclitaxel), Pepherics™ and Lutonix™ DCBs
- *Application:* Widely used for in-stent stenosis and also preferred for native FP lesions, restenotic lesions, and its use is increasing in IP segments

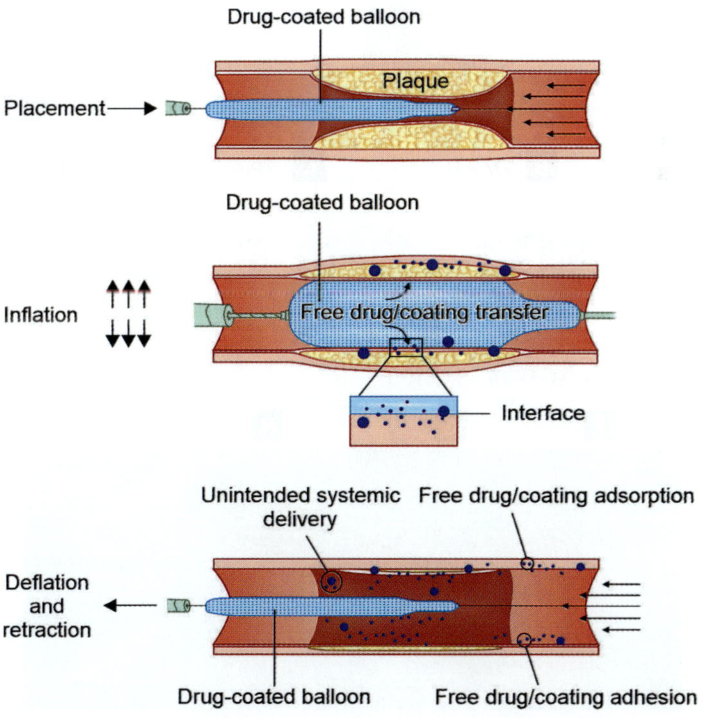


**Fig. 7:** Mechanism of drug-coated balloon.

in CLTI. DCBs are more effective in reducing restenosis as compared to POBA.

- *Outcomes:* The IN. PACT SFA trial demonstrated 12-month primary patency of 82.2% for DCBs versus 52.4% for POBA. Five-year data show sustained benefits, with reduced target lesion revascularization (TLR) rates.[7]
- *Challenges:* Drug loss during delivery and variable efficacy in heavily calcified lesions.

## Stenting

Stenting provides mechanical support to maintain vessel patency when POBA is followed by a recoil, dissection, or suboptimal luminal gain.

### *Bare-metal Stents*

- *Technique*: Self-expanding (nitinol) or balloon-expandable (stainless steel) stents are deployed post-angioplasty as a scaffold to maintain vessel patency. Precise sizing is critical to avoid undersizing or overstretching.
- *Device examples*: Absolute Pro™ (Nitinol), LifeStent™ and EverFlex™ stents **(Figs. 8A to J)**.

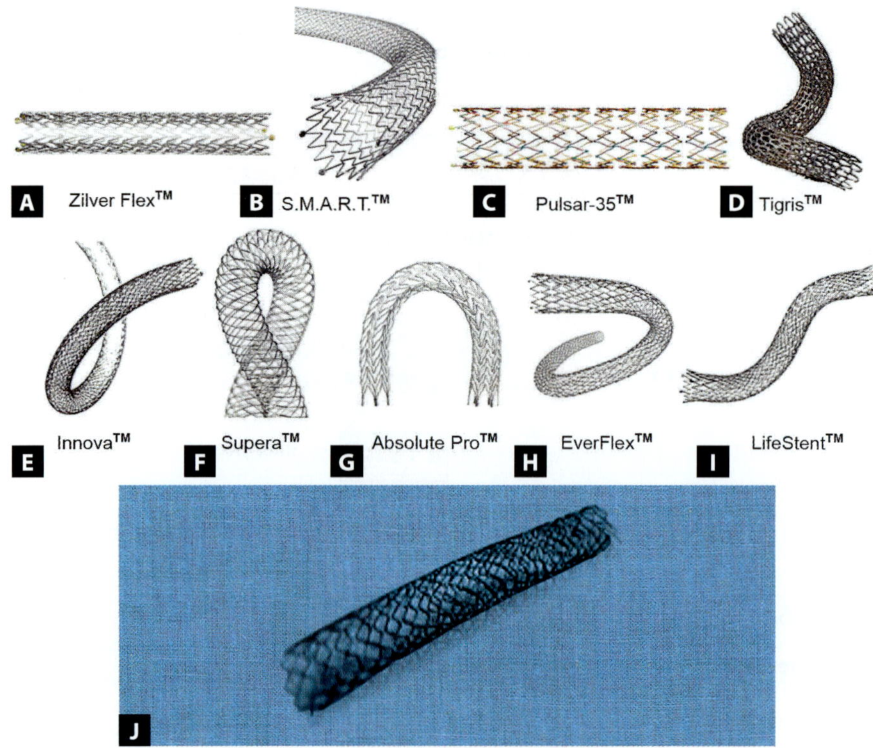


**Figs. 8A to J:** Various types of self-expanding stents.

- *Applications:* FP lesions with elastic recoil, dissection, or residual stenosis post-angioplasty. Less commonly used in IP segments due to small vessel diameters.
- *Outcomes:* In-stent restenosis (ISR) rates of 20–30% at 2 years, higher in longer lesions or CTOs.
- *Challenges:* ISR, stent fracture in mobile FP segments, and thrombosis risk.[8]

### *Drug-eluting Stents*

- *Technique:* DES release antiproliferative drugs (e.g., paclitaxel and sirolimus) to reduce ISR, deployed similarly to BMS. Postdilation ensures optimal apposition **(Fig. 9)**.
- *Device examples:* Zilver PTX™ (Paclitaxel) and Eluvia™ (Sirolimus) and Xience™ coronary DES used off-label for IP lesions.[9]
- *Applications:* FP lesions, short IP lesions in CLTI, and restenotic lesions. DES are preferred over BMS for improved patency.
- *Outcomes:* The Zilver PTX trial reported 5-year primary patency of 66.4% for DES versus 43.4% for BMS, with reduced TLR.[8]
- *Challenges:* Higher cost and potential for late thrombosis.

### *Covered Stents*

- *Technique:* Stents covered with polytetrafluoroethylene (PTFE) or other materials are deployed to exclude aneurysms, thrombus, or perforations.
- *Device examples:* Viabahn™, Fluency™, Solaris™ and I-cover™ **(Fig. 10)**.
- *Applications:* Complex FP lesions, perforations, pseudoaneurysms, or lesions with high thrombus burden.

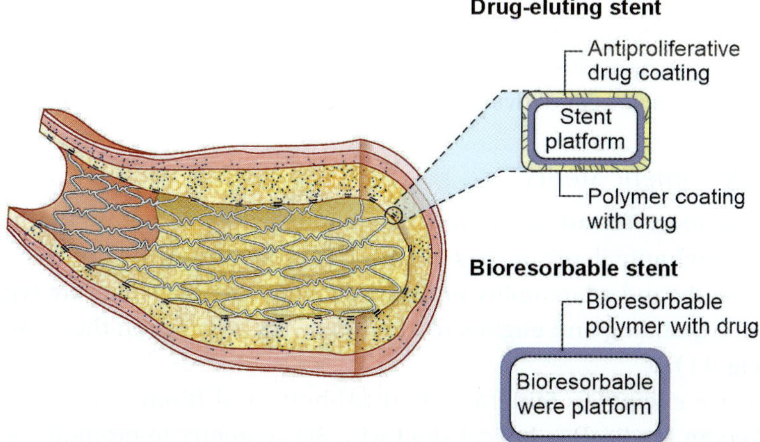


**Fig. 9:** Drug-eluting stent versus bioresorbable stent.

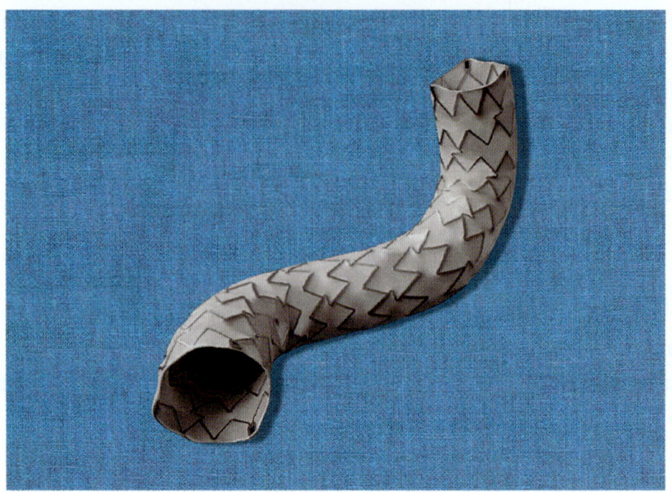

**Fig. 10:** Covered stents (I-cover™).

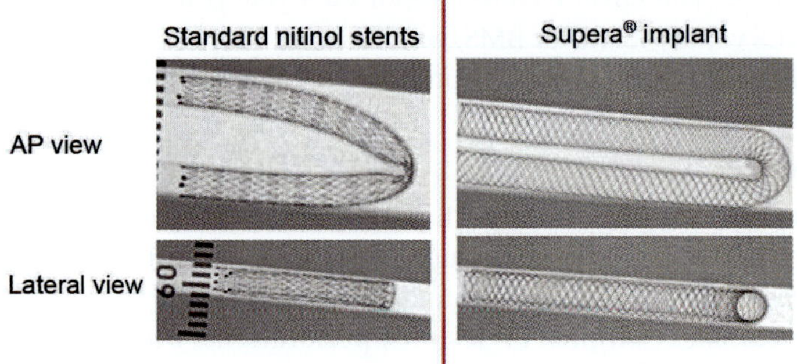


**Fig. 11:** Standard versus vasculomimetic stent (interwoven wires of Nitinol).

- *Outcomes:* Superior patency in long lesions (e.g., >15 cm) but risk of edge restenosis or occlusion.
- *Challenges:* Larger delivery systems and potential for graft thrombosis.[10]

## *Vasculomimetic Stents*

- *Technique:* Vasculomimetic stents are designed to mimic the natural biomechanical properties of arteries, combining flexibility, radial strength, and adaptability to vessel dynamics. These stents are typically self-expanding and engineered to reduce shear stress on the vessel wall **(Fig. 11)**.
- *Device examples:* Supera™ stent (Abbott) and Biomimics 3D™ stent (Veryan Medical), a helical stent with 3D geometry to promote swirling blood flow and reduce neointimal hyperplasia.[11]

- *Applications:* FP lesions, particularly in the superficial femoral artery (SFA), where vessel movement, twisting, torsion, and flexion are significant. Vasculomimetic stents are under investigation for IP use.
- *Outcomes:* The MIMICS-2 trial reported 12-month primary patency of 81.5% for BioMimics 3D, comparable to DES, with lower rates of stent fracture in dynamic FP segments.[12]
- *Advantages:* Reduced vessel wall stress, improved hemodynamic flow, and lower ISR compared to traditional BMS.

## Atherectomy

- *Technique:* Atherectomy devices are intravascular debulking devices that remove or modify atherosclerotic plaques to facilitate angioplasty or stenting. Types include:
  - *Directional atherectomy:* Uses a cutting blade to excise plaque (e.g., HawkOne™)
  - *Rotational atherectomy:* Employs a rotating burr to ablate plaque (e.g., Jetstream™ and Rotarex™).[13]
  - *Laser atherectomy:* Vaporizes plaque with laser energy (e.g., Turbo-elite™ and Excimer).[14] **(Fig. 12)**
- *Device examples:* HawkOne™, Jetstream™ and Rotarex™ **(Fig. 13)**.
- *Applications:* Calcified lesions, CTOs, and in-stent restenosis. Atherectomy is often used as an adjunct to angioplasty or stenting.
- *Outcomes:* Adjunctive atherectomy achieves >90% procedural success but lacks consistent long-term patency benefits in randomized trials.
- *Challenges:* Distal embolization (mitigated with embolic protection devices), vessel perforation, and high device costs.

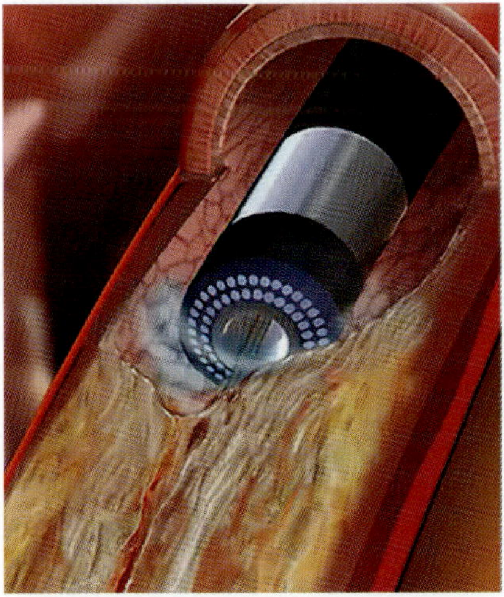

**Fig. 12:** Excimer laser atherectomy.

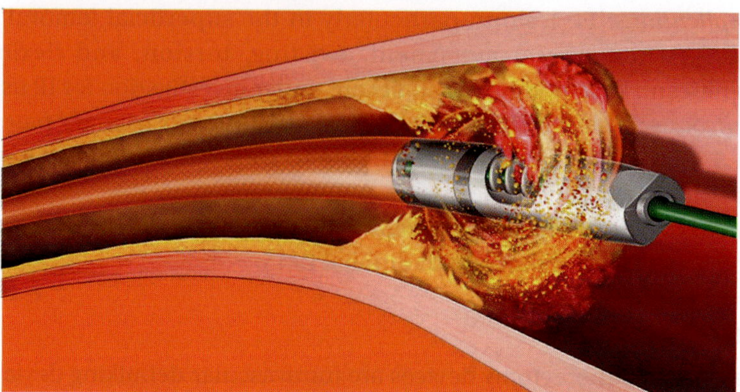

**Fig. 13:** Rotarex™ Atherectomy device (Rotational).

## Thrombectomy

- *Technique:* Aspiration or mechanical thrombectomy removes thrombus from the vessel using suction or fragmentation devices.
- *Device examples:* Penumbra's Indigo™ (aspiration), AngioJet™ (rheolytic) and FlowTriever™ system.[15]
- *Applications:* ALI, acute-on-chronic occlusions, or acute embolic events in FP or IP segments.
- *Outcomes:* Success rates >90% for thrombus removal, with reduced distal embolization when embolic protection is used.
- *Challenges:* Risk of vessel injury, hemolysis (with AngioJet), and incomplete thrombus removal in chronic lesions.

## Thromboaspiration

- Thromboaspiration is a cornerstone technique for managing thrombus in ALI and acute-on-chronic occlusions, rapidly restoring flow and reducing embolization risk.
- A specialized aspiration catheter is advanced over a 0.014- or 0.035″ guide wire to the thrombus site. Negative pressure, applied via a syringe or pump, extracts thrombus under fluoroscopic guidance (often with $CO_2$ angiography in CKD patients).
- The procedure may be standalone or combined with thrombolytic agents [e.g., recombinant tissue-type plasminogen activator (rtPA)] for large thrombus burdens. Pre- and postprocedural angiography confirms thrombus clearance and flow restoration.

## Devices

- *Penumbra's Indigo™ system:* High-powered aspiration for soft, fresh thrombus. Features flexible catheters (4–8 Fr) and a separator to prevent clogging, ideal for FP and IP vessels[16] **(Fig. 14)**.

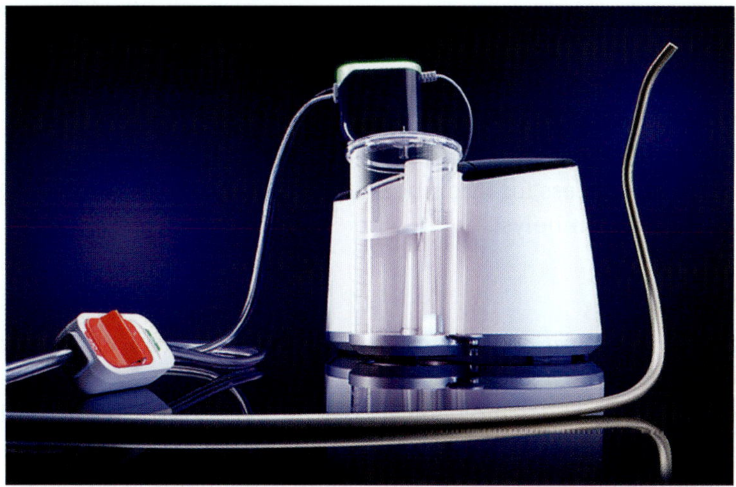

**Fig. 14:** Penumbra's Indigo™ thromboaspiration device.

- *AngioJet™ (Boston Scientific):* Rheolytic thrombectomy uses saline jets to fragment and aspirate thrombus, effective for larger clots in FP segments.[17]
- *Triever™ (Inari Medical):* FlowTriever System with large-bore (12–24 Fr) aspirations for massive thrombus in ALI, suitable for aortoiliac or proximal FP lesions.
- *Export™ AP (Medtronic):* Simple, cost-effective aspiration catheter for smaller thrombi in IP vessels.
- *Aspirex™ (Straub Medical):* Rotational aspiration catheter combining mechanical disruption and suction, effective for mixed thrombus types.

## Applications

- *ALI:* Rapid thrombus removal to restore flow within 6–12 hours of symptom onset, critical for limb salvage.
- *Acute-on-chronic occlusions:* Addresses thrombus superimposed on chronic lesions, common in CLTI with FP or IP involvement.
- *In-stent thrombosis:* Clears acute stent occlusions to prevent limb loss.
- *Postprocedure embolization:* Removes distal emboli after angioplasty or stenting, often with embolic protection devices.
- *Venous thrombosis:* Emerging use in deep vein thrombosis (DVT) with large-bore systems, such as FlowTriever.

## Outcomes

- *Success rates:* The *PRISM trial (Penumbra Indigo)* reported >90% thrombus removal success, with 80–85% vessel patency at 30 days.[18]
- *ALI outcomes:* Limb salvage in 85–90% of ALI cases when performed promptly, with 70–80% success in acute-on-chronic occlusions.

- *Embolization prevention:* Reduces distal embolization by 50–60% with protection devices (e.g., SpiderFX™).
- *CLTI:* Improves flow in 75–80% of thrombus-laden lesions, often followed by stenting or DCB.
- *Real-world data:* Vascular quality initiative (*VQI) registry* shows 85% procedural success for thromboaspiration in ALI, with 10–15% requiring adjunctive thrombolysis.[19]

### Advantages

- *Rapid flow restoration:* Minimizes ischemia time in ALI, critical for tissue preservation.
- *Reduced thrombolytic use:* Lowers bleeding risk compared to prolonged thrombolytic therapy.
- *Versatility:* Effective in FP, IP, and aortoiliac segments, with catheter sizes tailored to vessel diameter.
- *Compatibility:* Combines with angioplasty, stenting, or IVL for comprehensive treatment.
- *Safety in CKD:* Guided by $CO_2$ angiography, avoiding contrast nephropathy.

### Challenges

- *Vessel injury:* Dissection or perforation risk (2–5%), especially in calcified vessels.
- *Hemolysis:* AngioJet-related hemolysis in 5–10% of cases, requiring monitoring for hemoglobinuria.
- *Incomplete removal:* Chronic, organized thrombi may resist aspiration, necessitating mechanical thrombectomy or surgery.
- *Cost:* Advanced systems (e.g., FlowTriever) are expensive, limiting use in resource-constrained settings.
- *Technical skill:* Requires endovascular training to navigate through tortuous vessels and optimize aspirations.

## INTRAVASCULAR LITHOTRIPSY

- *Technique:* IVL uses sonic pressure waves delivered via a balloon catheter to fracture calcified plaque, improving vessel compliance for subsequent angioplasty or stenting.[20]
- *Devices:* Shockwave IVL (Shockwave Medical) **(Fig. 15)**.
- *Applications:* Heavily calcified FP and IP lesions, particularly in CLTI patients with rigid vessels.
- *Outcomes:* The *Disrupt PAD III trial* reported 95% procedural success, with low rates of dissection or perforation.[20]

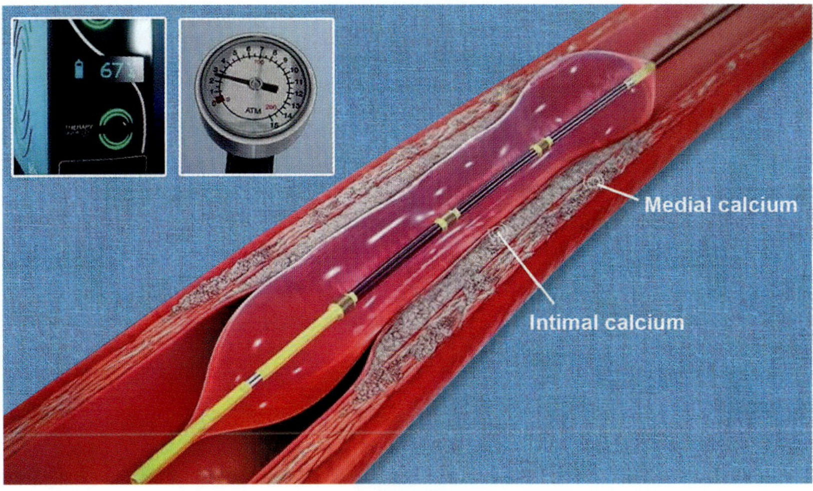


**Fig. 15:** Intravascular lithotripsy (IVL).

- *Advantages:* Effective for calcified lesions resistant to high-pressure balloons, with minimal vessel trauma.
- *Challenges:* Limited to calcified lesions, high cost, and need for additional interventions (e.g., stenting) in complex cases.

## PERCUTANEOUS FEMOROPOPLITEAL BYPASS (PQ BYPASS)

- *Technique:* A stent graft (e.g., TORUS) is deployed from the SFA to the popliteal artery via the femoral vein, bypassing long FP lesions or CTOs **(Fig. 16)**.
- *Devices:* TORUS stent graft (PQ Bypass)[17]
- *Applications:* Long (>20 cm), calcified CTOs are unsuitable for standard endovascular techniques.
- *Outcomes:* The *DETOUR I study* reported 84% primary patency at 12 months for lesions averaging 37.1 cm in length.[21]
- *Challenges:* Complex procedure requiring advanced skills, risk of graft thrombosis, and limited long-term data.

## BIORESORBABLE VASCULAR SCAFFOLDS

- *Technique:* Bioresorbable vascular scaffolds (BVS) provide temporary vessel support before dissolving over 1–3 years, reducing long-term complications associated with permanent implants.
- *Devices:* Motiv BVS™, Absorb GT1™ (used off-label in peripheral applications).
- *Applications:* IP lesions in CLTI, where small vessel diameters and high restenosis rates pose challenges.

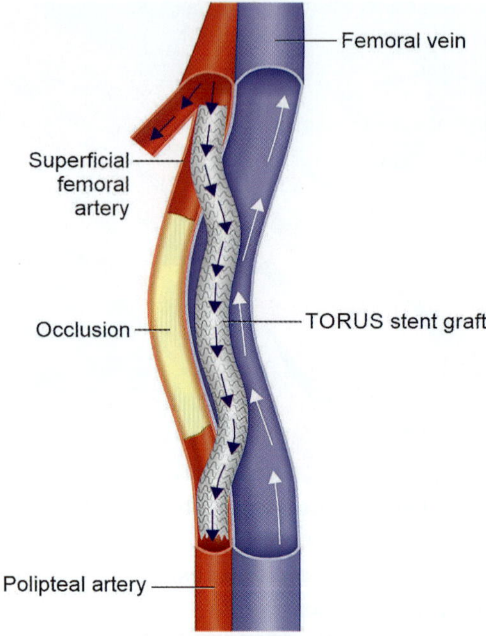


**Fig. 16:** Percutaneous femoropopliteal bypass (TORUS) stent graft.[21]

- *Outcomes:* 5-year data from early trials show patency rates comparable to DES, with the advantage of no permanent implant.[22]
- *Challenges:* Risk of early scaffold thrombosis, prolonged dual antiplatelet therapy, and limited commercial availability.

## HYBRID PROCEDURES

- *Technique:* Hybrid procedures combine endovascular and open surgical techniques in a single setting, often in a hybrid operating suite equipped with cath lab capabilities.[1]
- *Applications:* Multilevel disease in CLTI, such as SFA stenting combined with iliac endarterectomy or profundaplasty.[23]
- *Outcomes:* Effective for complex anatomies, with reduced morbidity compared to full surgical bypass. Patency rates vary based on lesion complexity.
- *Challenges:* Requires coordination between vascular surgeons and interventionalists, as well as advanced imaging capabilities.

## IMAGING AND GUIDANCE IN THE CATHETERIZATION LABORATORY

Advanced imaging is critical for procedural success, providing real-time visualization and precise guidance.

## Fluoroscopy

- *Role:* Fluoroscopy uses X-rays to provide real-time imaging of catheters, guidewires, and lesions, with contrast agents highlighting arterial anatomy.
- *Applications:* Guides all endovascular procedures, from diagnostic angiography to complex interventions.
- *Challenges:* Radiation exposure to patients and operators, and contrast nephrotoxicity in CKD patients (mitigated with $CO_2$ angiography).

## Intravascular Ultrasound

- *Technique:* A catheter-mounted ultrasound probe provides cross-sectional images of the vessel wall, plaque composition, and stent apposition **(Figs. 17A to C)**.
- *Devices:* Eagle eye platinum™ (Philips), Visions PV™ (Philips) and Opticross™ (Boston Scientific).

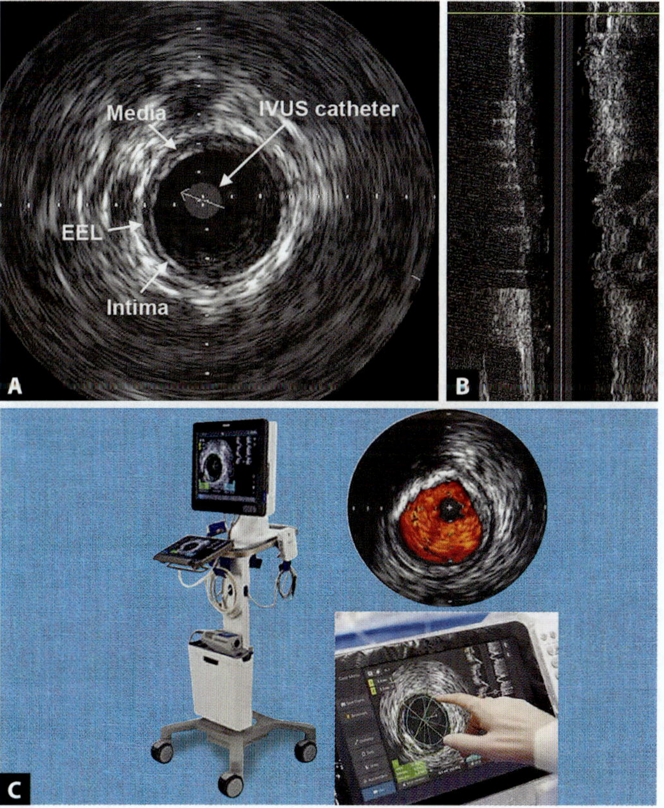


**Figs. 17A to C:** Intravascular ultrasound (IVUS).

- *Applications:* Optimizes stent sizing, detects dissection or incomplete expansion, and assesses calcification. IVUS is particularly valuable in complex CTOs and calcified lesions.
- *Outcomes:* IVUS-guided interventions reduce TLR rates by 20–30% in FP disease, as shown in the Society for Cardiovascular Angiography and Interventions (*SCAI) study.*[24]
- *Challenges:* Additional procedural time and cost, requiring operator expertise.

## ADVANCED VISUALIZATION SYSTEMS

- *Technique:* Systems such as Philips LumiGuide or GE's Innova provide 3D and color-enhanced imaging for detailed lesion mapping and navigation.
- *Applications:* Complex CTOs, calcified lesions, and multilevel disease, where precise anatomic delineation is critical.
- *Outcomes:* Reduces contrast use by 30–50% and improves procedural success rates in challenging cases.
- *Challenges:* High cost and limited availability in some centers.

### Guidelines

- *2024 ACC/AHA guideline:* Recommends endovascular therapy as first-line treatment for claudication and many CLTI cases, guided by WIfI and GLASS. Emphasizes DCBs and DES for FP lesions.
- *ESVS 2024 guidelines:* Endorse cath lab interventions for FP and IP lesions, with hybrid procedures for complex anatomies. Highlight $CO_2$ angiography for CKD patients.
- *Global vascular guidelines (2019):* Advocate WIfI and GLASS for tailoring endovascular strategies, with a focus on limb salvage in CLTI.[25]

### Real-World Evidence

Registry data (e.g., VQI registry) confirm the efficacy of endovascular interventions, with 1-year patency rates of 70–85% for FP lesions and 50–70% for IP lesions. $CO_2$ angiography has increased adoption in CKD patients, reducing nephropathy rates. Vasculomimetic stents show promise in reducing ISR in real-world FP cohorts, though further trials are needed.[11]

### Complications and Management

Endovascular procedures, while safer than open surgery, carry risks that require prompt recognition and management:

- *Restenosis:* Managed with DCBs, DES, or atherectomy. Vasculomimetic stents may reduce ISR rates in FP segments.
- *Dissection/perforation:* Treated with covered stents, prolonged balloon inflation, or rarely, surgical repair.

- *Embolization:* Addressed with aspiration of thrombectomy or embolic protection devices.
- *Access site complications:* Mitigated with ultrasound-guided access and closure devices (e.g., Angio-Seal).
- *Contrast-induced nephropathy:* Virtually eliminated with $CO_2$ angiography in CKD patients.[26]
- *Device-related complications:* Stent fracture (minimized with vasculomimetic stents), thrombosis, or infection require tailored interventions.

## TRAINING AND SKILL DEVELOPMENT

For surgical postgraduate students, learning endovascular techniques, which involve minimally invasive procedures to treat blood vessel problems, requires a well-organized training approach. Using advanced simulators, trainees can practice skills such as accessing blood vessels, navigating guidewires, and deploying devices in a safe, controlled environment. Hands-on experience in the cath lab under the guidance of experienced mentors helps build technical skills and confidence in making critical decisions. Collaborating with experts from other fields, such as interventional radiologists and cardiologists, provides valuable insights and improves procedural skills. Trainees must also become familiar with various tools, including balloons, stents, atherectomy devices (used to remove plaque), and newer technologies such as thromboaspiration devices (for clearing blood clots) and vasculomimetic stents (which mimic natural blood vessels). Additionally, learning how to handle complications, such as using covered stents to fix vessel perforations, is crucial for ensuring patient safety during procedures.

The treatment of PVD using endovascular methods, which involve minimally invasive procedures to treat blood vessel issues, is advancing quickly. New devices such as sirolimus-eluting stents and improved BVS are being developed to keep blood vessels open longer, especially in the iliac-popliteal (IP) region. Researchers are also testing vasculomimetic stents, which mimic natural blood vessels, to see if they work well for different types of blockages. Advances in $CO_2$ angiography, a technique using carbon dioxide for imaging, combined with tools like IVUS, are making it easier to see small blood vessels clearly. Artificial intelligence (AI) is being used to analyze images in real time and help plan procedures. Robotic systems are also being developed to guide catheters more precisely, especially for tough blockages called CTOs, while reducing radiation exposure for doctors and patients. Ongoing studies, such as BEST-CLI (Best Endovascular Versus Best Surgical Therapy in Patients With Critical Limb Ischemia) and BASIL-3 (Bypass Versus Angioplasty in Severe Ischemia of the Leg-3), are comparing endovascular treatments to surgery to figure out which works best.

Lastly, personalized medicine, using biomarkers and genetic information, could help create treatments tailored to each patient's unique needs.

## CONCLUSION

Endovascular treatment of PVD in the cath lab has evolutionized vascular surgery, offering minimally invasive, effective solutions for a wide range of lesions. Techniques such as balloon angioplasty, stenting, atherectomy, IVL, and novel approaches such as atherectomy and thromboaspiration devices have expanded treatment options, particularly for high-risk patients. For surgical postgraduates, mastering these procedures—supported by advanced imaging and evidence-based guidelines—is essential for delivering optimal patient care. As technology advances, including AI, robotics, and innovative devices, the cath lab will continue to drive improvements in PVD outcomes, reducing morbidity and enhancing limb salvage.

## REFERENCES

1. Authors, Clark M, Horton J. Hybrid Operating Room Suites. Hybrid Oper Room Suites CADTH Horiz Scan. Ottawa (ON): Canadian Agency for Drugs and Technologies in Health; 2023.
2. Lazar A, Morrissey N. Recent advances in endovascular treatment of peripheral arterial disease. F1000Research. 2020;9:F1000 Faculty Rev-122.
3. Norgren L, Hiatt WR, Dormandy JA, Nehler MR, Harris KA, Fowkes FG, et al. Inter-society consensus for the management of peripheral arterial disease (TASC II). J Vasc Surg. 2007;45(Suppl S):S5-67.
4. Ho C-F, Chern M-S, Wu M-H, Wu H-M, Lin W-C, Chang C-Y, et al. Carbon Dioxide Angiography in Lower Limbs: A Prospective Comparative Study With Selective Iodinated Contrast Angiography. Kaohsiung J Med Sci. 2003;19(12):599-606.
5. Coffey R, Quisling RG, Mickle JP, Hawkins IF Jr B. The cerebrovascular effects of intraarterial CO2. Radiology. 1984;(151):405-10.
6. Baerlocher MO, Kennedy SA, Rajebi MR, Baerlocher FJ, Misra S, Liu D, et al. Meta-analysis of drug-eluting balloon angioplasty and drug-eluting stent placement for infrainguinal peripheral arterial disease. J Vasc Interv Radiol. 2015;26(4):459-73.e4.
7. Tepe G, Laird J, Schneider P, Brodmann M, Krishnan P, Micari A, et al. Drug-coated balloon versus standard percutaneous transluminal angioplasty for the treatment of superficial femoral and popliteal peripheral artery disease 12-month results from the IN. PACT SFA randomized Trial. Circulation. 2015;131(5):495-502.
8. Dake MD, Ansel GM, Jaff MR, Ohki T, Saxon RR, Smouse HB, et al. Durable Clinical Effectiveness with Paclitaxel-Eluting Stents in the Femoropopliteal Artery: 5-Year Results of the Zilver PTX Randomized Trial. Circulation. 2016;133(15):1472-83.
9. Grant AJ, Yang N, Moore MJ, Lam YT, Michael PL, Chan AHP, et al. Selective NLRP3 Inflammasome Inhibitor MCC950 Suppresses Inflammation and Facilitates Healing in Vascular Materials. Adv Sci. 2023;10(20).

10. Piazza M, Squizzato F, Spolverato G, Milan L, Bonvini S, Menegolo M, et al. Outcomes of polytetrafluoroethylene-covered stent versus bare-metal stent in the primary treatment of severe iliac artery obstructive lesions Presented at the Forty-third Annual Symposium of the Society for Clinical Vascular Surgery, Miami, Fla, March 29-April 2, 2015. J Vasc Surg. 2015;62(5):1210-8.e1.
11. Salamaga S, Stępak H, Żołyński M, Kaczmarek J, Błaszyk M, Stanišić MG, et al. Three-Year Real-World Outcomes of Interwoven Nitinol Supera Stent Implantation in Long and Complex Femoropopliteal Lesions. J Clin Med. 2023;12(14):4869.
12. Sullivan TM, Zeller T, Nakamura M, Gaines PA. Treatment of Femoropopliteal Lesions With the BioMimics 3D Vascular Stent System: Two-Year Results From the MIMICS-2 Trial. J Endovasc Ther. 2021;28(2):236-45.
13. Franzone A, Ferrone M, Carotenuto G, Carbone A, Scudiero L, Serino F, et al. The role of atherectomy in the treatment of lower extremity peripheral artery disease. BMC Surg. 2012;12(Suppl_1):S13.
14. Dippel EJ, Makam P, Kovach R, George JC, Patlola R, Metzger DC, et al. Randomized controlled study of excimer laser atherectomy for treatment of femoropopliteal in-stent restenosis: Initial results from the EXCITE ISR Trial (EXCImer laser randomized controlled study for treatment of FemoropopliTEal in-stent restenosis). JACC Cardiovasc Interv. 2015;8(1):92-101.
15. Maldonado TS, Powell A, Wendorff H, Rowse J, Nagarsheth KH, Dexter DJ, et al. Safety and efficacy of mechanical aspiration thrombectomy for patients with acute lower extremity ischemia. J Vasc Surg. 2024;79(3):584-92.e5.
16. Rossi M, Tipaldi MA, Tagliaferro FB, Pisano A, Ronconi E, Lucertini E, et al. Aspiration Thrombectomy with the Indigo System for Acute Lower Limb Ischemia: Preliminary experience and analysis of parameters affecting the outcome. Ann Vasc Surg. 2021;76:426-3.
17. Li GQ, Wang L, Zhang XC. AngioJet Thrombectomy Versus Catheter-Directed Thrombolysis for Lower Extremity Deep Vein Thrombosis: A Meta-Analysis of Clinical Trials. Clin Appl Thromb. 2021;27:10760296211005548.
18. Benenati J, Saxon R, Teigen C, Adams G. Penumbra/Indigo System provides a novel aspiration thrombectomy tool in treatment of peripheral and visceral arterial occlusions: final results of the PRISM trial. J Vasc Interv Radiol. 2016; 27(3):S96.
19. Vascular Quality Initiative. (2022). Peripheral Vascular Intervention: The Vascular Quality Initiative. [Online]. Available from https://www.vqi.org/vqi-registries/peripheral-vascular-intervention/ [Last accessed November, 2025].
20. Holden A. The use of intravascular lithotripsy for the treatment of severely calcified lower limb arterial CTOs. J Cardiovasc Surg (Torino). 2019;60(1):3-7.
21. Scheinert D, Savlovskis J, Szopiński P, Krämer A, Ouriel K, Schmidt A. Percutaneous Femoropopliteal Bypass: 2-Year Results of the DETOUR System. J Vasc Surg. 2021;74(6):2114-5.
22. Drelich JW, Goldman J. Bioresorbable vascular metallic scaffolds: Current status and research trends. Curr Opin Biomed Eng. 2022;24:100411.
23. Dosluoglu HH, Lall P, Cherr GS, Harris LM, Dryjski ML. Role of simple and complex hybrid revascularization procedures for symptomatic lower extremity occlusive disease. J Vasc Surg. 2010;51(6):1425-35.e1.

24. Secemsky EA, Aronow HD, Kwolek CJ, Meissner M, Muck PE, Parikh SA, et al. Intravascular Ultrasound Use in Peripheral Arterial and Deep Venous Interventions: Multidisciplinary Expert Opinion From SCAI/AVF/AVLS/SIR/SVM/SVS. J Soc Cardiovasc Angiogr Interv. 2024;35(3):335-48.
25. Varcoe RL, DeRubertis BG, Kolluri R, Krishnan P, Metzger DC, Bonaca MP, et al. Drug-Eluting Resorbable Scaffold versus Angioplasty for Infrapopliteal Artery Disease. N Engl J Med. 2024;390(1):9-19.
26. Chaudhuri A, Dey R. Early experience of CO2 angiography using the CO2mmander system. [Online]. Available from https://www.researchgate.net/publication/312133902_Early_experience_of_CO2_angiography_using_the_CO2mmander_system [Last accessed November, 2025].
27. Conte MS, Bradbury AW, Kolh P, White J V, Dick F, Fitridge R, et al. Global vascular guidelines on the management of chronic limb-threatening ischemia. J Vasc Surg. 2019;69(6):3S-125S.e40.

CHAPTER 14

# Negative Pressure Wound Therapy

*Rohit Kumar Singh, Vivek Katiyar, Satyendra Kumar Tiwary, Puneet*

## INTRODUCTION

The concept of applying controlled subatmospheric pressure to wounds is relatively recent in the history of surgical care. The earliest systematic description came from Fleischmann and colleagues in 1993,[1] when they reported the use of a vacuum-sealed dressing in patients with open fracture wounds. Their observations were striking: the application of negative pressure not only facilitated continuous evacuation of exudate but also seemed to accelerate the formation of granulation tissue. Subsequent reports from the same group demonstrated similar benefits in the management of contaminated traumatic wounds and fasciotomy sites of the lower limb, conditions that traditionally posed formidable challenges to the surgeon.

Building on these principles, Argenta and Morykwas in 1997 popularized the concept of vacuum-assisted closure (VAC),[2] a device-based system that provides subatmospheric pressure across the entire wound site that promotes wound healing and has transformed the practical application of negative pressure wound therapy (NPWT). It is an innovative method of wound healing with secondary intention. Since then, the technology has undergone successive refinements—smaller, more portable pumps; improved foam interfaces; and the addition of instillation features—such that NPWT has become an indispensable component of the modern surgeon's repertoire. Indeed, it is now widely regarded as one of the most versatile tools available to the reconstructive and trauma surgeon.

## DESIGN AND BASIC CONCEPT

At its core, NPWT involves the application of controlled negative pressure to the wound bed through a sealed dressing system. The typical device comprises **(Figs. 1A and B)**:

- A porous interface material, usually polyurethane (black) foam with pores of 400–600 μm, which can be trimmed to conform to irregular wound geometry. Denser polyvinyl alcohol (white) foam is preferred where tissues are fragile or delicate structures, such as vessels, nerves, or exposed bone, must be protected.

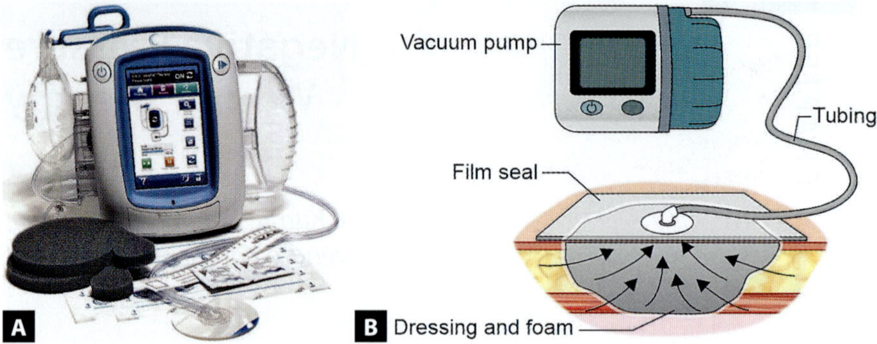


**Figs. 1A and B:** (A) Vacuum device; (B) Functioning of negative pressure wound therapy, foam covering the wound connected to the vacuum pump.

- A semiocclusive adhesive drape that creates an airtight seal with surrounding intact skin.
- A suction interface (track pad and tubing) connected to a reservoir and vacuum source.
- A pump unit capable of delivering continuous or intermittent subatmospheric pressure, usually between –50 and –200 mm Hg.

The open structure of the foam ensures even distribution of negative pressure across the wound surface, while preventing occlusion of the suction channels. Continuous suction provides consistent drainage and stabilization, whereas intermittent suction (commonly cycles of five minutes on and two minutes off) has been shown to enhance microstrain and stimulate tissue proliferation.[3,4]

From its initial application in orthopedic trauma, NPWT rapidly expanded into acute and chronic wound management. It is now used in diabetic foot ulcers, pressure injuries, venous ulcers, infected surgical wounds, dehisced sternotomies, abdominal wall defects, traumatic soft-tissue losses, and as an adjunct for skin grafts and flaps. In selected high-risk closed incisions, such as after joint replacements, vascular procedures in the groin, or midline laparotomies—closed-incision NPWT has been advocated to reduce seroma formation and surgical site infection (SSI).

Early reports suggested faster wound closure and improved graft take, and favorable outcomes in patients with chronic wounds. Further studies extended its use to radiation ulcers, pressure sores, and complex infected wounds following trauma. Despite these encouraging results, the literature is marked by heterogeneity in methodology and outcome measures.

Negative pressure wound therapy has become widely adopted in both hospital and community settings. Systematic reviews have pointed out methodological inconsistencies and the paucity of large-scale, definitive trials. Regulatory and reimbursement agencies differ in their appraisal of available evidence, further complicating universal guideline development.

Negative pressure wound therapy represents a major advancement in modern wound management. From its origins in experimental vacuum dressings in the early 1990s to the sophisticated, portable systems of today, NPWT has altered our approach to both acute and chronic wounds. While its widespread use reflects the confidence of clinicians in its clinical benefits—improved granulation, faster wound closure, better graft take—robust evidence is still evolving. As surgeons, it is our responsibility to employ NPWT judiciously: Selecting the right patient, preparing the wound meticulously, and aligning our practice with emerging evidence to optimize outcomes.[5-7]

## PRINCIPLES OF NEGATIVE PRESSURE WOUND THERAPY

### Mechanism of Action

Negative pressure wound therapy works through a combination of mechanical, physiological, and biochemical mechanisms that together create an optimal environment for healing. The four core mechanisms are:

1. Macrodeformation
2. Fluid drainage and exudate management
3. Stabilization of the wound environment
4. Microdeformation and mechanotransduction

#### *Macrodeformation*

Application of subatmospheric pressure causes the foam dressing to shrink by nearly 80% of its volume. Because the foam is in intimate contact with the wound's margins, this shrinkage exerts centripetal traction, pulling wound edges closer together. This phenomenon reduces wound surface area and depth, decreases dead space, and accelerates wound closure.[6-8] The shrinkage occurs in three dimensions and depends upon the surrounding tissue deformability, such as loose tissues (e.g., trunk and extremity wounds with skin laxity) are approximated at a much faster rate than high tension (e.g., scalp and tibia).[9]

#### *Drainage of Fluids*

One of the most important contributions of NPWT is its ability to continuously remove interstitial and inflammatory fluid.

- *Edema reduction:* By reducing tissue swelling, NPWT relieves compression of small vessels and restores perfusion at the wound base.
- *Biochemical clearance:* Exudate is rich in deleterious enzymes and cytokines such as tumor necrosis factor-alpha (TNF-$\alpha$), interleukin-6 (IL-6), and matrix metalloproteinases (MMPs). Continuous suction helps clear these, shifting the wound from a destructive inflammatory phase toward constructive repair.

- *Shear forces and ionic movement:* The flow of fluid through the foam produces subtle shear stresses and electric gradients, both of which stimulate cellular activity and proliferation.
- *Bacterial control:* By removing exudate and contaminants, NPWT reduces bacterial burden, especially when combined with instillation therapy.

The result is a wound bed that is cleaner, better perfused, and more receptive to subsequent grafting or closure.

### Stabilization of the Wound Environment

The closed, sealed system of NPWT creates a protected and physiologically favorable wound environment:

- *Barrier protection:* The polyurethane drape provides a near-airtight, bacteria-proof cover. This prevents external contamination and limits the spread of resident flora, including resistant organisms, such as Methicillin-resistant *Staphylococcus aureus* (MRSA).[10]
- *Moisture and temperature control:* The semiocclusive membrane maintains a moist environment and reduces evaporative cooling, preserving normothermia—an established promoter of cellular repair.
- *Fewer dressing changes:* Unlike conventional gauze that requires daily changes, NPWT dressings are typically changed every 48–72 hours. This minimizes wound bed disruption, improves patient comfort, and reduces nursing workload.
- *Odor and hygiene:* The closed system eliminates leakage, odor, and soiling of clothes or bedding, all of which improve patient dignity and mobility.

By stabilizing the microenvironment, NPWT converts a hostile, unstable wound into a controlled and predictable field for healing.

### Microdeformation and Mechanotransduction

At the cellular level, NPWT exerts micromechanical strain on the wound bed. The porous foam transmits negative pressure to individual cells, stretching their cytoskeleton, and altering integrin attachments.[11,12] The term "Mechanotransduction" is used to describe the effect of mechanical forces modifying the cellular function.

This mechanotransduction process:

- Stimulates fibroblast proliferation and extracellular matrix production.
- Increases angiogenesis and capillary sprouting.
- Enhances granulation of tissue formation, even over poorly vascularized structures such as tendon or bone.
- Inhibits apoptosis and upregulates growth-promoting gene expression.

The studies have demonstrated up to a 60% increase in granulation tissue compared with standard dressings, which clinically translates into faster readiness for grafting and improved rates of graft/flap take.[2,13]

## Additional Mechanisms

### *Biochemical Modulation*

Negative pressure wound therapy reduces the levels of destructive proteases [matrix metalloproteinase-1 (MMP-1), MMP-2, MMP-9, and MMP-13] and proinflammatory cytokines [interferon-gamma (IFN-γ) and IL-6] while supporting growth factor signaling. This biochemical "rebalancing" creates conditions for sustained tissue repair.

## Perfusion Effects

Although debated, most studies suggest that NPWT enhances periwound blood flow at moderate pressures (around –125 mm Hg), thereby improving oxygenation, leukocyte delivery, and antibiotic penetration. Excessive pressures, however, may compromise perfusion; hence the importance of titrating pressure settings in ischemic or fragile wounds.[14-16]

### *Reduction of Bacterial Load*

Experimental and clinical data consistently show that NPWT lowers bacterial counts more effectively than gauze dressings. With instillation of solution (detail discussed below in this chapter), this effect is amplified by periodic lavage, which dilutes and removes biofilm and debris. Instillation therapy in NPWT involves the controlled delivery of topical solutions, such as saline and antiseptics, into the wound bed, followed by a dwell phase before suction resumes. This technique enhances wound cleansing, reduces bacterial load, promotes granulation, and is particularly beneficial in infected or heavily exudative wounds.[17-19]

The principles of NPWT can be summarized in practical terms:

- *Mechanical:* Wound contraction and edge approximation.
- *Fluidic:* Continuous clearance of edema, toxins, and exudates.
- *Environmental:* Sealed, moist, warm, and protected wound bed.
- *Cellular:* Micromechanical stimulation of fibroblasts and angiogenesis.
- *Biochemical:* Favorable shift in protease and cytokine balance.
- *Microbials:* Reduction of bacterial burden and risk of infection.

## INDICATIONS OF NEGATIVE PRESSURE WOUND THERAPY

Negative pressure wound therapy is primarily indicated for wounds that are either nonhealing or at risk of impaired healing, especially when conventional closure techniques are unsuitable or contraindicated. Its versatility has expanded from initial use in complex open wounds to a wide range of acute, chronic, and prophylactic applications.

## Acute Wounds

Negative pressure wound therapy is often employed when primary closure is not feasible due to contamination, tissue loss, edema, or skin tension.

- *Traumatic wounds:* Open fractures, complex lacerations, degloving injuries, and lower-limb trauma with exposed soft tissue.
- *Burns and scalds:* Partial thickness burns with significant exudation or contamination.
- *Fasciotomy/dermatofasciotomy wounds:* To manage edema, protect exposed structures, and promote granulation.
- *Open abdomen:* As part of temporary abdominal closure following trauma, peritonitis, or damage-control surgery.[20]

## Chronic Wounds

Negative pressure wound therapy has proven particularly useful for *nonhealing or recalcitrant wounds* where standard dressings have failed.

- *Diabetic foot ulcers* (including postdebridement for necrotizing fasciitis or infected heel ulcers).
- *Venous leg ulcers and arterial ulcers* with impaired healing.
- *Pressure ulcers* (category 2 and 3, especially with heavy exudation).
- *Leg ulcers of mixed etiology.*
- *Wounds with exposed tendon, bone, or orthopedic implants,* where granulation coverage is otherwise slow.
- *Osteomyelitis-related wounds,* in selected cases, after adequate debridement and antibiotic therapy.[21-23]

## Surgical Wound Complications

Negative pressure wound therapy is a valuable adjunct in managing surgical wounds at risk of dehiscence or infection **(Figs. 2A and B)**.

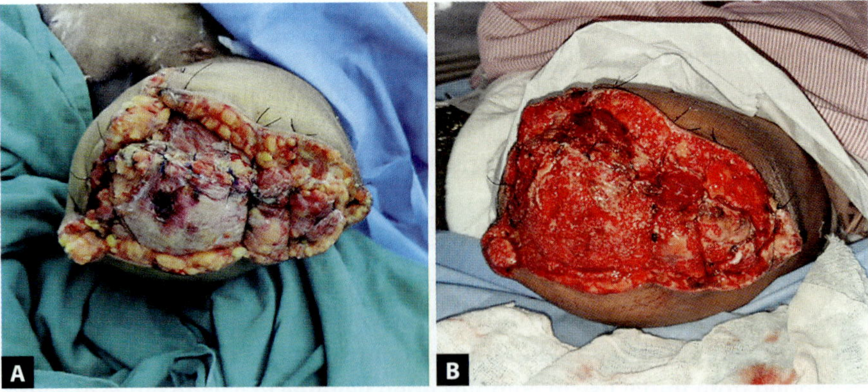

**Figs. 2A and B:** Amputation of the lower limb following a road traffic accident. (A) Unhealthy wound before negative pressure wound therapy (NPWT) and (B) Healthy granulation tissue after one cycle of NPWT for 3 days.

- *Dehisced incisions* and soft-tissue defects following abdominal, orthopedic, or vascular procedures.
- *Postmesh or prosthesis infection:* In selected cases, NPWT can assist in wound control around vascular grafts or prosthetic material.
- *Postreconstructive surgery:* Useful after breast or abdominal wall reconstruction for managing skin breakdown.[24-26]

### Flaps and Grafts

- *Skin grafts:* NPWT serves as an excellent bolster, securing grafts, minimizing shear, reducing seroma/hematoma formation, and enhancing graft take.
- *Local or free flaps:* Applied to reduce edema, stabilize the flap, and improve perfusion during the early postoperative phase.
- *Preparation of wound beds:* NPWT creates an optimal granulating surface for subsequent grafting or flap coverage.

### Therapeutic Objectives of Negative Pressure Wound Therapy

Across these diverse indications, the objectives remain consistent:

- *Exudate management:* Continuous drainage to reduce edema and wound bioburden.
- *Granulation promotion:* Enhanced angiogenesis and fibroblast activity for faster tissue coverage.
- *Bacterial control:* Reduced colonization and lower infection risk.
- *Perfusion improvement:* By decreasing interstitial pressures.
- *Temporary wound coverage:* As a bridge to definitive surgical closure (skin grafts, flaps, or delayed suturing).
- *Patient comfort and hygiene:* Reduced dressing frequency and improved mobility.

## CONTRAINDICATIONS TO NEGATIVE PRESSURE WOUND THERAPY

Although NPWT has transformed the management of complex wounds, it is not universally applicable. Careful patient selection and meticulous wound assessment are essential to avoid potentially serious complications.[27] Contraindications to NPWT can be divided into *absolute and relative*, with a further group of *practical cautions* that require attention during clinical use.

### Absolute Contraindications

These are situations where NPWT should not be applied under any circumstances:

- *Presence of malignancy in the wound bed:* Negative pressure is known to promote angiogenesis and cellular proliferation—the same biological processes that can theoretically accelerate tumor growth and facilitate malignant spread. Complete oncological clearance must therefore be ensured before NPWT is considered.

- *Untreated osteomyelitis:* Application of NPWT over an infected bone without prior debridement or appropriate antimicrobial therapy risks worsening the infection. Definitive treatment of osteomyelitis is a prerequisite.
- *Exposed vital structures:* Direct application of negative pressure over unprotected organs, major blood vessels, or vascular grafts carries the danger of erosion, fistula formation, or catastrophic hemorrhage. Adequate tissue, flap, or protective interface must cover these structures before NPWT use.
- *Necrotic tissue with eschar:* NPWT should not be applied over dry eschar or grossly devitalized tissue. Debridement is necessary first to expose a viable wound bed.
- *Unexplored or high-output fistulas:* Unexplored or high-output fistulas risk uncontrolled fluid loss, electrolyte imbalance, and progressive tissue breakdown when exposed to suction.[26-28]

## Relative Contraindications

These situations require *caution and individualized judgment* rather than absolute avoidance:

- *Ischemic tissue:* In critically ischemic wounds, the transient reduction in perfusion associated with suction may exacerbate tissue compromise. Revascularization should precede NPWT wherever feasible.
- *Active bleeding or high bleeding risk:* Patients with uncontrolled hemorrhage, coagulopathy, or those on anticoagulants require close monitoring. While NPWT has been used successfully in such settings, the risk of bleeding must be weighed carefully against potential benefits.
- *Fragile skin:* Elderly patients, those on long-term corticosteroids, or individuals with connective tissue disorders often have delicate skin prone to avulsion during dressing changes. Proper protective barriers and gentle technique are essential. In cases where fragility outweighs benefits, NPWT may be avoided.[28]

## Practical Considerations and Precautions

- Ensure *vital structures* such as bowels, large vessels, and nerves are protected with tissue or a suitable interface before applying NPWT.
- Avoid *overpacking foam* into cavities, which may generate excessive pressure and impair tissue viability.
- Monitor closely for *complications* such as bleeding, infection, maceration of periwound skin, or autonomic dysreflexia (particularly in patients with spinal cord injury).

- Ensure therapy is instituted by *trained personnel*, with regular reassessment of wound progress and device function.

Negative pressure wound therapy is a powerful adjunct in wound management, but its benefits are realized only when applied judiciously. While acute trauma, infected surgical wounds, ulcers, grafts, and high-risk incisions are well-validated indications, clinicians must remain vigilant about absolute contraindications—especially untreated infection, necrotic tissue, and exposed vital structures. Relative contraindications such as ischemia and fragile skin require individualized assessment, careful monitoring, and, in some cases, avoidance. A thoughtful, evidence-informed approach ensures that NPWT serves as a tool for healing rather than a source of harm.[29-32]

## TECHNIQUE OF APPLICATION OF NEGATIVE PRESSURE WOUND THERAPY

The success of NPWT depends less on the device itself and more on the discipline with which it is applied. A carefully executed application ensures effective suction, reduces complications, and enhances patient comfort. The technique can be divided into sequential steps: Patient preparation, wound bed optimization, selection of interface material, sealing, pressure settings, and maintenance.

### Patient Preparation

- *Assessment:* Begin with a thorough evaluation of the wound—its size, depth, anatomical location, degree of contamination, and presence of exposed structures. Assess systemic factors, such as glycemic control, nutrition, and vascular status.
- *Analgesia and sedation:* The first application, especially in painful wounds (burns, debridement sites, and fasciotomies), may require systemic analgesia or even short anesthesia. Subsequent dressing changes can often be managed with oral analgesics or local anesthesia.
- *Infection control:* Ensure that gross infection and necrotic tissue have been addressed by adequate debridement and appropriate antimicrobial therapy before initiating NPWT.[33]

### Wound Bed Preparation

- *Debridement:* Remove all necrotic, devitalized, or infected tissue. NPWT applied over eschar or slough is ineffective and may worsen the wound.
- *Hemostasis:* Achieve meticulous hemostasis; negative pressure can exacerbate bleeding if small vessels are left unsecured.
- *Irrigation:* Copious saline wash helps reduce bacterial burden and clears debris, optimizing the bed for granulation of tissue formation.

## Protection of Vital Structures

- *Exposed structures:* If tendon, bone, joint capsule, or vascular grafts are exposed, cover them with a *nonadherent layer* (e.g., paraffin gauze, petroleum-impregnated dressing, or a protective biologic interface).
- *Prevention of erosion:* This step prevents erosion, fistula formation, or direct suction injury over fragile tissues.[34,26,27].

## Selection of Interface Material

- *Polyurethane foam (black foam):* Highly porous (400–600 µm), promotes tissue ingrowth and robust granulation. Suitable for most acute and chronic wounds.
- *Polyvinyl alcohol foam (white foam):* Denser, less adherent, used over delicate structures (e.g., tendons, vessels, and nerves) or in painful wounds.
- *Gauze dressings:* Used as an alternative interface in shallow or irregular wounds where foam cannot conform adequately. Gauze may be premoistened or used with antiseptic or antimicrobial solutions in NPWT with instillation therapy.
- *Antimicrobial foams:* Silver- or polyhexamethylene biguanide (PHMB)-impregnated foams are valuable in wounds with high bioburden.

## Placement of the Foam and Drape

- *Sizing:* Trim the foam to fit the wound dimensions precisely, ensuring gentle contact without overpacking. Excess compression can impair perfusion.
- *Application:* Insert the foam into the wound cavity, ensuring contact with all wound surfaces. Avoid leaving multiple fragments—count pieces in and out.
- *Sealing:* Cover the foam with a transparent polyurethane drape extending 2–3 cm beyond the wound edges on intact skin. Eliminate wrinkles and secure the margins with gentle pressure to maintain an airtight seal.
- *Tubing/track pad*: Position the suction port over the foam but away from bony prominences or pressure areas. For multiple wounds, bridging with foam strips can permit a single suction source.

## Setting Negative Pressure

- *Pressure levels:*
  - *Standard*: *–125 mm Hg* continuous suction, effective for most acute wounds.
  - *Grafts/flaps*: *–75 to –125 mm Hg*, often continuous for 3–5 days to ensure secure take.
  - *Fragile tissue, pediatrics, or painful wounds*: Start at *–50 to –75 mm Hg*.

- *Mode of application:*
  - *Continuous mode:* Preferred during the initial 48 hours and in highly exudative or contaminated wounds, ensuring steady drainage and wound stabilization.
  - *Intermittent mode (e.g., 5 minutes on, 2 minutes off):* Enhances microdeformation and granulation once the wound is clean and pain is controlled.

## Dressing Change and Maintenance

- *Frequency:* Every *48–72 hours* in clean wounds. For infected or heavily exudating wounds, change every *24–48 hours.*
- *Inspection:* At each change, reassess wound dimensions, tissue quality, exudate volume, odor, and periwound skin condition. Document findings meticulously.
- *Seal integrity:* Regularly monitor for air leaks, blocked tubing, or canister overfilling. Patient education is vital to recognize alarms and maintain seal integrity.
- *Adjunctive care*: Combine NPWT with systemic antibiotics (when infection is present), nutritional support, glucose control, and appropriate off-loading or compression as required.

## Practical Tips from Clinical Experience

- *First dressing change* is often the most painful—plan adequate analgesia and reassurance.
- *Protect the periwound* with barrier films or hydrocolloid strips to reduce maceration.
- *Avoid overnegative pressures* in ischemic limbs; lower settings with careful monitoring are safer.
- *Plan ahead for closure:* NPWT is a bridge, not an endpoint—always define when and how definitive closure (secondary suturing, graft, or flap) will be attempted.

Application of NPWT is a *stepwise, meticulous process* rather than a mechanical ritual. Proper wound bed preparation, careful interface selection, airtight sealing, and tailored pressure settings are essential for success. Regular reassessment and attention to detail—hallmarks of sound surgical practice—ensure that NPWT fulfills its promise: creating a stable, well-vascularized wound environment that accelerates healing and facilitates timely closure.[35-40]

# NEWER MODALITIES IN NEGATIVE PRESSURE WOUND THERAPY

Since its introduction in the 1990s, NPWT has undergone significant refinement. The success of conventional VAC therapy encouraged further innovation, leading to *advanced modalities* that expand its indications, improve efficacy, and address specific clinical challenges. The most widely recognized newer modalities include NPWT with instillation and dwell (NPWTi-d), specialized cleansing dressings (Cleanse Choice systems), and closed incision negative pressure wound therapy (ciNPWT).[40-42]

## Negative Pressure Wound Therapy with Instillation and Dwell Time

It combines conventional negative pressure therapy with the intermittent instillation of topical solutions into the wound bed, followed by a controlled dwell phase before suction resumes. This technique harmonizes the benefits of NPWT, such as enhanced granulation and exudate management, with the cleansing and antimicrobial properties of irrigating agents. Commonly used instillation solutions include normal saline, antiseptic agents such as polyhexamethylene hydrochloride biguanide (PHMB) and hypochlorous acid, as well as antimicrobial and enzymatic debriding solutions. The therapy allows customization of key parameters such as the type of solution, dwell time, negative pressure level, and frequency of instillation cycles, enabling individualized wound management.

Evidence demonstrates that NPWTi-d significantly enhances healing outcomes compared to standard NPWT. Studies have shown a 43% increase in granulation tissue formation, with clinical series reporting up to 95% healing in chronic, previously nonhealing wounds. The addition of antiseptic instillation has been associated with a measurable reduction in bacterial load, disruption of biofilm, and improved graft or flap salvage rates. Furthermore, NPWTi-d has been shown to reduce hospital stay, the number of operative interventions, and the time required for definitive wound closure. This modality is particularly valuable for infected, heavily colonized, or exudative wounds, as it integrates mechanical wound management with active wound cleansing. While NPWTi-d is cost-effective in selected cases, the optimal soak times, choice of solutions, and standardized protocols continue to evolve.[42-44]

## Cleanse Choice Systems

Certain complex wounds, such as those associated with necrotizing infections, burns, and extensive sloughing, produce thick exudate and viscous debris that cannot be effectively managed using standard NPWT foams. To address this limitation, the VERAFLO™ Cleanse Choice dressing was developed as a specialized reticulated open-cell polyurethane ester foam with reduced hydrophobicity, allowing for more uniform distribution of instillation fluids across the wound bed. This design enhances the mechanical cleansing action during NPWTi-d. The dressing offers several advantages: it promotes efficient removal of fibrin, slough, and bacterial contaminants; its high tensile strength prevents foam fragmentation and allows for safe, intact removal; and it supports granulation tissue formation, particularly in cases where surgical debridement is not feasible. The Cleanse Choice system is therefore particularly beneficial for wounds with heavy bioburden, thick exudate, or incomplete debridement, effectively bridging the gap between mechanical cleansing and advanced wound healing.

## Closed Incision Negative Pressure Wound Therapy

Closed-incision negative pressure wound therapy differs from conventional NPWT in that it is applied over primarily closed surgical incisions rather than open wounds. The principle behind ciNPWT is to protect closed incisions from postoperative complications such as infection, seroma, hematoma, or wound dehiscence by maintaining a controlled sub-atmospheric pressure that stabilizes the incision edges, removes subcutaneous fluid, and promotes microvascular perfusion.

Clinical evidence supports its effectiveness across various surgical settings. Condé-Green et al. reported that patients undergoing abdominal wall reconstruction treated with ciNPWT experienced significantly fewer complications compared with those receiving standard dressings (22% vs. 65.9%), with dehiscence rates notably reduced (9% vs. 39%).[32] Similarly, Stannard et al.[33] demonstrated that ciNPWT decreased postoperative infections following high-risk lower extremity trauma surgeries. In obstetric applications, ciNPWT has been shown to lower wound complication rates in obese women undergoing cesarean section.

Overall, ciNPWT has been associated with a reduction in SSIs, seroma and hematoma formation, as well as improved scar quality and cosmetic outcomes. It is particularly beneficial in high-risk patient groups such as those with obesity, diabetes, immunosuppression, or those undergoing vascular and colorectal surgeries. While the current evidence is promising, further research is required to refine patient selection criteria, optimize pressure parameters, and establish cost-effectiveness for broader clinical use.

## Evidence in Specific Wound Types

- *Diabetic foot ulcers:* NPWT improves closure rates, reduces secondary amputations, and shortens healing time compared with advanced moist therapy.
- *Pressure ulcers:* Studies show fewer hospitalizations and reduced long-term care requirements when NPWT is used.
- *Chronic wounds:* Meta-analyses confirm faster wound size reduction and shorter healing times compared with conventional therapy.
- *Skin grafts:* NPWT functions as an effective bolster, with significantly improved graft survival and reduced need for repeat grafting.

## CLINICAL OUTCOMES AND EVIDENCE

Since its introduction, NPWT has been extensively studied across diverse wound types, from chronic ulcers to complex surgical and traumatic wounds. Although methodological variations and limited sample sizes are common challenges in wound research, a consistent body of evidence supports NPWT's role in accelerating healing, reducing complications, and improving cost-effectiveness when compared with conventional dressings.[43-46]

### Chronic Wounds

- *Diabetic foot ulcers (DFUs):* A large comparative study demonstrated significantly higher wound closure rates with NPWT (43.2%) compared to advanced moist wound therapy (28.9%), along with a reduction in secondary amputation rates. Subsequent clinical trials have also shown faster granulation of tissue formation and shorter overall healing times in diabetic foot ulcers managed with NPWT.
- *Pressure ulcers:* Studies show NPWT reduces hospitalization rates, shortens the duration of home-care support, and lowers the risk of chronic infection compared with standard moist wound care.
- *Venous and arterial ulcers:* Meta-analyses confirm that NPWT reduces wound size more rapidly and decreases overall healing time compared to conventional modalities.

### Surgical and Traumatic Wounds

- *Dehisced wounds and SSI prevention:* Closed incision NPWT (ciNPWT) has shown reduced incidence of wound dehiscence, seroma, and SSI, particularly in high-risk patients (e.g., obese, diabetic, colorectal, or orthopedic surgeries) **(Figs. 2 and 3)**.
- *Open abdomen therapy:* NPWT for temporary abdominal closure in trauma and sepsis improves fluid management, protects viscera, and facilitates staged repair with lower mortality compared to traditional methods.
- *Orthopedic and trauma wounds:* NPWT has been shown to promote limb salvage in severe crush injuries, support revision arthroplasty, and reduce infection rates in contaminated wounds.

### Skin Grafts and Flaps

Negative-pressure wound therapy used as a bolster dressing improves graft adherence, reduces seroma/hematoma formation, and enhances graft survival. Clinical studies report significantly fewer repeat grafting procedures compared with conventional bolster techniques.

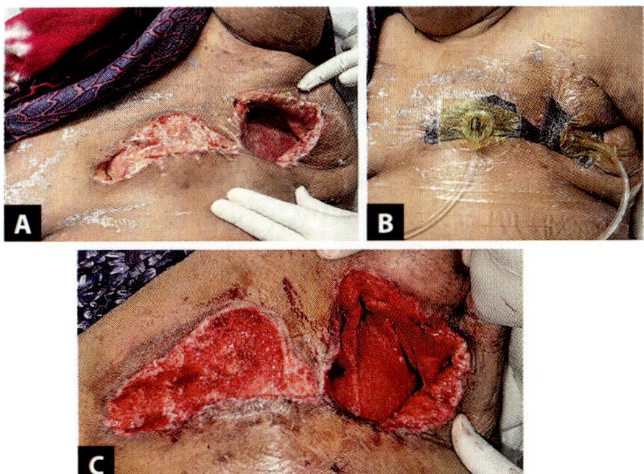

**Figs. 3A to C:** (A) Postmastectomy flap necrosis leading to a large wound in the left anterior chest wall; (B) Application of negative-pressure wound therapy (NPWT) with foam dressing in the wound; (C) Post-NPWT healthy wound, secondary suturing performed.

### Negative-pressure Wound Therapy with Instillation and Dwell

Randomized and observational studies indicate that NPWTi-d enhances granulation tissue formation, accelerates wound cleansing, and decreases bacterial bioburden more effectively than standard NPWT. In infected or biofilm-heavy wounds, NPWTi-d has been associated with shorter hospital stays and fewer operative interventions.[47,48]

### Cost-effectiveness and Quality of Life

Several analysts suggest that while the upfront cost of NPWT is higher, reduced length of hospital stay, fewer surgical procedures, and faster wound closure make it cost-effective overall. Patients also benefit from fewer dressing changes, reduced pain, and improved mobility, enhancing quality of life.

The clinical evidence for NPWT, while heterogeneous, consistently supports its efficacy in accelerating wound closure, reducing infection rates, improving graft and flap outcomes, and lowering overall healthcare costs. Advanced modalities such as ciNPWT and NPWTi-d further broaden its application. Future large-scale, randomized controlled trials will help refine protocols and strengthen guideline recommendations, but NPWT is already firmly established as a cornerstone in modern wound management.[44-48]

## SPECIAL CONSIDERATIONS IN NEGATIVE PRESSURE WOUND THERAPY

While NPWT has become an integral component of wound management, its application must be tailored to the unique clinical circumstances of each patient. Beyond standard indications and contraindications, several *special considerations* influence the safe and effective use of this therapy[49-51].[4]

## Patient Selection and Comorbidities

- *Diabetes and peripheral vascular disease:* Careful monitoring is needed, as impaired perfusion can limit NPWT benefits and increase the risk of ischemia. Optimization of glycemic control and vascular status is essential before initiation.
- *Elderly and frail patients:* Thin, fragile skin increases the risk of periwound maceration or avulsion during drape changes. Barrier films or hydrocolloid strips can help protect the surrounding tissue.
- *Anticoagulated patients:* Although not an absolute contraindication, there is a heightened risk of bleeding. Close observation and lower pressure settings are advisable.

## Anatomical Considerations

- *Exposed structures:* Direct application over vessels, nerves, bowel, or grafts should be avoided. Protective nonadherent layers or biological dressings must be placed before applying foam.
- *Difficult locations:* Areas such as the scalp, perineum, or axilla pose challenges in achieving airtight seals. Customized dressing techniques, bridging, or adjunctive adhesives may be required.
- *Orthopedic settings:* When NPWT is used around fixation devices or prostheses, care must be taken to minimize contamination risk while ensuring adequate coverage.

## Pediatric and Neonatal Use

Negative-pressure wound therapy has been increasingly reported in children, including neonates. While beneficial in congenital defects, traumatic wounds, and postoperative infections, pressure settings must be adjusted to lower ranges (–50 to –75 mm Hg) to avoid complications. Dressing changes should be performed under analgesia or anesthesia when required.

## Home-based and Outpatient Therapy

The development of lightweight, portable NPWT devices has expanded use beyond hospitals. Patient and caregiver education is critical to maintaining seal integrity, recognizing alarms, and ensuring timely follow-up. Remote monitoring and telemedicine support may further improve safety and compliance in the home-care setting.

## Infection Control and Biofilm Management

Although NPWT can reduce bacterial burden, its use on inadequately debrided wounds or in the presence of uncontrolled infection may worsen outcomes. In such cases, NPWTi-d and antiseptic solutions may provide added benefits. Strict aseptic technique during dressing changes remains essential to avoid iatrogenic contamination.

### Multidisciplinary Approach

Optimal results often require collaboration among surgeons, wound care nurses, infectious disease specialists, and nutritionists. A structured, interdisciplinary care pathway ensures that NPWT is not viewed as a standalone solution but as part of a comprehensive wound healing strategy.[44-52]

## COMPLICATIONS AND LIMITATIONS OF NEGATIVE PRESSURE WOUND THERAPY

Although NPWT has transformed modern wound care, it is not devoid of risks. Awareness of potential complications and limitations is essential for safe and effective application. Complications may arise from improper patient selection, technical errors during application, or the inherent physiological effects of negative pressure.[53-55] The common adverse events arising from NPWT are preventable.

### Local Wound-related Complications

- *Bleeding and hemorrhage:* Perhaps the most serious complication, bleeding, can occur due to erosion of exposed vessels, inadequate hemostasis at the time of dressing application, or use in anticoagulated patients. Life-threatening hemorrhage has been reported, particularly in wounds overlying vascular grafts, sternotomy sites, or irradiated tissue. The bleeding may also be encountered if foam is left in place for a prolonged time or if rapid granulation occurs (in children). Thus, while removing the foam, bleeding may occur, which can usually be controlled with manual pressure.
- *Tissue damage and necrosis:* Excessive suction or overpacking of foam may impair perfusion, leading to ischemia at wound edges. Fragile periwound skin in elderly or steroid-treated patients is susceptible to avulsion during drape removal. Other minor complications of skin such as irritation, allergic rashes, and maceration, are also reported.
- *Infection and sepsis:* While NPWT reduces bacterial burden in many cases, improper use—especially over inadequately debrided or necrotic tissue—can worsen infection. There are a few case reports of Toxic Shock syndrome following the application of VAC therapy. Retained foam fragments may also act as nidus.
- *Pain and discomfort:* Patients often report pain during dressing changes, particularly when foam adheres to granulating tissue. This can limit

compliance if not addressed with analgesia or alternative dressing materials (e.g., white foam or application of saline or xylocaine). Pain due to pressure can be overcome by reducing the starting pressure to –50 mm Hg and later may be gradually increased (up to –125 mm Hg). Continuous suction can cause less pain and discomfort as compared with intermittent suction.

## Systemic and Technical Complications

- *Fluid and electrolyte imbalance:* The application of NPWT in a large-sized wound may result in suctioning of a large quantity of fluid on the first day, causing hemodynamic instability. High-output wounds may also lead to significant electrolyte disturbances if not carefully monitored.
- *Fistula formation:* Direct suction applied over the bowel or other hollow viscera may induce fistulization. Thus, a synthetic mesh or absorbable biological dressing should be placed as an interface between the foam and the organ to prevent fistulation. Similarly, prolonged application over unprotected vascular grafts or nerves risks erosion and functional loss.
- *Device malfunction or seal failure:* Air leaks, blocked tubing, or loss of suction compromise therapy effectiveness, leading to maceration of surrounding skin and delayed healing.

## Limitations of Negative Pressure Wound Therapy

- *Not a substitute for debridement or antibiotics:* NPWT is an adjunct, not a replacement, for surgical debridement and appropriate antimicrobial therapy. In infected wounds, failure to address underlying sepsis results in poor outcomes.
- *Contraindications:* Malignancy in the wound bed, untreated osteomyelitis, necrotic eschar, unexplored fistulas, and exposed unprotected organs or vessels remain in strict contraindications.
- *Evidence limitations:* Despite widespread use, much of the supporting evidence for NPWT arises from small, randomized trials, retrospective studies, or industry-sponsored research. Heterogeneity in study design, endpoints, and patient populations limits the strength of guideline recommendations.
- *Cost considerations:* NPWT is more expensive than traditional dressings, and while long-term savings may be realized through reduced complications and shorter hospital stays, upfront costs remain a barrier in resource-limited settings.
- *Training and expertise:* Effective NPWT requires skilled application, ongoing monitoring, and interdisciplinary collaboration. Inadequate training can lead to misuse and higher complication rates.

While NPWT offers significant benefits, clinicians must be vigilant about its potential complications—including bleeding, infection, fistula formation, and skin injury—and remain mindful of its limitations as an adjunctive therapy rather than a substitute for basic surgical principles. Cost, evidence of heterogeneity, and technical expertise remain in ongoing challenges.[55-60] Careful patient selection, meticulous technique, and regular monitoring are key to maximizing benefits while minimizing risks.

## CONCLUSION

Negative pressure wound therapy has revolutionized modern wound management, evolving from an experimental concept to a widely adopted therapeutic modality. Its effectiveness lies in its ability to simultaneously reduce edema, improve perfusion, remove exudates, and stimulate granulation of tissue formation—creating an optimal environment for wound healing. Over the past three decades, innovations such as NPWTi-d, Cleanse Choice dressings, and ciNPWT have broadened its clinical applications, from chronic ulcers and traumatic wounds to complex surgical incisions and reconstructive procedures. Looking forward, integration with digital monitoring systems, portable devices, and combination therapies promises to make NPWT even more accessible and effective, particularly in outpatient and resource-limited settings. Further high-quality trials are needed to refine protocols, standardize instillation parameters, and strengthen evidence across diverse wound types. In summary, NPWT is not merely a dressing but a dynamic adjunct to surgical practice, offering a versatile, evidence-based approach that continues to shape the landscape of wound management. When applied thoughtfully within a multidisciplinary framework, it can significantly improve outcomes, reduce complications, and enhance the quality of life for patients with complex wounds.

## REFERENCES

1. Fleischmann W, Strecker W, Bombelli M, Kinzl L. Vakuumversiegelung zur Behandlung des Weichteilschadens bei offenen Frakturen. Unfallchirurg 1993;96(09):488-92
2. Argenta LC, Morykwas MJ. Vacuum-assisted closure: a new method for wound control and treatment: clinical experience. Ann Plast Surg. 1997;38(06):563-76.
3. Venturi ML, Attinger CE, Mesbahi AN, Hess CL, Graw KS. Mechanisms and clinical applications of the vacuum-assisted closure (VAC) Device: a review. Am J Clin Dermatol. 2005;6(03):185-94.
4. OrgillDP, Manders EK, SumpioBE, Lee RC, Attinger CE, Gurtner GC, et al. The mechanisms of action of vacuum assisted closure: More to learn. Surgery. 2009;146(01):40-51.
5. Scherer SS, Pietramaggiori G, Mathews JC, Prsa MJ, Huang S, Orgill DP. The mechanism of action of the vacuum-assisted closure device. Plast Reconstr Surg. 2008;122(03):786-97.
6. Stechmiller JK, Kilpadi DV, Childress B, Schultz GS. Effect of vacuum-assisted closure therapy on the expression of cytokines and proteases in wound fluid of adults with pressure ulcers. Wound Repair Regen 2006;14(03):371-4.

7. Agarwal P, Kukrele R, Sharma D. Vacuum assisted closure (VAC)/negative pressure wound therapy (NPWT) for difficult wounds: A review. J Clin Orthop Trauma. 2019;10(05):845-8.
8. Kloth LC, Berman JE, Nett M, Papanek PE, Dumit-Minkel S. A randomized controlled clinical trial to evaluate the effects of noncontact normothermic wound therapy on chronic full-thickness pressure ulcers. Adv SkinWound Care 2002;15(06):270-6.
9. Saxena V, Hwang CW, Huang S, Eichbaum Q, Ingber D, Orgill DP. Vacuum-assisted closure: microdeformations of wounds and cell proliferation. Plast Reconstr Surg. 2004;114(05):1086-96.
10. McNulty AK, Schmidt M, Feeley T, Kieswetter K. Effects of negative pressure wound therapy on fibroblast viability, chemotactic signaling, and proliferation in a provisional wound (fibrin) matrix. Wound Repair Regen 2007;15(06):838-46.
11. McNulty AK, Schmidt M, Feeley T, Villanueva P, Kieswetter K. Effects of negative pressure wound therapy on cellular energetics in fibroblasts grown in a provisional wound (fibrin) matrix. Wound Repair Regen 2009;17(02):192-9.
12. Urschel JD, Scott PG, Williams HT. The effect of mechanical stress on soft and hard tissue repair; a review. Br J Plast Surg. 1988;41 (02):182-6
13. Morykwas MJ, Argenta LC, Shelton-Brown EI, McGuirt W. Vacuum-assisted closure: a new method for wound control and treatment: animal studies and basic foundation. Ann Plast Surg. 1997;38(06):553-62
14. Garcia-Cardeña G, Comander J, Anderson KR, Blackman BR, Gimbrone MA Jr. Biomechanical activation of vascular endothelium as a determinant of its functional phenotype. Proc Natl Acad Sci U S A. 2001;98(08):4478-85.
15. Huang S, Chen CS, Ingber DE. Control of cyclin D1, p27(Kip1), and cell cycle progression in human capillary endothelial cells by cell shape and cytoskeletal tension. Mol Biol Cell. 1998;9(11): 3179-93.
16. Huang S, Ingber DE. Shape-dependent control of cell growth, differentiation, and apoptosis: switching between attractors in cell regulatory networks. Exp Cell Res. 2000;261(01):91-103.
17. Nishimura K, Blume P, Ohgi S, Sumpio BE. Effect of different frequencies of tensile strain on human dermal fibroblast proliferation and survival. Wound Repair Regen. 2007;15(05):646-56.
18. Greene AK, Puder M, Roy R, Arsenault D, Kwei S, Moses MA, et al. Microdeformational wound therapy: effects on angiogenesis and matrix metalloproteinases in chronic wounds of 3 debilitated patients. Ann Plast Surg. 2006;56(04):418-22.
19. Shi B, Chen SZ, Zhang P, Li JQ. Effects of vacuum-assisted closure (VAC) on the expressions of MMP-1, 2, 13 in human granulation wound [in Chinese]. Zhonghua Zheng XingWai Ke Za Zhi. 2003;19(04):279-81.
20. Norbury K, Kieswetter K. Vacuum-assisted closure therapy attenuates the inflammatory response in a porcine acute wound healing model. Wounds. 2007;19(04):97-106.
21. Kairinos N, Voogd AM, Botha PH, Kotze T, Kahn D, Hudson DA, et al. Negative-pressure wound therapy II: negative-pressure wound therapy and increased perfusion. Just an illusion? Plast Reconstr Surg. 2009;123(2):601-12.
22. Kim PJ, Attinger CE, Steinberg JS, Evans KK, Powers KA, Hung RW, et al. The impact of negative-pressure wound therapy with instillation compared with

standard negative-pressure wound therapy: a retrospective, historical, cohort, controlled study. Plast Reconstr Surg. 2014;133(03):709-16.

23. Gwan-Nulla DN, Casal RS. Toxic shock syndrome associated with the use of the vacuum-assisted closure device. Ann Plast Surg. 2001;47(05):552-4.
24. Rao M, Burke D, Finan PJ, Sagar PM. The use of vacuum-assisted closure of abdominal wounds: a word of caution. Colorectal Dis. 2007;9(03):266-8.
25. Fischer JE. A cautionary note: the use of vacuum-assisted closure systems in the treatment of gastrointestinal cutaneous fistula may be associated with higher mortality from subsequent fistula development. Am J Surg. 2008;196(01):1-2
26. White RA, Miki RA, Kazmier P, Anglen JO. Vacuum-assisted closure complicated by erosion and hemorrhage of the anterior tibial artery. J Orthop Trauma. 2005;19(01):56-9.
27. Cai SS, Gowda AU, Alexander RH, Silverman RP, Goldberg NH, Rasko YM. Use of negative pressure wound therapy on malignant wounds - a case report and review of literature. Int Wound J. 2017;14(04):661-5.
28. Gupta S, Gabriel A, Lantis J, Téot L. Clinical recommendations and practical guide for negative pressure wound therapy with instillation. Int Wound J. 2016;13(02):159-74.
29. Téot L, Boissiere F, Fluieraru S. Novel foam dressing using negative pressure wound therapy with instillation to remove thick exudate. Int Wound J. 2017;14(05):842-8.
30. Matthews MR, Hechtman A, Quan AN, Foster KN, Fernandez LG. The use of V.A.C. VERAFLO CLEANSE CHOICE in the burn population. Cureus. 2018;10(11):e3632.
31. Fernandez L, Ellman C, Jackson P. Initial experience using a novel reticulated open cell foam dressing with through holes during negative pressure wound therapy with instillation for management of pressure ulcers. J Trauma Treat. 2017;6:410.
32. Condé-Green A, Chung TL, Holton LH III, et al. Incisional negative pressure wound therapy versus conventional dressings following abdominal wall reconstruction: a comparative study. Ann Plast Surg. 2013;71(04):394-7.
33. Stannard JP, Volgas DA, McGwin G 3rd, Stewart RL, Obremskey W, Moore T, et al. Incisional negative pressure wound therapy after high-risk lower extremity fractures. J Orthop Trauma. 2012;26(01):37-42.
34. Hyldig N, Vinter CA, Kruse M, Mogensen O, Bille C, Sorensen JA, et al. Prophylactic incisional negative pressure wound therapy reduces the risk of surgical site infection after caesarean section in obese women: a pragmatic randomised clinical trial. BJOG. 2019;126(05):628-35.
35. Riot S, de Bonnecaze G, Garrido I, Ferron G, Grolleau JL, Chaput B. Is the use of negative pressure wound therapy for a malignant wound legitimate in a palliative context? "The concept of NPWT ad vitam": a case series. Palliat Med. 2015;29(05):470-3.
36. Kairinos N, Solomons M, Hudson DA. Negative-pressure wound therapy I: the paradox of negative-pressure wound therapy. Plast Reconstr Surg. 2009;123(02):589-98.
37. Hopf HW, Humphrey LM, Puzziferri N, West JM, Attinger CE, Hunt TK. Adjuncts to preparing wounds for closure: hyperbaric oxygen, growth factors, skin substitutes, negative pressure wound therapy (vacuum-assisted closure). Foot Ankle Clin. 2001;6(04):661-82.

38. Whelan C, Stewart J, Schwartz BF. Mechanics of wound healing and importance of Vacuum Assisted Closure in urology. J Urol. 2005;173(05):1463-70.
39. Riou JP, Cohen JR, Johnson H. Factors influencing wound dehiscence. Am J Surg. 1992;163(3):324-30.
40. Fernandez R, Griffiths R. Water for wound cleansing. Cochrane Database Syst Rev. 2008;2:CD003861.
41. Ford CN, Reinhard ER, Yeh D, Syrek D, De Las MA, Bergman SB, Williams S, Hamori CA. Interim analysis of a prospective, randomized trial of vacuum-assisted closure versus the HealthPoint system in the management of pressure ulcers. Ann Plast Surg. 2002;49(1):55-61.
42. Moues CM, Van Den Bemd GJ, Heule F, Hovius SE. Comparing conventional gauze therapy to vacuum-assisted closure wound therapy: a prospective randomised trial. J Plast Reconstr Aesthet Surg. 2007;60(6):672-81.
43. Braakenburg A, Obdeijn MC, Feitz R, van Rooij IA, van Griethuysen AJ, Klinkenbijl JH. The clinical efficacy and cost effectiveness of the vacuum-assisted closure technique in the management of acute and chronic wounds: a randomized controlled trial. Plast Reconstr Surg. 2006;118(2):390-7; discussion 398-400.
44. Goss SG, Schwartz JA, Facchin F, Avdagic E, Gendics C, Lantis JC II. Negative pressure wound therapy with instillation (NPWTi) better reduces postdebridement bioburden in chronically infected lower extremity wounds than NPWT alone. J Am Coll Clin Wound Spec. 2014;4(4):74-80.
45. Boone D, Braitman E, Gentics C, Afthinos J, Latif J, Sordillo E, et al. Bacterial burden and wound outcomes as influenced by negative pressure wound therapy. Wounds. 2010;22(2):32-7.
46. Bernstein BH, Tam H. Combination of subatmospheric pressure dressing and gravity feed antibiotic instillation in the treatment of post-surgical diabetic foot wounds: a case series. Wounds. 2005;17(2):37-48.
47. McNulty AK, Nguyen K. What is the benefit of instillation therapy? Int J Low Extrem Wounds. 2010;9(2):68-9.
48. Rycerz AM, Slack P, McNulty AK. Distribution assessment comparing continuous and periodic wound instillation in conjunction with negative pressure wound therapy using an agar-based model. Int Wound J. 2013;10(2):214-20.
49. Brinkert D, Ali M, Naud M, Maire N, Trial C, Teot L. Negative pressure wound therapy with saline instillation: 131 patient case series. Int Wound J. 2013;10(Suppl 1):56-60.
50. Fluieraru S, Bekara F, Naud M, Herlin C, Faure C, Trial C, et al. Sterile-water negative pressure instillation therapy for complex wounds and NPWT failures. J Wound Care. 2013;22(6):293-4,296,293-9.
51. Gabriel A. Integrated negative pressure wound therapy system with volumetric automated fluid instillation in wounds at risk for compromised healing. Int Wound J. 2012;9(Suppl 1):25-31.
52. Kim PJ, Attinger CE, Steinberg JS, Evans KK, Lehner B, Willy C, et al. Negative-pressure wound therapy with instillation: international consensus guidelines. Plast Reconstr Surg. 2013;132(6):1569-79.
53. Gabriel A, Shores J, Heinrich C, Baqai W, Kalina S, Sogioka N, et al. Negative pressure wound therapy with instillation: a pilot study describing a new method for treating infected wounds. Int Wound J. 2008;5(3):399-413.

54. In: Myers BA (Ed). Wound management: principles and practice. Prentice Hall: Upper Saddle River; 2004.
55. Warriner R, Burrell R. Infection and the chronic wound: a focus on silver. Adv Skin Wound Care. 2005;18(Suppl 1):2-12.
56. Costerton JW, Stewart PS, Greenberg EP. Bacterial biofilms: a common cause of persistent infections. Science. 1999;284(5418):1318-22.
57. Schultz GS, Sibbald RG, Falanga V, Ayello EA, Dowsett C, Harding K, et al. Wound bed preparation: a systematic approach to wound management. Wound Repair Regen. 2003;11(Suppl 1):S1-28.
58. Dow G, Browne A, Sibbald RG. Infection in chronic wounds: controversies in diagnosis and treatment. Ostomy. Wound Manage. 1999;45(8):23-40.
59. Schultz GS, Barillo DJ, Mozingo DW, Chin GA. Wound bed preparation and a brief history of TIME. Int Wound J. 2004;1(1):19-32.
60. Attinger CE, Janis JE, Steinberg J, Schwartz J, Al-Attar A, Couch K. Clinical approach to wounds: débridement and wound bed preparation including the use of dressings and wound-healing adjuvants. Plast Reconstr Surg. 2006; 117(7 Suppl):72S-109.

# Index

Page numbers followed by *b* refer to box, *f* refer to figure, *fc* refer to flowchart, and *t* refer to table.

## C

## F

## I

## J



## K



## L

## M



## N

## Q



## R

## S